Medical Decision Making

Medical Decision Making

Third Edition

Harold C. Sox
Geisel School of Medicine at Dartmouth, Hanover, NH, USA

Michael C. Higgins
Stanford Center for Biomedical Informatics Research, Stanford University, Stanford, CA, USA

Douglas K. Owens
Department of Health Policy, School of Medicine, and Center for Health Policy, Freeman-Spogli Institute for International Studies, Stanford University, Stanford, CA, USA

Gillian Sanders Schmidler
Department of Population Health Sciences, Medicine, and Duke-Margolis Institute for Health Policy, Duke University, Durham, NC, USA

WILEY Blackwell

Edition History
Butterworth Publishers (1e, 1988); John Wiley & Sons, Ltd (2e, 2013)

Registered Offices
John Wiley & Sons, Inc., 111 River Street, Hoboken, NJ 07030, USA
John Wiley & Sons Ltd, The Atrium, Southern Gate, Chichester, West Sussex, PO19 8SQ, UK

For details of our global editorial offices, customer services, and more information about Wiley products visit us at www.wiley.com.

Wiley also publishes its books in a variety of electronic formats and by print-on-demand. Some content that appears in standard print versions of this book may not be available in other formats.

Library of Congress Cataloging-in-Publication Data
Names: Sox, Harold C., author. | Higgins, Michael C. (Michael Clark),
    1950–author. | Owens, Douglas K., author. | Sanders Schmidler, Gillian,
    author.
Title: Medical decision making / Harold C. Sox, Michael C. Higgins, Douglas
    K. Owens, Gillian Sanders Schmidler.
Description: Third edition. | Hoboken, NJ : Wiley-Blackwell, 2024. |
    Includes bibliographical references and index.
Identifiers: LCCN 2023017110 (print) | LCCN 2023017111 (ebook) |
    ISBN 9781119627807 (paperback) | ISBN 9781119627845 (adobe pdf) |
    ISBN 9781119627722 (epub)
Subjects: MESH: Clinical Decision-Making | Diagnosis, Differential |
    Decision Support Techniques
Classification: LCC RT48 (print) | LCC RT48 (ebook) | NLM WB 142.5 |
    DDC 616.07/5–dc23/eng/20230703
LC record available at https://lccn.loc.gov/2023017110
LC ebook record available at https://lccn.loc.gov/2023017111

Cover Design: Wiley
Cover Image: © VectorKid/Shutterstock

Set in 9.5/12pt PalatinoLTStd by Straive, Pondicherry, India

SKY10073889_042624

Dedications for Medical Decision Making, 3rd edition

To Jean and Kathleen
To Sara, Rachel, and Christopher
To Carol, Colin, and Lara
To Scott, Gib, Oliver, Edgar, and Irving

Their support has meant everything.

Contents

Foreword

The diagnostic tools available to today's clinicians are breathtaking. Scans explore previously inaccessible life-threatening disorders and space-occupying lesions. Scopes invade nearly every tubular structure, finding tumors and inflammatory diseases. Panels of antigen tests identify a panoply of microscopic invaders. PCRs and genome sequencers seek out the rarest of the rare. Given the accuracy provided by scanning, our thin biopsy needles and our drainage catheters can be safely inserted; even our invasive procedures are less invasive and less risky. Biopsying the pancreas or the heart is no longer science fiction.

These technical advances are dramatically altering our time-honored approach to diagnosis. Whereas we previously delved deeply into a patient's illness history and meticulously carried out a physical examination looking for salient clues to guide our next diagnostic or therapeutic recommendation, now, bolstered with merely a chief complaint or a cursory examination, clinicians scan the chest, or abdomen, or head (or all three); send for panels of tests; and wait for the results for further guidance. To old-time doctors, this process feels like a violation, yet it often yields answers more efficiently, achieves earlier treatment, and reduces hospital stays.

The new era in diagnostic expertise ushered in by technical innovations should be satisfying to the profession and the public, but it has not been. Within the profession, we battle over how to use prostate-specific antigen (PSA) and bone density tests; we argue whether prediabetes and long COVID really exist. We offer conflicting advice to the public on when to get a colonoscopy or when to wear masks. We confuse our trainees by repurposing diagnostic criteria from controlled trials into clinical entities and by using lists of numerical diagnostic summations, as if a single calculated number is meaningful. But we fail even more fundamentally when we make diagnostic mistakes that cost patients not just their peace of mind but their lives. Outcomes researchers tell us that thousands of costly medical errors occur every year and that many are attributable to faulty diagnosis. The problem of errors became so acute several years ago that expert panels convened by the National Academy of Medicine issued reports highly critical of existing medical practices.

Therapeutics have shared scientific progress in diagnosis. New diseases have appeared, some diseases have been reclassified based on new pathophysiologic understanding, transplants are commonplace, and a substantial fraction of the population became immunosuppressed for one reason or another. A pharmacopeia of new powerful drugs came into wide use, replete with its vast benefits and its inevitably troublesome risks and costs. Practice also evolved. Over the years, the choice of one treatment or another was based primarily on individual doctors' experiences and personal preferences or the opinion of experts. For better or worse, the profession did recognize that this chaotic method had to be replaced by greater standardization, itself based on available rigorous clinical research. Data from research studies today are combined, analyzed, and packaged for everyday use. The choice of alternative treatment regimens has been rigorously subjected to probabilistic reasoning and decision science, thus illuminating the basic principles of therapy.

The public also became engaged. Diagnosis and therapeutics are no longer the exclusive purview of professionals; they are the talk of the town. Access to case reports in the Sunday newspapers, clinical image entries on social media, talking stool-testing boxes on television, and endless, often authoritative, data on easily accessible search engines have helped make the public our partners in all things medical. And for that, we should be grateful.

Needless to say, medical researchers have not been inattentive to the persistence of medical diagnostic and therapeutic errors. During most of the twentieth century, only a few lone voices were offering new ideas, but during the past five decades, clinical decision-making has been a prime focus, particularly in divisions of General Internal Medicine in Departments of Medicine. Investigators have clarified the language and stages of the diagnostic process, illuminated causal reasoning, defined the inextricable association between testing on one hand and the risks and benefits of treatment on the other, clarified the role of probabilistic thinking, applied mathematical formulations to decision-making, and pressed physicians on the merits of making all judgments on a hierarchy of solid data. Professional societies have embraced diagnostic sections in their national meetings, several major journals feature an array of medical images, and medical schools have introduced clinical reasoning courses.

Diagnosis and therapy selection are physicians' fundamental tasks, principal skills, and awesome responsibility. Many believed that by now, artificial intelligence or machine learning would take over medical diagnosis and therapy.

Regrettably, waiting for this transition is like waiting for Godot: it hasn't happened and it won't happen soon: we're still on our own.

Many of the concepts and language in *Medical Decision Making* have already seeped into day-to-day medical practice. Decisions on which scan to use for suspected pulmonary embolism are couched in probabilities, likelihood ratios, false positives, and false negatives. Terms such as Bayes' Rule, decision analysis, utility theory, and decisional toss-ups, though uncommon, are used by clinicians as rationales for clinical decision-making. Slow seeping is fine, but it is not sufficient.

Fortunately, the basic principles and practices of clinical diagnostics and therapeutics have come a long way, and they are superbly described in *Medical Decision Making*. This new edition contains much new and advanced material: decision models, clinical prediction models, survival analysis, patients' utility assessment, the threshold approach to testing and treating, and cost-effectiveness analysis, to name only a few. In many ways, the breadth and extent of these approaches represent a mathematics of medical thinking. The third edition of *Medical Decision Making* will be the reference standard of the field for decades.

For physicians eager to improve their abilities, for teachers of clinical medicine, and for medical students trying to comprehend the basic concepts of clinical reasoning and decision-making, *Medical Decision Making* is the "go-to" book. Becoming comfortable with the concepts in the book will require concentration, discipline, and persistence, but the effort will be well worth it.

Jerome P. Kassirer, M.D.
Distinguished Professor, Tufts University School of Medicine
Editor-in-Chief Emeritus, *New England Journal of Medicine*

Preface

The textbook *Medical Decision Making* (MDM) took form in the mid-1980s as an extension of the notes for an introductory course for medical students. The notes and slides became the draft of a book. The draft found a publisher and, eventually, readers from everywhere. Thanks to leaders like Barbara McNeil, Ron Howard, Stephen Pauker, Jerome Kassirer, Amos Tversky, and Daniel Kahneman, the foundations of decision science were in place at the time of the first edition. But the field has continued to grow, and a standard textbook must keep pace with change.

The ultimate measure of the field of medical decision making is its effect on medical education, decision making in clinical practice, and clinical policies.

In education, Bayes' theorem is a gift to clinical teachers, especially in its odds ratio form. Think of a patient with high pre-test odds of a clinical condition and a negative result on a test with low sensitivity. The students are stunned by how little the odds change. A teachable moment.

Do clinicians use decision analysis in day-to-day care? I suspect that opportunities are infrequent, given the high-pressure conditions of office practice. When they do arise, clinicians need quick access to the evidence. Posting a list of frequently used tests and their likelihood ratios on the wall of each examination room would be one way to address that need. More complicated decision making would require a smartphone app built around a decision model like the one for pulmonary embolism in Chapter 13.

Practice guidelines do affect the world of office practice, and some guidelines were shaped by advanced decision models like those described in Chapter 14. The US Preventive Services Task Force relies on sophisticated decision models to inform their cancer screening recommendations.

This volume addresses these needs. Chapters 1 and 2 set the stage: uncertainty is everywhere in clinical practice, yet clinical reasoning depends on logical deduction as exemplified by differential diagnosis. Chapters 3, 4, and 5 are about defining and navigating uncertainty: determining probability, updating probability, and the determinants of post-test probability, all basic tools of the clinician. Chapters 6 and 7 are about modeling the factors that shape decisions. Chapters 8–12 explore in-depth the measurement of utility, both the basics and the underlying theory. Topics include attitudes toward taking risks, the quality of life, and the length of life. The last three chapters are about making decisions: deciding when to treat, when to test, and when to wait (Chapter 13); the advanced modeling methods that inform policy (Chapter 14); and cost-effectiveness analysis (Chapter 15).

This book describes how to translate subjective judgements about events into numbers—probabilities and utilities—with which to identify the best decision—treat, test, or do nothing—for an individual. While the book uses a numerical framework to guide decision making, the actual math is straightforward except for parts of Chapters 8–12. Even there, the text surrounding the math will explain the basic concepts. Bottom line: when the reader finds the math challenging, read on. The text will explain what it means.

A brief update on the authors: Mike Higgins teaches a high-level course on medical decision analysis for Stanford University graduate students and medical students. The middle chapters are an outgrowth of his lectures. Doug Owens has continued to do advanced decision modeling to inform clinical policy making while adding several academic leadership responsibilities to his portfolio at Stanford. We welcome Gillian Schmidler, PhD, as a co-author. She is a member of the faculty at Duke University. She co-led the Second Panel on Cost-Effectiveness, a group of experts that has literally set the standards for study in that field. Chapter 15 is an outgrowth of her work with the Panel. I retired recently after 9 years developing a peer review program for the Patient-Centered Outcomes Research Institute (PCORI), an organization that funds clinical comparative effectiveness research.

A word about artificial intelligence and the contents of this book: In the past year, advances in machine learning analysis of very large observational data sets has raised the possibility that clinical reasoning could evolve toward a model in which clinician and machine collaborate. This possibility raises questions. How will observations based on machine learning and artificial intelligence interface with clinical reasoning based on good science such as that described in this book? Will clinical outcomes reflect decisions that incorporates the preferences of a specific patient for potential downstream health states? In a vast observational data set, the patient characteristics, treatments, and outcome as well as the relationships between them are all subject to the biases described in this book and elsewhere. While the way forward is uncertain, readers of this book should be well-placed to evaluate AI-based input against a reference standard based upon scientific observation and reasoning.

We thank the following individuals who read chapters at our request and gave us good advice, both clinical and technical: John Wong, Ross Schacter, and Marc Dewey. Many thanks also to Jerome P. Kassirer, internist, editor, and pioneer in our field whose Introduction sets the stage for the third edition of MDM and to Jeremy Goldhaber-Fiebert for advice about medical decision analysis in the age of artificial intelligence.

We hope that this book achieves two goals. The first is to introduce readers to basic concepts that may enrich their lives in the practice of medicine or their experiences as a patient. The second is to attract leaders – present and future – who will take these ideas into their field – medicine, policy making, and research – and advance it to the next level. We'll be watching!

H.C.S.

Introduction

> *"Proof," I said, "is always a relative thing. It's an overwhelming balance of probabilities. And that's a matter of how they strike you."*
> *(Raymond Chandler in Farewell, My Lovely, 1940)*

Thoughtful clinicians ask themselves many difficult questions during the course of taking care of patients. Some of these questions are as follows:

- How may I be thorough yet efficient when considering the possible causes of my patient's problem?
- How do I characterize the information I have gathered during the medical interview and physical examination?
- How should I interpret new diagnostic information?
- How do I select the appropriate diagnostic test?
- How do I choose among several risky treatments?

The goal of this book is to help clinicians answer these important questions.

The first question is addressed with observations from expert clinicians "thinking out loud" as they work their way through a clinical problem. The last four are addressed from the perspective of medical decision analysis, a quantitative approach to medical decision making.

The goal of this introductory chapter is to preview the contents of the book by sketching out preliminary answers to these five questions.

1.1 How may I be thorough yet efficient when considering the possible causes of my patient's problems?

Trying to be efficient in thinking about the possible causes of a patient's problem often conflicts with being thorough. This conflict has no single solution. However, much may be learned about medical problem-solving by listening to expert diagnosticians discuss how they reasoned their way through a case. Because the single most powerful predictor of skill in diagnosis is exposure to patients, the best advice is "see lots of patients and learn from your mistakes." How to be thorough, yet efficient, when thinking about the possible causes of a patient's problem is the topic of Chapter 2.

1.2 How do I characterize the information I have gathered during the medical interview and physical examination?

The first step toward understanding how to characterize the information one gathers from the medical interview and physical examination is to realize that information provided by the patient and by diagnostic tests usually does not reveal the patient's true state. A patient's signs, symptoms, and diagnostic test results are usually representative of

Medical Decision Making, Third Edition. Harold C. Sox, Michael C. Higgins, Douglas K. Owens, and Gillian Sanders Schmidler.
© 2024 John Wiley & Sons Ltd. Published 2024 by John Wiley & Sons Ltd.

more than one disease. Therefore, distinguishing among the possibilities with absolute certainty is not possible. A 60-year-old man's history of chest pain illustrates this point.

Mr. Costin, a 60-year-old bank executive, walks into the emergency room complaining of intermittent substernal chest pain that is "squeezing" in character. The chest pain is occasionally brought on by exertion but usually occurs without provocation. When it occurs, the patient lies down for a few minutes, and the pain usually subsides in about 5 minutes. It never lasts more than 10 minutes. Until these episodes of chest pain began 3 weeks ago, the patient had been in good health, except for intermittent problems with heartburn after a heavy meal.

Although there are at least 60 causes of chest pain, Mr. Costin's medical history narrows down the diagnostic possibilities considerably. Based on his history, the two most likely causes of Mr. Costin's chest pain are coronary artery disease or esophageal disease.

However, the cause of Mr. Costin's illness is uncertain. This uncertainty is not a shortcoming of the clinician who gathered the information; rather, it reflects the uncertainty inherent in the information provided by Mr. Costin. Like most patients, his true disease state is hidden within his body and must be inferred from imperfect external clues.

How do clinicians usually characterize the uncertainty inherent in medical information? Most clinicians use words such as "probably" or "possibly" to characterize this uncertainty. However, most of these words are imprecise, as seen as we hear more about Mr. Costin's story:

The physician who sees Mr. Costin in the emergency room tells Mr. Costin, "I cannot rule out coronary artery disease. The next step in the diagnostic process is to examine the results of a stress ECG." She also says, "I cannot rule esophageal disease either. If the stress ECG is negative, we will work you up for esophageal disease."

Mr. Costin is very concerned about his condition and seeks a second opinion. The second physician who sees Mr. Costin agrees that coronary artery disease and esophageal disease are the most likely diagnoses. He tells Mr. Costin, "Coronary artery disease is a likely diagnosis, but to know for certain we'll have to see the results of a stress ECG." Concerning esophageal disease, he says, "We cannot rule out esophageal disease at this point. If the stress ECG is normal, and you don't begin to feel better, we'll work you up for esophageal disease."

Mr. Costin feels reassured that both clinicians seem to agree on the possibility of esophageal disease, since both have said that they cannot rule out esophageal disease. However, Mr. Costin cannot reconcile the different statements concerning the likelihood that he has coronary artery disease. Recall that the first clinician said "coronary artery disease can't be ruled out," whereas the second clinician stated, "coronary artery disease is a likely diagnosis." Mr. Costin wants to know the difference between these two different opinions. Mr. Costin explains his confusion to the second clinician and asks him to speak to the first clinician.

The two clinicians confer by telephone. Although they expressed the likelihood of coronary artery disease differently when they talked with Mr. Costin, it turns out that they had similar ideas about the likelihood that he has coronary artery disease. Both believe that about one patient out of three with Mr. Costin's history has coronary artery disease.

From this episode, Mr. Costin learns that clinicians may choose different words to express the same judgment about the likelihood of an uncertain event.

To Mr. Costin's surprise, the clinicians have different opinions about the likelihood of esophageal disease, despite the fact that both described its likelihood with the same phrase, "esophageal disease can't be ruled out." The first clinician believes that among patients with Mr. Costin's symptoms, only one patient in ten would have esophageal disease. However, the second clinician thinks that as many as one patient in two would have esophageal disease.

Mr. Costin is chagrined that both clinicians used the same phrase, "can't be ruled out," to describe two different likelihoods. Mr. Costin learns that clinicians commonly use the same words to express different judgments about the likelihood of an event.

The solution to the confusion that can occur when using words to characterize uncertainty with words is to use a number: a probability. Probability expresses uncertainty precisely because it is the likelihood that a condition is present or will occur in the future. When one clinician believes the probability that a patient has coronary artery disease is 1 in 10, and the other clinician thinks that it is 1 in 2, the two know that they disagree and that they must talk about why

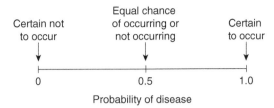

Figure 1.1 A scale for expressing uncertainty.

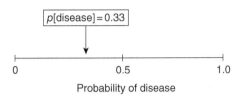

Figure 1.2 A clinician can visualize the level of certainty about a disease hypothesis on a probability scale. Thirty-three is marked on this certainty scale to correspond to a clinician's initial probability estimate that Mr. Costin had coronary artery disease.

their interpretations are so disparate. The precision of numbers to express uncertainty is illustrated graphically by the scale in Figure 1.1. On this scale, uncertain events are expressed with numbers between 0 and 1.

To understand the meaning of probability in medicine, think of it as a fraction. For example, the word "one-third" means 33 out of a group of 100. In medicine, if a clinician states that the probability that a disease is present is 33%, it means that the clinician believes that if they see 100 patients with the same findings, 33 of them will have the disease in question (Figure 1.2).

Although probability has a precise mathematical meaning, a probability estimate need not correspond to a physical reality, such as the prevalence of disease in a defined group of patients. We define probability in medicine as a number between zero and 1 that expresses a clinician's opinion about the likelihood of a condition being present or occurring in the future. The probability of an event a clinician believes is certain to occur is equal to 1. The probability of an event a clinician believes is certain not to occur is equal to 0.

A probability may apply to the present state of the patient (e.g., that they have coronary artery disease), or it may be used to express the likelihood that an event will occur in the future (e.g., that they will experience a myocardial infarction within 1 year).

When should a clinician use probability in the diagnostic process? The first time that probability is useful in the diagnostic process is when the clinician feels the need to synthesize the medical information in the medical interview and physical examination into an opinion. At this juncture, the clinician wants to be precise about their uncertainty because they are poised to make decisions about their patient. They may decide to act as if the patient is not diseased. They may decide that they need more information and will order a diagnostic test. They may decide that they know enough to start the patient on a specific treatment. To decide between these options, they do not need to know the diagnosis. They do need to estimate the probability that the patient has, as in the case of Mr. Costin, coronary artery disease as the cause of his chest pain.

A clinician arrives at a probability estimate for a disease hypothesis by using their personal experience and the published literature. Advice on how to estimate probability is found in Chapter 3.

1.3   How do I interpret new diagnostic information?

New diagnostic information often does not reveal the patient's true state, and the best a clinician can do is to estimate how much the new information has changed their uncertainty about it. This task is difficult if one is describing uncertainty with words. However, if the clinician is expressing uncertainty with probability, they can use Bayes' theorem to estimate how much their uncertainty about a patient's true state should have changed. To use Bayes' theorem, a

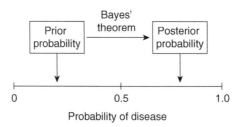

Figure 1.3 The pre-test probability and the post-test probability of disease.

clinician must estimate the probability of disease before the new information was gathered (the *prior probability* or pre-test probability) and know the accuracy of the new diagnostic information. The probability of disease that results from interpreting new diagnostic information is called the *posterior probability* (or post-test probability). These two probabilities are illustrated in Figure 1.3.

Chapter 4 explains about how to use Bayes' theorem to estimate the post-test probability of a disease.

1.4 How do I select the appropriate diagnostic test?

Although the selection of a diagnostic test is ostensibly straightforward, the reasoning must take into account several factors. In the language of medical decision analysis, the selection of diagnostic tests depends on the patient's feelings about states of disease and health, the physician's estimate of the prior probability of disease, and the accuracy of the diagnostic tests that the physician is trying to choose between.

A logical approach to selecting diagnostic tests depends on three principles:
- Diagnostic tests are imperfect and therefore seldom reveal a patient's true state with certainty.
- Choose tests whose results could change your mind about what to do for your patient.
- Clinicians often start treatment when they are uncertain about the true state of the patient.

These three principles lead to an important concept: the selection of diagnostic tests depends on the level of certainty at which a physician is willing to start treatment. This level of certainty is known as the treatment threshold probability. How to use the treatment-threshold probability to make decisions is the topic of Chapter 9.

A clinician must take two steps to assess the treatment-threshold probability of disease. The first step is to list the harms and benefits of treatment. The second step is to assess the patient's feelings about these harms and benefits. A decision analyst assesses a patient's attitudes toward the risks and benefits of treatment using a unit of measure called *utility*. Measuring a patient's utilities is covered in Chapter 8.

1.5 How do I choose among several risky treatment alternatives?

Choosing among risky treatment alternatives is difficult because the outcome of most treatments is uncertain: some people respond to treatment but others do not. If the outcome of a treatment is governed by chance, a physician cannot know in advance which outcome of the treatment will result. Under these circumstances, the best way to achieve a good outcome is to choose the treatment alternative whose average outcome is best. This concept is called *expected value decision making*. Expected value decision making is the topic of Chapters 6, 7, and 10.

Summary

The care of patients is difficult in part because of the uncertainty inherent in the nature of medical information: tests are imperfect, and treatments have unpredictable consequences. The application of probability, utility, and expected value decision making provides a framework for making the right decision despite the uncertainty of medical practice. Medical decision analysis helps clinicians and patients to cope with uncertainty.

Differential diagnosis

This chapter is about differential diagnosis, a systematic process for narrowing the range of possible explanations for a patient's problem. The goal of this chapter is to describe a thorough, yet efficient, approach to this process.

2.1 An introduction

Differential diagnosis is the process of considering the possible causes of a patient's symptoms or physical findings and narrowing the list of possibilities. Differential diagnosis is a safeguard against premature conclusions as well as a time-proven method for attacking what can be a supremely difficult intellectual challenge. All clinicians, regardless of their specialty, use differential diagnosis and strive to master it. For many clinicians, to be called a superb diagnostician is the highest form of praise.

The challenge of differential diagnosis: A patient visits your office on a busy afternoon because of a symptom. They want you to discover the reason for the symptom and then cure it quickly and painlessly. You must discover its cause or at least assure yourself that it is not due to a serious, treatable disease. This task can be difficult, especially when the symptom has many possible causes. Recalling a long list of possible causes or the features of even one cause of the symptom is a difficult feat. Moreover, these key features typically occur in more than one disease. Time pressure often adds to intellectual difficulties.

The purposes of the interview: The medical interview has many purposes. The first goal is to establish a relationship of mutual trust with the patient. Another goal is to observe the patient closely for clues that may help focus your investigation. A third goal is to narrow the list of diseases that could be causing the patient's problem and focus the physical examination on a few possible diagnoses. Later, comes the physical examination and decisions about whether to perform diagnostic tests.

2.2 How clinicians make a diagnosis

We know more about how clinicians *should* reason than about how they *do* reason. This book is about how physicians should reason in specific situations, such as selecting and interpreting diagnostic tests or choosing between two treatments. These normative methods are based on first principles of logical reasoning and take full advantage of all sources of information. This chapter is about how physicians *do* reason as they strive to narrow the list of possible causes of a patient's symptoms.

Medical Decision Making, Third Edition. Harold C. Sox, Michael C. Higgins, Douglas K. Owens, and Gillian Sanders Schmidler.
© 2024 John Wiley & Sons Ltd. Published 2024 by John Wiley & Sons Ltd.

This chapter describes a logical framework for diagnosis, but we cannot claim that it is based on first principles of logical reasoning. We can claim that expert clinicians use the process. However, while the path to expertise starts with a good process, research shows that expert clinicians got that way by seeing lots of patients. Moreover, they are skillful at recalling what they learned from past experiences and using it to solve the problem of the patient of the moment.

The process that we will describe is based on listening to expert diagnosticians think aloud as they solve a diagnostic problem. Diagnosticians, expert or not, use a similar process. The expert has a larger, more accessible fund of knowledge than the average clinician. Some of this knowledge comes from textbooks and articles, but most of it comes from having seen similar patients and recalling the details (pattern recognition).

The message for the beginning student is twofold. First, they will learn a process that is the foundation of excellence in diagnosis. Second, the pathway to excellence is open to those who constantly strive to enlarge their experience by immersing themselves in clinical medicine and the important details of individual patients and their ultimate fate. The more you challenge yourself, the more you will learn and the more expert you will become. You do not get better by playing it safe and avoiding exposure to the possibility of being wrong. In fact, experts will tell you that they learn more from when they are wrong than when they are right.

The central mystery of medical education is how students acquire skills in differential diagnosis. This topic is seldom taught as a formal discipline. Most learn it while discussing specific patients with a clinical teacher. This gap in the medical curriculum is easily understood: our understanding of the methods used by skilled diagnosticians would scarcely sustain an hour's lecture. What we do know about differential diagnosis is the result of research in which clinicians "think out loud" as they work their way through a diagnostic problem. These observations may be summarized in five conclusions:

1. Hypotheses are generated early in the interview.
2. Only a few hypotheses are being actively considered at any moment.
3. Newly acquired information is often used incorrectly.
4. Clinicians often fail to take full advantage of their experience with similar patients.
5. A clinician's skill in differential diagnosis varies from topic to topic; more experience usually means greater expertise.

Each of these conclusions requires additional comment.

1. *Hypotheses are generated early:* Beginning students are often instructed to obtain all relevant data before starting to exclude diseases from the list of possible causes of the patients' complaints. They soon outgrow this mistaken teaching. Experienced clinicians observe the patient closely while introducing themselves and often begin to draw tentative conclusions before the patient has spoken. As soon as they identify the patient's main complaint, they use the patient's age and gender to help identify the main diagnostic possibilities. Good interviewers will ask the patient to tell the story of their main complaint while they listen, observe, and formulate hypotheses. These hypotheses determine their first specific questions, and the replies bring other hypotheses to mind.

Conclusion: Data collection is hypothesis-driven.

2. *Only a few hypotheses are considered simultaneously:* Research about cognition shows that the human mind has limited working memory. Just as a juggler can keep only a few objects in the air at once, the clinician can consider only a few hypotheses simultaneously.

The clinician begins to evaluate a hypothesis by matching the patient's findings with the clinician's internal representation, or model, of the disease. Sometimes this internal representation is the pathophysiology of the condition. One pathophysiological derangement causes another, as inferred by logical deduction, which leads to another and eventually to the expected clinical manifestations. Reasoning backward along this chain of logical deductions may lead to the cause of the patient's problem. One way to remember the differential diagnosis of low serum sodium is to reason deductively from the pathophysiology of the condition. Research indicates that expert diagnosticians use pathophysiological reasoning mainly for difficult, atypical cases. Expert diagnosticians typically have an excellent understanding of pathophysiology.

More often, the clinician uses an associative model of disease, also known as pattern recognition. Associative models consist of clinical findings, illness progression, predisposing characteristics, and complications that are associated with a disease. The clinician asks about the typical features of a disease and is often able to eliminate hypotheses solely from the patient's responses. Hypotheses that cannot be readily discarded are further tested during the physical examination. Another mark of an expert diagnostician is the ability to quickly match the patient's findings to a pattern of disease manifestations. Often, the patient's findings remind the clinician of a similar patient seen many years earlier. Expert clinicians retain these experiences and can recall details of specific patients from many decades earlier.

The supreme mystery of clinical reasoning is the cognitive process that clinicians use to discard or confirm a hypothesis. Several models of this process have been proposed. These models are based on analyzing what clinicians say about how they test hypotheses.

- *Additive model:* In a linear model, clinicians assign a positive weight to findings that tend to confirm a diagnosis and negative weights to findings that disconfirm the diagnosis. In some unknown cognitive process, the clinician decides to discard or accept a hypothesis based on the sum of the diagnostic weights. Clinical prediction rules use this model (see Chapter 3). Physicians probably assign weights subjectively and subconsciously.
- In the context of this chapter, the analog of the diagnostic weight of a finding might be the likelihood ratio of the finding, which indicates whether the odds of the target condition go up or down and by how much. It is, therefore, an empirical, quantitative measure of the changes in the probability of the target condition (see Chapters 4 and 5). Aspiring experts in diagnosis should make a list of the likelihood ratios of key findings and diagnostic tests.
- *Bayesian model:* Bayes' theorem is the method to calculate the post-test probability of the target condition. Bayes' theorem tells the clinician how much new information should change the probability. By analogy, clinicians may change their belief in a hypothesis with each new item of information and conclude at some point that the probability is low enough to discard the hypothesis. Bayes' theorem is the topic of Chapter 4.
- *Algorithmic model:* Algorithms are commonly used to represent the logic of diagnosis. Do clinicians follow an internal flow sheet with branching logic as they test a hypothesis? Does a series of "no" branches eventually lead to discarding a hypothesis? We do not know.
- Undoubtedly, clinicians use features of these admittedly speculative models as they consider a diagnostic hypothesis, but the essence of diagnostic reasoning eludes understanding.

3. *Newly acquired information is often used inappropriately:* Mistakes happen when a clinician begins to believe in a diagnostic hypothesis. The clinician may ignore conflicting information or misinterpret it as confirming an existing hypothesis when the correct action is to disregard it, use it to reject the hypothesis or use it as a clue to a new hypothesis. The clinician may exaggerate the importance of findings that fit with a preconceived idea or accommodate inconsistent data by reformulating a hypothesis to the point where it is too general to be tested parsimoniously.

Example: These errors are illustrated by the story of the medical student who offered a diagnosis of leishmaniasis in a patient with diffuse lymphadenopathy. The patient had taken a steamship cruise to a South American port many years before. When the attending physician asked him to justify this arcane diagnosis, the student replied, "What else causes lymphadenopathy?" Unable to remember any other causes of lymphadenopathy, the student exaggerated the importance of a rather dubious travel history in order to support a far-out hypothesis.

Conclusion: Placing too much weight on data to support a low-probability hypothesis leads to mistakes.

4. *Past experience can be used inappropriately:* Clinicians use rules of thumb (heuristics) for using experience to estimate probability from the match between the patient's case history and patients from their past. These heuristics include representativeness (the goodness of fit between the patient's case and past cases) and availability (how easily past cases come to mind). Thoughtless use of these heuristics can lead to mistakes (as discussed at length in Chapter 3).

5. *Skill in clinical reasoning varies from topic to topic:* Students of cognitive psychology have assumed that individuals who are able to reason well about one topic should be equally proficient with other topics. In fact, clinicians' reasoning skills vary from topic to topic. Associations between hypotheses and clinical findings are learned by experience. Therefore, mastery of a topic requires experience with a wide variety of cases. A good memory and cognitive facility are not enough.

Conclusion: Expertise requires deep clinical experience.

Summary: Descriptive studies of clinical reasoning provide helpful insights for the beginning clinician. However, despite dogged efforts by researchers, we do not understand many aspects of clinical reasoning. Meanwhile, all agree that experience is the best teacher.

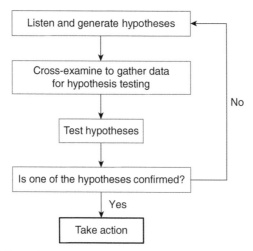

Figure 2.1 The cyclic process of differential diagnosis.

2.3 The principles of hypothesis-driven differential diagnosis

The most important conclusion from research on how experts make a diagnosis is that the questions they are asking at any moment are intended to test the small number of diagnostic hypotheses that they are considering at that moment. In other words, the main function of the interview and physical examination is to test diagnostic hypotheses. Thinking of this principle may help the clinician steer the interview back on topic when it threatens to get side-tracked.

While reading this chapter, imagine that you are evaluating a patient with a chief complaint of "nocturnal anterior chest pain for one week." The pain is a sensation of tightness that begins an hour or so after lying down. A complete evaluation of this complaint will include the following steps:

1. Taking the history
2. Doing a physical examination
3. Selecting and interpreting diagnostic tests
4. Choosing a treatment.

This book will cover the principles underlying each of these steps in considerable detail. The purpose of this chapter is to describe the thinking processes that guide the history and physical examination. Subsequent chapters prepare the reader to choose diagnostic tests and therapy.

Differential diagnosis is a cyclic process consisting of three steps which ultimately lead to a fourth step, to act (Figure 2.1).

These three steps are repeated many times as hypotheses are considered and either rejected, confirmed, or put on hold for testing later. Steps 2 and 3 are repeated during the physical examination. The following four sections follow the cyclic process shown in Figure 2.1.

2.3.1 The first step in differential diagnosis: listening and generating hypotheses

This process begins as the patient voices the chief complaint. Most clinicians ask the patient to provide a chronologic account of their illness from its beginning. This approach provides valuable information and perspective on the patient's illness. It also respects the patient. As patients tell their story, the clinician has time to think, write down some diagnoses to consider, and observe the patient for diagnostic clues.

Hypothesis generation begins at the start of the interview. The first catalyst for hypothesis generation is usually the chief complaint, although the patient's appearance and agility as they take their seat in the examining room also provide a context for interpreting the history. As shown in Figure 2.2, the patient's history generates the most hypotheses. The physical examination is usually a time to gather objective clues to confirm or discard a hypothesis. For example, an older patient complaining of shortness of breath usually evokes the hypothesis of heart failure. If the patient does not have pulmonary rales, elevated neck veins, cardiac enlargement, or a third heart sound, heart failure is much less likely.

After the physical examination, a skilled clinician usually has only a few remaining hypotheses to evaluate further. The next step may be to start treatment, do a diagnostic test, or simply wait a few days to see if the complaint is resolving spontaneously.

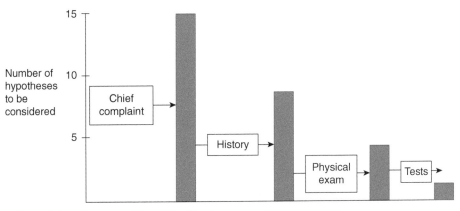

Figure 2.2 Number of diagnostic hypotheses remaining during the steps of evaluating a symptom.

Recall that our patient's complaint is "nocturnal anterior chest pain for one month." This complaint might elicit several of the following hypotheses:

Lung:	**Bony Thorax:**	**Esophageal:**
– pneumonia	– rib fracture	– reflux esophagitis
– pulmonary embolus	– muscle strain	– esophageal spasm
– tuberculosis	– costochondritis	– esophageal rupture
– tumor		– esophageal cancer
– pneumothorax		
Pericardial or pleural:	**Great vessels:**	**Cardiac**
– Pericarditis	– dissecting	– coronary artery disease
– pleuritis	aneurysm	– aortic stenosis
Mediastinal:	**Referred pain:**	
– mediastinitis	– cholecystitis	
– tumor	– peptic ulcer	
	– pancreatitis	
	– cervical arthritis	

As you generate the first few hypotheses, you may ask these questions:
1. Which hypothesis should I test first?
2. What should I do when I am unable to think of possible diagnoses?

1. *Which hypothesis should I test first?* Start with *common* diseases that are *important to treat*.
- *Common diseases*: Think of them first. These hypotheses are more likely to be true – when supported by confirmatory evidence – than hypotheses about rare diseases. However, hypotheses about common diseases are harder to disconfirm (rule out) than hypotheses about rare diseases (If this point puzzles you, go to Chapter 4, which explains how new information changes probability).

   Example: Because coronary artery disease is a common disease, consider it before pericarditis, which is less common.

- *Importance of treatment*: Consider diagnoses for which delay in starting treatment could lead to death or serious disability. These are "the diseases that you cannot afford to miss."

   Example: Be sure to consider two relatively uncommon but treatable causes of our patient's chest pain, pneumonia, and pneumothorax (a pocket of air within the thorax and outside the lung). You can safely delay testing hypotheses about diseases that benefit relatively little from treatment, such as muscular strain.

   This example is a reminder that always adhering to the usual sequence of history taking followed by physical examination can endanger the patient. Some diagnoses, such as pneumothorax, are very important to treat promptly, do not have a characteristic history, but do have characteristic physical findings. If the patient is in severe distress, you should do a targeted physical examination first in order to rule out diseases, like pneumothorax. Likewise, gently palpating the abdomen of someone complaining of severe abdominal pain can provide clues about serious diseases that move quickly, like peritonitis or a ruptured abdominal aneurysm. The physical examination in such patients provides context and focus for taking the history.

2. *What should I do when I cannot think of possible diagnoses?* Beginning students are the main victims of this problem. Even an experienced clinician has trouble when the patient's complaint is vague.

- *Vague, nonspecific complaints:*

  Hypotheses can be slow in coming to mind when the patient's chief complaint is nonspecific, such as weakness or fever, which can be caused by many different illnesses. While most clinicians have difficulty remembering long lists of possible diagnoses, reliance on memory is unnecessary in the era of hand-held computers.

  When the chief complaint is nonspecific, ask the patient about other symptoms that started at about the same time as their main complaint. One of these may have a much smaller list of possible causes of the patient's illness. For example, a patient with low-grade fever may volunteer that their right knee has been bothering them since the fever began. Localized joint pain, especially with fever, suggests a relatively small number of diagnoses.

  If this approach fails, many clinicians fall back on a time-honored technique: doing the review of systems immediately, rather than at the end of the interview. Several findings may merge into a pattern that suggests a syndrome or disease. Another, more specific, complaint may emerge. This technique has an inherent risk: you may forget the original complaint as you focus on more easily solved problems.

  Example: If our patient with chest pain instead presented with a chief complaint of excessive intestinal gas, an experienced clinician might do the review of systems rather than try to think of causes of this very nonspecific main complaint. This strategy might elicit the patient's chest pain, which would become the starting point for the differential diagnosis.

- *Memory failure:*

  To overcome a temporary lapse of memory, think of categories of disease rather than trying to recall specific diseases. First, think of anatomy. Try to identify the organ system that is the probable source of the patient's symptoms. Then, focus on diseases of that organ system. This strategy usually reduces the number of diseases to consider. Once you have identified a body system, think of *categories of etiology*. Most diseases are in one of the following categories: congenital, infectious, neoplastic, degenerative, or metabolic.

  Example: In our patient, first evaluate the hypothesis that the patient's chest pain is caused by chest wall disease rather than considering the many possible musculoskeletal causes of chest pain individually. If the pain has the characteristics of chest wall pain (pain on deep breathing or movement; pain on palpating the thorax), think of the anatomic components of the chest wall and the diseases that affect them (bone, nerve, cartilage, and muscle).

  In the era before hand-held computers, one coat pocket held a notebook listing common chief complaints and their causes. The other pocket held a stethoscope. Now the stethoscope is draped around the neck, and the coat pocket holds a hand-held computer. The principle is the same across generations of clinicians: relying on memory is poor practice.

2.3.2 The second step in differential diagnosis: gathering data to test hypotheses

After accumulating a few hypotheses through listening to the patient tell the story of their chief complaint, ask specific questions to test each hypothesis. This phase of history taking is sometimes called the cross-examination. Cross-examination is the most active part of history taking because several diagnostic hypotheses are being considered in rapid succession. The answers to several hypothesis-testing questions may exclude one diagnosis while elevating another to the "active list." Some diagnostic hypotheses are under active consideration only briefly, while others survive the cross-examination and are retested during the physical examination and beyond.

Data gathering can be quite time-consuming. Here is a discussion of several efficient strategies for history taking and the physical examination.

1. Screen and branch
2. Use pathognomonic findings

3. Consider the cost of additional information
4. Avoid getting information simply to reassure yourself.

1. *Screen and branch*: In screening and branching, the clinician moves from one hypothesis to another with one or two screening questions, rather than exploring each hypothesis in depth. The clinician asks about a clinical finding that is nearly always present in patients with a disease (*screening*). If the finding is not present, the clinician eliminates the diagnostic hypothesis and moves on to other hypotheses (*branching*).

Example: If our patient with chest pain denies having fever or cough, the clinician rapidly excludes pneumonia and moves on to screening questions for other hypotheses. If the clinician can press on the chest without eliciting pain, they decide that the patient does not have musculoskeletal chest pain.

Screening and branching are efficient but risky. If a finding is truly present in all patients with a disease, screening is a reliable method for excluding a hypothesis. However, effective screening questions are the exception rather than the rule. Few findings are always present in a disease. Clinicians seldom know exactly how often a finding is absent in patients with a disease because the information is unknown or easily forgotten.

Errors in screening may be avoided by using the following principle: *do not try to eliminate a common disease with a single screening question*. If you believe that a hypothesis is likely to be true, a negative response to a screening question should not eliminate the hypothesis. On the other hand, you can eliminate a "long shot," low-probability hypothesis if the patient answers no to a screening question. This reasoning is based on principles to be described in Chapter 4.

Screening and branching is a basic strategy in the physical examination. As a student, clinicians learn a "screening physical examination." If the screening examination of an organ shows an abnormality, clinicians perform a more detailed examination. If no abnormalities are found, the examiner moves on to the next part of the screening physical exam.

When to avoid the screening and branching strategy:

* When the hypothesized diagnosis has serious consequences if untreated (the disease you cannot afford to miss), focus on the manifestations of that disease.
* The disease is very common and therefore difficult to exclude with a single screening question.
* Effective screening questions do not exist.
* The patient may be an unreliable source of information. Best practice would be to do a complete review of systems and to do a physical examination.

2. *Pathognomonic findings*: A good screening question excludes disease; a pathognomonic finding establishes a diagnosis. A pathognomonic finding occurs in only one disease. Pathognomonic findings improve diagnostic efficiency, but very few such findings exist. Verifying a claim that a finding is pathognomonic of a disease is very difficult because the claimant must show that all patients with the finding have one and only one disease. Unquestioning belief in pathognomonic findings can lead the clinician to prematurely terminate a diagnostic search. A so-called pathognomonic finding is strong evidence in favor of a hypothesis, but supporting evidence should be sought.

Example: If cardiac auscultation in our patient with chest pain showed an easily audible pericardial friction rub, you should conclude that they have pericarditis. A pericardial friction rub is one of the few examples of a pathognomonic finding (this claim is, of course, subject to dispute!).

3. *Consider the cost of information*: The pursuit of evidence starts with the history and physical exam. As the pursuit of additional diagnostic information becomes more difficult, weigh the risk and costs of getting the information against its potential contribution to a secure diagnosis.

4. *Avoid getting information simply to reassure yourself*: When you know enough about the patient to formulate a plan, pause and think: "do I need more information?"

Get additional information only if it could change the plan. Chapter 13 provides evidence that the diagnostic search should stop when further information would not change the decision to act.

2.3.3 Hypothesis testing

Hypothesis testing is the most important but least understood part of differential diagnosis. In this section, we consider principles for evaluating hypotheses. These include:

1. Principles for comparing two hypotheses
2. Principles for reducing the list of active hypotheses
3. *The final step*: testing the adequacy of the proposed explanation for the patient's complaint.

1. *Principles for comparing two hypotheses:* Hypotheses are often evaluated in pairs. In this direct comparison, the less likely hypothesis is discarded. The remaining hypothesis is retained on the list of active hypotheses and then matched against another hypothesis. The rules in schoolyard pick-up basketball games are similar: The winner plays the next challenger. If it wins, it plays the next challenger and then the one after that until it finally loses. Then it sits and waits its turn to be a challenger.

Typically, clinicians compare hypotheses by how well each one matches up with the features of the patient's history. Whether they also take account of the relative prevalence of the hypothesized diseases is not known.

Several principles apply when deciding which hypothesis to discard:

- When deciding between evenly matched hypotheses, favor the diagnosis that is most prevalent in the population. This principle is a direct consequence of Bayes' theorem, which is the subject of Chapter 4. Clinicians typically do not know the exact prevalence in their practice and rely on impressions from personal experience and textbooks.

  Example: In patients with chest pain, coronary artery disease is common, and pericarditis is very uncommon. If the patient's findings match up equally well with the typical features of both diagnoses, favor coronary artery disease. Perhaps the patient has some features of coronary artery disease and some features of pericarditis. In that case, favor coronary artery disease.

- If the patient's pattern of findings is more likely to occur in diagnosis A than diagnosis B, favor diagnosis A.

  Example: In a patient with chest pain that is aggravated by breathing, signs of pulmonary consolidation are more common in pneumonia than in a fractured rib. When deciding between pneumonia and a fractured rib, we should favor pneumonia if consolidation is present. This statement is equivalent to saying that pulmonary consolidation is more representative of pneumonia than of fractured rib. It is an example of the *representativeness heuristic*, which we will discuss in Chapter 3. This principle also follows from the definition of the likelihood ratio, which is the single number that best characterizes the value of the information contained in a clinical finding (see Chapters 4 and 5).

- Strong evidence against one hypothesis increases the probability that another hypothesis is correct. This principle follows from the requirement that the sum of the probabilities of a set of mutually exclusive findings must add up to 1.0. Therefore, if the patient does not have a finding that is usually present in diagnosis A, diagnosis A becomes less likely and diagnosis B more likely. This principle underlies the "diagnosis of exclusion," in which we assume that a disease is present because we have excluded all other diseases.

After taking the history, several hypotheses often remain. By using the principles just described, the clinician can reduce this list still further during the physical examination. Often, however, more than one hypothesis may remain after performing the physical examination. Diagnostic tests or re-evaluation a short time later may resolve a diagnostic impasse, but one should first try to reduce the number of active hypotheses, if only to reduce the number of tests to choose between.

2. *Principles for reducing the list of active hypotheses:*
- Rank the remaining hypotheses and list the evidence for each and against each.
- *Consider the rule of parsimony*: One diagnosis is probably responsible for the patient's complaint.
- Combine diagnoses which require the same treatment.
  1. *Rank the remaining active hypotheses*: Rank the active hypotheses from the most likely to the least likely. List the evidence for each hypothesis. Committing your ideas to paper may remind you of some needed data, help eliminate some hypotheses, and put the situation in perspective.

     Example: Our patient has anterior chest pain that is squeezing in character and occurs principally at night. These findings are consistent with either an atypical form of coronary artery disease or esophageal spasm. Pericarditis and musculoskeletal disease are much less likely, and other possibilities have no supporting evidence.

  2. *The Rule of Parsimony*: According to the rule of parsimony, one disease is the cause of the patient's complaint, with rare exceptions. This rule implies that the clinician should eventually reduce the list of active hypotheses to a single disease.

     The Rule of Parsimony is based on a basic theorem of probability theory: the probability that two unrelated events occur simultaneously is the probability of one event multiplied by the probability of the other event. The product of the two probabilities is a much lower number than the probability of either event occurring by itself. The Rule of Parsimony is probably reliable in previously healthy people but may be less reliable in persons with several chronic diseases. In this case, two diagnostic hypotheses are less likely to be independent of each other, which increases the probability that both are present.

The rule of parsimony should occasionally be ignored. First, the probability that two common diseases occur simultaneously may be greater than the probability of a single rare disease. Second, when a delay in treating two hypothesized diseases might have serious consequences, it is better to treat both until it is possible to make a definitive diagnosis.

Example: If our patient with chest pain presented with fever, cough with blood-streaked sputum, a pleural friction rub, and a pulmonary infiltrate on a chest x-ray, they most likely have either pulmonary embolism or pneumonia. A suspected diagnosis of pneumonia requires twenty-four hours to confirm by culturing sputum or blood. Tests to diagnose suspected pulmonary embolism may not be available. An experienced clinician will start therapy for both these life-threatening diseases while awaiting more information.

3. *Combine diagnoses with the same consequences*: "Clustering" is acting as if two diseases were really one disease because both have the same treatment. One should always consider whether to cluster several diseases on the list of active hypotheses in order to reduce the number of them that require independent evaluation.

Example: If our patient had nocturnal chest pain that is relieved by antacids, they might have either esophagitis or esophageal spasm. Distinguishing between these two hypotheses is unnecessary because both diseases require treatment to reduce gastric acid secretion.

3. *A final step: Testing how well the active hypotheses explain the patient's complaint*: At this point, in differential diagnosis, one or two diagnostic hypotheses are still active. The next step is to decide between starting treatment, getting more information, or taking no immediate action (the subject of Chapter 13). One last step remains before deciding. After reviewing the patient's findings and the active hypothesis, the clinician should ask two questions:
- Do the hypothesized diagnoses account for the principal clinical features of the case? Put differently, does the patient's clinical picture match the features of the hypothesized diagnoses?
- Are any of the major clinical features of the case inconsistent with the hypothesized diagnoses?
  The purpose of these last questions is to assure a coherent and consistent explanation for the patient's findings. In effect, they remind the clinician to try to identify any "loose ends" that do not fit with the hypothesized diagnoses.

Example: Let us review the history of our patient with chest pain. The principal clinical features are:
- A chief complaint of "nocturnal chest pain for one month."
- The pain is tightness in the anterior chest that begins an hour or so after lying down.
- It is unrelated to exertion and unaffected by antacids.
- No recent injury and no fever or cough.
- The physical examination is normal.

We have discarded several categories of illness because the patient's history is inconsistent with key features of these categories. Musculoskeletal causes are unlikely because the history does not include recent trauma and pressing on the chest does not reproduce the pain. Infection is unlikely since fever, chills, cough, and signs of pulmonary disease are all absent. Finally, the pain is not relieved by antacids. This finding reduces the likelihood of esophagitis or esophageal spasm but does not entirely eliminate this hypothesis since the location and onset of the pain after lying down are consistent with this diagnosis. The remaining active hypothesis is an atypical form of coronary artery disease ("atypical angina pectoris").

Atypical coronary artery disease is a *coherent* explanation for the patient's complaint because it accounts for all of the features of the case. It is a *consistent* explanation because all findings are consistent with this hypothesis. Esophageal spasm and esophagitis are not a consistent explanation because antacids do not relieve the pain.

2.3.4 Selecting a course of action

When the active hypotheses have been ranked in order of plausibility, the clinician must decide what to do next. The three choices are:
- Treat
- Gather more information now
- Withhold treatment. Additional evidence may emerge as a hypothesized disease is allowed to follow its natural history.

The choice between these three alternatives is guided by probability (how likely is a disease?) and utility (how beneficial is prompt action and what are its harms?). The choice is obvious when a hypothesized illness is lethal, prompt treatment is safe and effective, and the patient is highly likely to have the disease. Despite a low probability of the disease, clinicians often begin treatment if therapy is safe, and failure to treat has dire consequences. If a disease requires treatment that is expensive or dangerous, they should require stronger evidence.

Treating a disease has two elements of uncertainty. First, some patients with the disease do not respond to the treatment. Second, the patient may not have the disease. The patient is then exposed to the risk of harm from the treatment with no possibility of benefit. When the clinician is uncertain that the patient has the disease but starts treatment anyway, some patients will receive treatment for a disease that they do not have, a recurring theme of Chapter 13.

Example: Our patient with chest pain has symptoms of two diseases – esophageal spasm and atypical coronary artery disease – that cannot easily be distinguished from one another by the history and physical examination. Further information must be obtained. The clinician has many options, ranging from performing a coronary arteriogram to initiating a therapeutic trial aimed at esophageal spasm.

The rest of this book is an exposition of the principles for making the best possible decision when the diagnosis and the consequences of taking action are uncertain. "Decision making under uncertainty" could be its subtitle.

2.4 An extended example

The following scenario is a transcript of an imaginary interview between a clinician and a patient. We present the scenario to illustrate the concepts we have just presented. The references list in this chapter includes the book by Jerome Kassirer and his colleagues, which contains many examples of physicians "thinking out loud" as they work through a difficult diagnostic problem.

Doctor: "How may I help you today?"
Patient: "It's these headaches I've been having."

Doctor thinks: I'll have to think about tension headaches, vascular headaches, headache due to medications, brain tumor, and infection.

Comment: The clinician begins forming hypotheses as soon as the patient voices her chief complaint. At this point, the clinician will ask the patient to tell her story. After hearing the narrative, she cross-examines the patient to supply needed details and to test hypotheses.

Doctor: "How long has this been going on?"
Patient: "For years, but it's worse now."
Doctor: "How often are you getting these headaches?"
Patient: "I used to get them a few times a month, but now it's almost every day."

Doctor thinks: This is a chronic problem that appears to have changed in severity. Either something has happened to exacerbate a pre-existing condition, or we are looking at a new process.

Comment: The clinician is beginning to ask screening questions that will help exclude some diagnoses (e.g., many kinds of meningitis are unlikely with a chronic headache) and will serve to increase the likelihood of other diagnoses (e.g., both tension and vascular headaches are suggested by the present pattern).

Doctor: "Have you noticed any other symptoms with the change in your headaches?"
Patient: "Well, yes. My vision has been rather blurry at times. Also, I don't think my appetite is as good, and I am not sleeping very well."

Doctor thinks: These are rather nonspecific symptoms. I'd better ask a few questions that relate to causes of headache that are serious and treatable.

Doctor: "Have you had any fever?"
Patient: "No."
Doctor: "Have you had a lack of coordination or weakness or paralysis?"
Patient: "No."

Doctor: "Have you noticed any numbness, weakness, or loss of sensation in a part of your body?"
Patient: "No."

Doctor thinks: Good. So far I see no evidence of any serious treatable disease, such as meningitis or brain tumor. Let's find out a little bit more about the headache itself.

Comment: With these initial screening questions, the clinician has efficiently tested and rejected several hypotheses. Tension headache and vascular headache remain likely explanations for the patient's complaint. Brain tumor and infection seem quite unlikely. As a result of responses to screening questions, the clinician has not pursued these hypotheses in depth. At this point, she will ask questions to test the hypotheses that the patient has a tension headache or vascular headache.

For the sake of brevity, we will not repeat this entire conversation. Suffice it to say, that as the clinician tests hypotheses, she asks questions about aggravating or precipitating factors, ameliorating factors, and the relationship between the headaches to time of day and physical activity. Of course, the clinician also ascertains the location and nature of the headache, as well as its response to medications. Finally, she obtains a brief past medical history, including allergies and medication consumption, and use of alcohol, tobacco, or drugs of abuse.

At this point, the clinician moves to the physical examination. Because many hypotheses have already been rejected, she can focus her attention on seeking evidence for the remaining active hypotheses. She will take the blood pressure and will pay particular attention to the head, ears, eyes, nose, and throat. In addition, she will do a screening neurologic examination to look for evidence of brain tumor.

After completing the physical examination, the clinician reflects on what she has learned and lists the remaining active hypotheses. While she has been testing hypotheses throughout the examination, now she must weigh the evidence for the remaining active hypotheses and decide whether to do a diagnostic test, start specific treatment, or wait to see if the headache resolves spontaneously.

Doctor thinks: Let's see. So far, I know that the patient has had headaches for many years and that they have increased in frequency and intensity in the last few months. Nonetheless, they do not awaken the patient from sleep, and there are no other symptoms except for some blurred vision and some loss of appetite. The patient has not lost weight, and the physical examination is completely normal, including normal visual acuity. The patient also tells me that the headaches are diffuse, occurring over the entire top, front, sides, and back of the head. The headache seems to be least severe in the morning and most severe by the end of the day. Aspirin partially relieves the headache. Finally, she took a new job approximately six months ago and now spends most of her day at a computer terminal.

Of my active hypotheses, which are the most likely? What is the commonest cause of headache? Tension headache is not only the commonest cause of headache, but her findings fit the classic description of tension headache quite well. What about other possibilities?

What are the diseases that I cannot afford to miss? With a normal neurologic exam and a history of many years of headache, brain tumor is extremely unlikely. Could she have a chronic infection, such as tuberculous or fungal meningitis? The absence of nocturnal headache or other associated systemic signs or symptoms of a chronic illness makes infection very unlikely. There's not enough evidence to pursue these diagnoses.

What about other common causes of headache, such as vascular headache? She has none of the typical prodromal symptoms. Moreover, her headache is diffuse rather than unilateral and is frequently relieved by simple analgesic medication. She also has no family history of migraine. Thus, her symptoms do not fit my concept of vascular headache at all. Furthermore, there is evidence of tension headache: her new job is monotonous and associated with increased visual strain. At this point, I think that tension headache is the most likely diagnosis.

Comment: In following the clinician's analysis, you can see several features of clinical reasoning. First, she gave special weight to tension headache because it is a common diagnosis. Second, she considered the more serious and treatable but rare causes of headache. In each case, she considered the data for and against those diagnoses and ended up eliminating them as possibilities. Of course, as any good clinician, she will reconsider these possibilities at a later date if new information appears or if the patient does not respond to therapy. Finally, she did a pairwise comparison of the two leading diagnostic hypotheses: tension headache and vascular headache.

Now, the clinician must select a course of action. She must gather more information, observe the patient without treatment, or begin treatment.

Doctor thinks: At this point, I am fairly comfortable with the diagnosis of tension headache. I don't think any further tests are necessary. Instead, I will learn a little bit more about the patient's work environment and see if I can identify anything that could be changed.

Doctor says to the patient: "I think there are some things we can do to help improve your headache problem. Let's review your daytime activities and begin to develop a plan of action. In addition, I want you to return to my office in a month to reevaluate the situation."

Patient: "Fine."

Comment: The clinician will try to help relieve the tension headaches, and she will use the "test of time" to re-evaluate other diagnostic possibilities. If the headache has not disappeared or has changed in character when the patient pays an office visit in one month, the clinician may repeat part of the physical exam or may obtain diagnostic tests.

The clinician has chosen a relatively risk-free approach. She has not irrevocably excluded the possibility of a serious cause of headache. In deciding to forego diagnostic tests, she has concluded that the likelihood of finding a treatable cause of headache is extremely low. Moreover, the expense and worry that diagnostic studies may engender appear to outweigh the remote possibility of a result that could benefit her patient.

Conclusion: Even the simplest of clinician-patient interactions contain the elements of rational decision making. Using these principles does not necessarily increase the amount of time required to evaluate the patient, especially if the screening and branching strategy is used to exclude hypotheses.

2.4.1 Clinical aphorisms

Clinical aphorisms are pithy, memorable distillates of clinical experience. Master diagnosticians rely on common-sense rules for clinical reasoning:

- If you hear hoofbeats, think of horses, not zebras.
- If a test result surprises you, repeat the test before taking action.
- Do a test only if the result could change your management plan.
- Infrequent manifestations of common diseases are often more likely than common manifestations of rare diseases.
- Your first priority is to think about the diseases you can't afford to miss.

When you have read this book, you should be able to explain each of these aphorisms.

Summary

1. Experienced clinicians formulate and test diagnostic hypotheses from the moment they first encounter the patient. At any moment, they actively consider only a few hypotheses.
2. Research on how clinicians evaluate diagnostic hypotheses has shown that they compare their patient's findings to similar cases from their experience. Expert diagnosticians appear to have a larger, more easily recalled body of cases.
3. The process of clinical reasoning has four steps. The first three steps comprise the process of differential diagnosis, which is a cyclic process that goes on throughout the history and physical examination. The last step occurs when the clinical evaluation is complete.
   Step 1: Generate alternative hypotheses.
   Step 2: Gather data.
   Step 3: Use data to test hypotheses.
   Step 4: Select a course of action: treat, test, or observe.
4. Clinicians who wish to become master diagnosticians should remember that a systematic approach to differential diagnosis is much preferred to brilliant leaps of intuition. That said, expertise in diagnosis is almost always associated with a wide exposure to patients. Seek contact with patients. Listen to their stories, first-hand from your experience and second-hand from the experiences of colleagues. Learn from your mistakes and your successes.

Bibliography

Elstein, A.S., Shulman, L.S., and Sprafka, S.A. (1978) *Medical Problem Solving: An Analysis of Clinical Reasoning*, Harvard University Press, Cambridge.

This book describes and analyzes experiments that were designed to uncover the basis for clinical reasoning. The authors propose a clinical problem solving method based on their observations.

Gorry, G.A., Pauker, S.G., and Schwartz, W.B. (1978) The diagnostic importance of the normal finding. *The New England Journal of Medicine*, **298**, 486–9.

A brief analytic paper showing how reducing the probability of one diagnosis increases the probability of all other active hypotheses.

Groopman, J. (2007) *How Doctors Think*, Houghton Mifflin, Boston, MA.

A physician wrote this engaging book for the general public. It uses extended examples to describe errors and triumphs of clinical cognition and judgment.

Kahneman, D. (2011) *Thinking: Fast and Slow*, Farrar, Straus & Giroux, New York.

Reflections on how the mind works with an emphasis on the perils of relying too much on a quick response.

Kassirer, J.P., Wong, J., and Kopelman, R. (2009) *Learning Clinical Reasoning*, 2nd ed., Lippincott, Williams and Wilkins, Baltimore, MD.

This book consists largely of analysis of case histories from the authors' experience. Excellent discussion of differential diagnosis.

National Academies of Sciences, Engineering, and Medicine (2015) *Improving Diagnosis in Health Care*, The National Academies Press, Washington, DC. https://doi.org/10.17226/21794.

The report of a National Academies of Science, Engineering, and Medicine study committee about the problem of diagnostic errors and strategies and policies to reduce diagnostic error. The report Summary is a concise description of the broad context of accurate diagnosis. The report can be downloaded from the National Academy of Medicine website at no charge.

Norman, G. (2005) Research in clinical reasoning. Past history and current trends. *Medical Education*, **39**, 418–27.

A survey of the body of evidence about how clinicians reason.

Slovic, P., Fischoff, B., and Lichtenstein, S. (1977) Behavioral decision theory. *Annual Review of Psychology*, **28**, 1–39.

A thorough exploration of why decision makers act as they do.

Probability: quantifying uncertainty

Uncertainty is the only certainty there is, and knowing how to live with insecurity is the only security.

John Allen Paulos

As we learned in Chapter 1, clinicians usually cannot directly observe the true state of the patient and must infer it from external, imperfect cues. These cues are the history, the physical examination, and diagnostic tests. In day-to-day clinical practice, the clinician relies on these imperfect indirect indicators of the patient's true state and accepts a degree of uncertainty when making decisions. Fortunately, many, perhaps most, decisions do not require certain knowledge of the true state of the patient.

Representing our uncertainty about the patient's true state as a probability is an essential first step in learning how to make decisions without certain knowledge. In this chapter, we will learn how to use the concept of probability to think clearly about the uncertainty inherent in most medical situations.

3.1 Uncertainty and probability in medicine

3.1.1 The uncertain nature of clinical information

Imagine a clinical finding that occurred in a disease in the following ways:

- **always** present in patients with the disease
  - Therefore, if the finding is absent, the disease is absent
- **never** present in patients who do not have the disease
  - Therefore, if the finding is present, the disease is present

We would not require clinical judgment to diagnose the disease; it would be sufficient to know if this finding were present.

Because no clinical finding has this perfect, one-to-one correspondence with a disease, clinicians must recognize the following bleak truth:

The true state of the patient lies hidden within the body, inaccessible to direct observation. The clinician must infer the patient's true state from external, imperfect cues.

Medical Decision Making, Third Edition. Harold C. Sox, Michael C. Higgins, Douglas K. Owens, and Gillian Sanders Schmidler.
© 2024 John Wiley & Sons Ltd. Published 2024 by John Wiley & Sons Ltd.

The following three examples illustrate typical clinical situations in which the clinician cannot directly observe the patient's true state and must infer it by imperfect clinical cues.

Example 1

The patient complains of left leg pain four days after hip surgery. The left leg is not warm or tender; its circumference is the same as the right leg. The clinician ignores these normal findings and obtains an ultrasound image of the leg veins, which shows a large blood clot.

Comment: Only one-third of patients with suspected deep venous thrombosis of the leg have physical signs of the disease.

Example 2

A 60-year-old man complains of retrosternal pain that radiates to the left arm. Exercise and emotional stress bring on the pain, which resolves promptly when the patient stops to rest or regains his composure. The patient's clinician initially believes the pain is due to myocardial ischemia and obtains an exercise electrocardiogram. Somewhat to their surprise, the exercise test is normal. The pain resolves after a trial of medication for ischemic cardiac pain

Comment: The patient's pain had the typical characteristics of ischemic pain, and his probability of coronary artery disease is at least 90%. In patients with this type of chest pain, the clinician knows that the probability of coronary artery disease is approximately 60% after a normal exercise electrocardiogram. The clinician could obtain a coronary arteriogram, which would resolve lingering uncertainty about the diagnosis. Instead, the patient receives a prescription for treating angina pectoris. The chest pain resolves after this therapeutic trial, providing enough evidence to justify a diagnosis of ischemic heart disease.

Example 3

James recently had close contact with someone who was later diagnosed as having COVID-19. Now, James is feeling achy and has a persistent cough. He gets tested for the virus at a drive-by testing station. The test comes back negative. He wonders if it is safe for him to visit his grandmother.

Comment: Suppose his pre-test probability of having COVID-19 illness is 50%. The polymerase chain reaction test for the virus appears to have a sensitivity of approximately 70%. Despite the negative test, his probability of COVID-19 illness is approximately 25%.

3.1.2 Definition and key concepts

Clinicians use language to express their uncertainty. In talking about a difficult decision, one clinician may say that treatment is needed because a disease is "possibly present" while another clinician withholds treatment for a disease because it is "probably not present." Clinicians often use "possibly" or "probably" to describe gradations of belief in a hypothesis. However, using these words may interfere with clear communication, for the following reasons:

- Clinicians choose different words to express the same judgment about the likelihood of a future event.
- Clinicians use the same word to express very different judgments about the likelihood of an event.
- Words cannot describe precisely how much one's belief in a diagnostic hypothesis has changed as new information becomes available.

Clinicians who use words to communicate their uncertainty may feel confident that they have conveyed their meaning. In fact, words are the enemy of clarity in expressing one's uncertainty. In a famous study by Bryant and Norman, clinicians assigned a wide range of probabilities of disease to the word "probably" (0.3–0.95) and "possibly" (0.05–0.80). Clearly, two people could agree despite using different words or could disagree despite using the same word. **Probability**, a quantitative expression of uncertainty, avoids this ambiguity.

Probability provides a model for talking about uncertainty. The foundation for that model is the three axioms that define what is meant by the probability of an event. These axioms are:

Axiom 1: The probability of a null event – an event that cannot occur – is zero.
Axiom 2: The probability of a certain event – an event that must occur – is one.
Axiom 3: If A and B are any two events, then the probability of the union of A and B is the sum of the probability of each event minus the probability that they both occur at the same time (p[A] + p[B] – p[A and B]).

What is the union of A and B? It is all the points that are either only in A or all the points that are only in B or all the points that are in both A and B. In other words, the union of A and B will occur when either A or B occurs. If there is no overlap between A and B, which means that A and B are mutually exclusive, the probability of the union of A and B is the sum of the probabilities that each will occur.

The union of A and B is an example of a *disjunctive* event: either A or B must be present to define the event. Another term for a disjunctive event is *probabilistic independence*. As an example of a disjunctive event, chest pain caused by EITHER physical exertion OR emotional distress defines the syndrome of angina pectoris.

The scale for probability is typically zero to 1.0. This scale is arbitrary but convenient. We could assign any number to the probabilities for the null event and the certain event; choosing zero and one makes the arithmetic simpler.

The third axiom is fundamental because it is the basis of the first tool that makes probability useful. With it, we can use probability to do useful tasks. For example, we can determine the probability of a disease if we know the probability that the disease occurs if a finding is present and the probability of the disease occurring if the finding is not present.

Independence is the other fundamental concept in probability theory. Two events, A and B, are independent if the occurrence of A does not affect the probability of B. Stated slightly differently:

Definition of independence

Events A and B are independent if the probability that they both occur is the product of the probability that each occurs.

The dependence of two events is an example of a *conjunctive*. Both A and B must be present to define a conjunctive event. Another term for it is *probabilistic dependence*. As an example of a conjunctive, cough productive of yellow sputum AND a chest radiograph showing an infiltrate in the lung are needed to make a clinical diagnosis of pneumonia. Neither alone is sufficient.

With the three axioms and the definition of independence, we can build the computational tools that make probability so useful in daily life.

3.1.3 The meaning of probability: the present state vs. a future event

Probability can refer to a "present state" or a "future event" because uncertainty in medicine can be about the present state of the patient or the occurrence of a future event. For example, the patient's history can provide clues about whether the patient *has* coronary artery disease or *will develop* coronary artery disease in the future.

The distinction between present state and future event applies to the design of studies to identify information with which to quantify uncertainty. Discovering the predictors of the present state would involve a systematic history and physical examination, performing a definitive test (e.g., a coronary arteriogram) on the same day, and using statistical techniques to identify the predictors of the result of the arteriogram. This is a *cross-sectional study design*. To discover the predictors of a future event, one would obtain a systematic history and physical examination of members of a population (a cohort) and then contact each of them periodically to see who had experienced the outcome event of interest (e.g., a myocardial infarction). This is a *cohort study design*.

In the next few chapters, we will focus on how to determine the probability of the patient's present state before and after obtaining a diagnostic test. We will use the term "probability of the target condition" to represent uncertainty about the patient's *present* state. The term "target condition" refers to the hypothesized disease that the test is intended to detect.

3.1.4 Odds: an alternative way to express a probability

Odds: some prefer to use odds rather than probability to express their uncertainty. They ask themselves, "For every time that a patient with these characteristics had cancer, how many times was cancer not present?" Figure 3.1 illustrates the concept of odds.

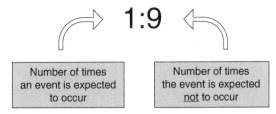

Figure 3.1 The meaning of the odds of an event.

> **Definition**
>
> *ODDS*: The probability that an event will occur divided by the probability that the event will not occur.

Odds and probability are equivalent. The relationship between the odds of an event and its probability is the following:

$$\text{odds} = \frac{p}{1-p}$$

where p is the probability that the event will occur.

Thus, if the probability of the event is 0.67, the odds of the event are 0.67 divided by 0.33, or 2 to 1. Another way to express the odds of an event is: p:[$1–p$]. Thus, writing 2:1 odds is equivalent to saying "2 to 1 odds," or expressed as a quotient: 2/1.

Facility in converting a probability to its equivalent expressed as odds is important, as we will see in Chapter 4 when we calculate post-test odds using the odds ratio form of Bayes' theorem.

Convert odds to probability with the following relationship:

$$p = \frac{o}{1+o}$$

where o is the odds that the event will occur.

Some find it especially useful to use odds to express their opinion about very infrequent events (1:99 odds, rather than a probability of 0.01) or very common events (99:1 odds, rather than a probability of 0.99).

3.2 How to determine a probability

3.2.1 Probability: a quantification of judgment about the likelihood of an event

This definition provides one of the foundations for this textbook. It captures two key properties of a probability.

- Probability reflects a judgment. It is subjective – different individuals can have different probabilities for the same event because they see the event somewhat differently.
- A probability also is a number.

How can these seemingly incompatible properties coexist? A number seems so concrete. How can it also represent something so intangible as a judgment? This duality can be hard to grasp. How does one attach a number to a subjective judgment?

An example may help. Imagine a person choosing between two gambles, as represented by Figure 3.2 (see next page). One is betting that it will rain later this afternoon, which relies on subjective judgment. The other is betting on drawing a white ball while blindfolded from an urn containing a known proportion of black vs. white balls: an objective probability. If the proportion of white balls is high, the person will prefer to bet on drawing a white ball. If the proportion of white balls is low, the person will prefer betting that it will rain. The choice between betting on rain or drawing a white ball is repeated with different proportions of white and black balls.

When the person is indifferent between the two gambles, the proportion of white balls to black balls – an objective, measurable probability – is that person's subjective probability that it will rain this afternoon. An intuitive sense about whether it will rain has been transmuted into a number, a probability.

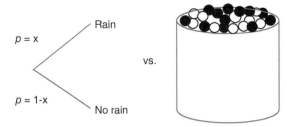

Figure 3.2 On the left is a gamble representing the possibility of rain; on the right is an urn with a mixture of black and white balls in a proportion that changes during the assessment of the subject's probability that it will rain.

This translation of an intuitive sense (low, intermediate, or high likelihood of rain) into a probability is fundamental. A probability, unlike an intuitive sense, can take advantage of a large body of knowledge, such as the sensitivity and specificity of tests, to make strong conclusions. Reread Section 3.2.1 again and come back to it until you have absorbed this concept.

3.2.2 Indirect probability assessment

The process just described for determining a person's probability of rain has a name: *indirect probability assessment*. This approach is seldom, if ever, used in clinical practice, but it may help some people choose a number to represent their opinion about a specific diagnosis given a patient's clinical presentation.

To embed the concept of indirect probability assessment solidly in your mind, consider a second example. Suppose you must assess a clinician's belief that cancer is the cause of a patient's weight loss. You ask the clinician to choose between two wagers: betting that cancer is present or making a wager at defined odds, such as buying a state lottery ticket. If the two wagers are equally attractive to the clinician, the clinician's probability that weight loss is due to cancer is the same as the probability of winning the lottery. Frank P. Ramsey, a pioneer in the concept of subjective probability, devised this method.

Indirect probability assessment is analogous to weighing an object. The event to be measured (the weight of the object) is compared with a standard of reference (a 1-kilogram weight). If the scale balances, the object weighs one kilogram. Indirect probability assessment allows the clinician to express a difficult concept (the probability of a disease) by comparing it to a more tangible event (the outcome of a lottery).

Although the lottery takes place only in the clinician's imagination, it should be treated seriously. Therefore, the prize should be truly desirable, such as a tuition rebate, the internship of one's choice, or a three-month paid vacation!

The following scenario depicts the steps in the indirect assessment of probability. Imagine that a clinician has seen a patient with high blood pressure and asks for your help in assessing the probability that the patient has a mineralocorticoid-secreting adrenal adenoma.

YOU: Which would you prefer?
- Betting that the patient has an adrenal adenoma (if they do, you win a paid vacation).
- Drawing a ball from an urn containing one red ball and 99 white balls (if you draw a red ball, you win the paid vacation).

CLINICIAN: I'd bet on the adenoma being present.

Interpretation: The clinician believes that the probability of the patient having an adenoma is higher than 0.01 and prefers to bet on the event that is more likely to occur.

YOU: Which would you prefer?
- Betting that the patient has an adenoma (if they have one, you win a paid vacation).
- Drawing a ball from an urn containing 10 red balls and 90 white balls (if you draw a red ball, you win the paid vacation).

CLINICIAN: I'd draw from the urn.

Interpretation: The clinician believes that the probability of an adenoma is less than 0.10 and prefers the gamble with the higher chance of winning.

YOU: Which would you prefer?
- Betting that the patient has an adenoma (if they do, you win the paid vacation).
- Drawing a ball from an urn that has five red balls and 95 white balls (if you draw a red ball, you win the paid vacation).

CLINICIAN: I really can't decide. The two wagers look equally good to me.

> *Interpretation: Since the prize for the two gambles is the same, the inability to choose between the two gambles means that the clinician believes that the chance of winning is the same for both gambles. Since the chance of drawing a red ball from the urn is 0.05, the clinician's subjective probability that this patient has an adrenal adenoma is 0.05.*

Probabilities obtained in this way must obey the laws of probability. Therefore, the probabilities of all possible causes of the patient's hypertension must add up to 1.0.

3.2.3   Direct probability assessment

Direct probability assessment: To assess a person's probability directly, ask for a number between zero and 1.0 that expresses the person's belief that an event will occur.

Experienced clinicians usually have little difficulty responding to this request, especially when they recall experiences with similar patients. For example, after hearing a patient describe their chest pain, the clinician may use the following frame of reference: "How often was the coronary arteriogram abnormal in patients from whom I have obtained a similar history?"

Matching the patient's findings to prior patients should, in principle, be effective, although subject to biases in using the representative heuristic (see Section 3.3.2). The reader may wonder how a clinician could estimate a probability so that it truly reflected many years of medical practice.

Disagreement about the next steps in the care of a patient has many causes. The first step is to identify the source of the disagreement. It may stem from differing opinions about the patient's probability of the target condition. Stating one's probability and discussing the reasons for differences may lead to an agreement on the next steps.

3.3   Sources of error in using personal experience to estimate the probability

Determining a subjective probability seems dangerously prone to error for an activity that is so central to medical practice. Clinicians base their probability assessments on personal experience with similar patients, which may be limited in many situations or subject to errors in reasoning. This section describes the cognitive processes for performing this mental task and the errors that can occur. The content is based on research done by two cognitive psychologists: Daniel Kahneman and Amos Tversky.

The discussion has four parts:
- Heuristics defined
- The representativeness heuristic
- The availability heuristic
- The anchoring and adjustment heuristic

3.3.1   Heuristics defined

Research shows that people use several types of cognitive processes (also called **heuristics**) for using prior experience to assess probability.

Definition

COGNITIVE HEURISTIC: A mental process used to learn, recall, or understand knowledge.

Research has identified several ways in which we misuse our cognitive heuristics for estimating probability and making systematic errors (bias). If clinicians understood these heuristics and learned how to avoid common mistakes in using them, their probability assessments might be more accurate.

We next define three heuristics and show how people misuse them. This material is easy to understand and very important in clinical medicine and in life. The heuristics are:

1. Representativeness
2. Availability
3. Anchoring and adjustment

3.3.2 Heuristic I: representativeness

Clinicians often ask: "What is the probability that patient A has disease B?" To answer such questions, they usually ask *how closely does patient A resemble the class of patients with disease B?*

Definition

REPRESENTATIVENESS HEURISTIC: a process for categorizing something by how closely its essential features resemble those of the parent population.

To evaluate the similarity of patient A to a typical member of class B, we use a stereotypical picture of disease B as our standard of reference. Consider a patient with symptoms of an inflamed gallbladder (cholecystitis). Our estimate of the probability of cholecystitis will depend on how closely the patient's findings resemble the textbook description of cholecystitis (or patients from our own clinical experience with cholecystitis).

Clinicians often use the representativeness heuristic and must be aware of several ways that it can lead to mistakes. To avoid these errors, the clinician should ask the questions depicted in Figure 3.3.

Errors in using the representativeness heuristic: ignoring the prior probability of the disease
The features of a case history that make it resemble the features of a disease are important but not the only characteristics that affect the probability that the disease is present. An additional, frequently forgotten, feature is the prevalence of the disease in clinical practice. As we will see in Chapter 4, the probability of disease, as new information becomes available, is strongly influenced by the prior probability of disease. By analogy, *the prevalence of a disease in the clinical setting affects its probability after the clinician has asked about the typical features of the disease.* Even if the patient's features are a close match, the disease is unlikely if it seldom occurs in the clinical setting. One of the authors studied patients presenting with chest pain in different clinical settings. The results showed that the probability of coronary artery disease in patients with a similar history depended on the overall prevalence of coronary artery disease in the clinical setting.

An interesting consequence of this finding is placing too much weight on the expected prevalence of a disease and too little weight on the patient's findings. A clinician might fail to diagnose an older patient with typical clinical features of a common disease that seldom occurs in older people.

The following examples illustrate the effects of ignoring the prior probability of disease.

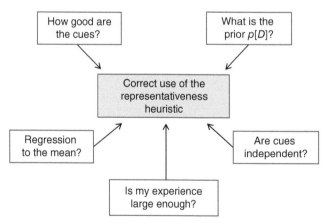

Figure 3.3 Factors that affect probabilities derived from using the representativeness heuristic.

Example 1

A long-time resident of Kansas presents to their community clinician with a history of intermittent shaking chills, sweats, and fever for one week. The physical examination is unrevealing. The examining clinician has just entered the private practice after having spent two years on the staff of a hospital in Southeast Asia, where malaria is very common. The clinician estimates that the probability of malaria in this patient is 0.90.

Comment: The clinician has ignored the rarity of malaria in the usual North American patient and has made a diagnosis strictly on the similarity between this patient and a typical patient with malaria. Based on their prevalence in North American patients, other diseases are far more likely than malaria to be the cause of fever, shaking chills, and sweats.

Example 2

A 35-year-old woman with mild hypertension is obese and has prominent striae and moderately excessive facial hair. She does not take corticosteroids. The medical student clerk has just completed an endocrinology elective. They immediately suspect Cushing's disease and tell their preceptor that there is a 30% chance that the patient has this disease. They had written an order for a complete battery of tests of adrenal function. Their preceptor cancels the order.

Comment: Cushing's disease is the cause of hypertension in fewer than one in 100 patients. Features of Cushing's disease occur in other conditions which are much more prevalent. Even when the patient's clinical features are quite representative of classic Cushing's, the diagnosis is still a long shot.

To avoid the mistake of ignoring prior probability, the clinician must ask, "How common is the hypothesized disease in my clinical setting?" The commonest error is to overestimate the prevalence of the disease.

Errors in using the representativeness heuristic: using clinical cues that do not accurately predict disease
The cues that make up the textbook description of a disease are imperfect indicators of who has the disease. Cues are sometimes absent in persons with the disease and sometimes present in persons who do not have the disease. One mark of an excellent diagnostician is to know how well clinical features predict disease.

Example

A previously healthy patient comes to the emergency department with the sudden onset of shortness of breath. The clinician on duty initially suspects a pulmonary embolism but discards the possibility because the patient shows no signs of blood clots in the leg veins. Furthermore, the patient does not complain of coughing blood or chest pain. The clinician sends the patient home. Two days later, the patient's shortness of breath worsens, and the patient goes to another hospital where the emergency department clinicians correctly diagnose pulmonary embolism.

Comment: The clinician who first saw the patient has underestimated the probability of pulmonary embolism because the patient did not have two of the classic features of pulmonary embolism. The clinician did not know that only one-quarter of patients with pulmonary embolism cough blood and only one-third have clinical evidence of blood clots in the leg veins. These findings, while part of the classic description of pulmonary embolism, are not reliable clues to the disease.

Knowing how well the classic features of commonly encountered diseases predict the disease is essential to a lean, safe style of medical practice. In the next two chapters, we will lay the foundation for understanding the *likelihood ratio*, which is the best single measure of predictivity. Past issues of the *Journal of the American Medical Association* are the best source of the likelihood ratios of common clinical findings. Since 1998, the journal has published many articles that summarize how well the clinical findings of common diseases predict the disease. The feature is called The Rational Clinical Examination, which is also the name of the book that summarizes this series of articles (see the Bibliography).

Errors in using the representativeness heuristic: being too sure of a diagnosis when redundant predictors are present

When a patient has many of the classic predictors of a disease, the clinician is often very confident of the diagnosis because "the story holds together pretty well."

However, internal consistency does not necessarily lead to accurate predictions. Consider this extreme case. If the classic predictors of disease *always* occur together, knowing that one predictor is present is the same as knowing that all are present. For purposes of diagnosis, the other predictors are redundant. They do not add information, and the clinician should not be any more confident of the diagnosis when several features are present than if only one feature is present. Clinicians often assume that each additional finding increases the probability of disease proportionately. In fact, clinical cues may be less predictive in combination than the clinician expects.

Example

A 40-year-old woman has chest pain that is retrosternal, radiates to the left arm and is crushing, squeezing, and pressure-like. The clinician concludes that the pain is indicative of coronary artery disease and admits the patient to the cardiac care unit. The patient is discharged the next day with an appointment for a test of her gallbladder function.

Comment: The patient appeared representative of coronary artery disease, and her pain is indeed anginal in quality. But the probability that she had coronary artery disease would have increased considerably if she had one or more of the following independent predictors of coronary artery disease. Each one adds information even when the others are present.

- A history of pain brought on by exertion and emotional stress
- Pain relieved promptly by rest or nitroglycerin
- Pain so severe that the patient had to stop all activities when the pain occurred
- A history of smoking cigarettes for many years

These findings are independent predictors of coronary artery disease. We know this because a multivariate regression analysis (a statistical method) of patients with chest pain showed that each of them increased the probability of coronary artery disease regardless of the presence of the others. In contrast, the location, radiation, and descriptors of anginal pain tend to occur together and are therefore highly correlated.

Empirical evidence about which disease cues are uncorrelated predictors of disease (i.e., independent) is increasingly available. This information often is presented in the form of models for using clinical findings to predict disease. We discuss these **clinical prediction models** later in this chapter.

Errors in using the representativeness heuristic: mistakenly using regression to the mean as diagnostic evidence

A change in the patient's condition is often used to test a diagnostic hypothesis:

A **therapeutic trial** consists of giving a treatment that relieves the symptoms of a hypothesized disease but is ineffective in other diseases. If the patient improves, the clinician's estimated probability of the disease increases accordingly. The drug's mechanism of action leads us to expect that it would affect the pathophysiology of the disease, and so the change in the patient's status becomes a diagnostic feature of the hypothesized disease. A response to specific treatment, therefore, increases the match between the patient's features and the classic features of the disease.

The test of time is another form of therapeutic trial. Here, the clinician withholds treatment to test the hypothesis that the patient does not have a serious disease. If the patient improves without treatment, the probability of serious disease goes down. The response to the test of time also improves the match between the patient's features and the typical features of a self-limited illness. This type of hypothesis testing is often used in clinical practice.

However, changes in disease status that coincide with a therapeutic trial may mislead the clinician because they are due to random variation in the course of the disease rather than cause-and-effect. The name of this relationship is **regression to the mean**.

Example

A patient has mild hyperglycemia on a single measurement of serum glucose. The clinician puts the patient on a diabetic diet. The patient's blood sugar falls, and the clinician concludes that the patient had diabetes.

Comment: The patient may not have diabetes. Hyperglycemia on the first blood glucose test could be a random variation in this biological measure. The second measurement was simply a less extreme sample from the same frequency distribution of serum glucose for this patient.

What is the basis for this example? Most biological measurements vary randomly over time in an individual. When these random values are symmetrically distributed about a mean value, the result is called the normal distribution curve (Figure 3.4).

The shape of the normal distribution curve shows that events whose value is close to the mean are much more common than events whose value is far from the mean. Therefore, an extreme value is more likely to be followed by a value that is closer to the mean than a value close to the initial value.

In the upper panel, a healthy person has an unlikely, surprisingly high, test result. A repeat test gives a much more likely value, given the shape of the distribution curve in healthy people. The lower panel depicts a surprisingly low value for a diseased person. A repeat test gives a much more likely, higher value. A high value is more likely than not to be followed by a low value. The clinician may therefore misinterpret a random event such as the fluctuations in symptoms of a minor illness as proving the success or failure of a therapeutic trial.

Errors in using the representativeness heuristic: comparing a patient to a small, unrepresentative experience with a disease

When clinicians use the representativeness heuristic to judge the probability that a patient has a disease, they often compare the patient to their personal experience with the disease. In doing so, they often neglect to account for the size of their personal experience. When personal experience with a disease is limited, the principles of statistical sampling tell us that it is likely to be atypical. A patient with atypical clinical features may match the clinician's small, atypical experience of patients with a disease, leading the clinician to conclude that the patient is highly likely to have the disease.

Why is a small experience likely to be atypical? A clinician's personal experience with an event is a sample of the universe of all such events. From statistical theory, we learn that a small sample is more likely to deviate from the parent population than a large sample. Thus, a small personal experience may be quite unrepresentative of the parent

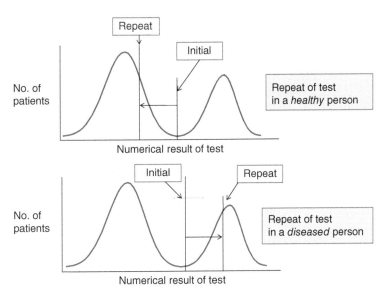

Figure 3.4 Two examples of regression to the mean: in normal individuals (top panel) and in diseased individuals (bottom panel). The curve on the left corresponds to the random distribution of results in a normal individual. The distribution on the right corresponds to results in a diseased individual.

population. An event which is unusual in the parent class, and therefore improbable, may be judged probable because it is representative of a clinician's small personal experience.

Example

Dr. V's patient has a heart rate of 100/min, has lost a little weight, and has been irritable of late. Although there is no enlargement of the thyroid gland, Dr. V estimates that the probability of hyperthyroidism is 0.50 because the patient closely resembles the only two cases of hyperthyroidism that Dr. V has diagnosed in ten years of primary care practice. When thyroid tests are all normal, Dr. V can scarcely believe the results and sends the patient to a consultant to help resolve this unusual case.

Comment: In a large population of hyperthyroid patients, 95% will have an enlarged thyroid gland. Dr. V's personal experience was too small to be representative of hyperthyroidism.

Mistakes in using the representative heuristic are avoidable. Clinicians should rely more on published accounts of the typical features of diseases and less on personal experience. Knowing more about the prevalence of diseases in one's practice would help, as would a wider exposure to patients and their resulting diagnoses. The best way to become an expert diagnostician is to see lots of patients.

This example concludes our discussion of the representativeness heuristic. Time spent on learning about the representativeness heuristic will be well repaid. Clinicians use this heuristic many times each day in clinical practice. Clinicians could improve their clinical reasoning skills by remembering these examples.

The next heuristic is much easier to understand than the representativeness heuristic.

3.3.3 Heuristic II: availability

Availability, the process by which repetition enhances recall, is a second heuristic for using personal experience to determine probability.

Definition

Availability Heuristic judging the probability of an event by how easily similar events come to mind.

Availability is a valid clue for judging probability, owing to experimental evidence that frequent events are easier to remember than infrequent events. However, other factors also affect the ease of recall. They include vividness, the consequences for the clinician or the patient, immediacy, recency, and, paradoxically, rarity. Making a difficult diagnosis is deeply satisfying, and its memory persists. For the same reason, clinicians remember the patient with a rare disease. When examining a patient with an unusual pattern of findings, a clinician may vividly recall a patient with similar findings and an unusual disease. Clinicians overestimate the frequency of these special events in their professional life because their memories of them are so vivid. They remember the patient with a rare or difficult-to-diagnose disease but forget the many patients with similar findings who had more commonplace diseases.

Example 1

A clinician overestimates the probability that a patient with diarrhea has amoebiasis because of a recent patient who had amoebiasis (which is an unusual cause of diarrhea in the United States).

Example 2

A clinician recently made a first-ever diagnosis of a subphrenic abscess by doing a white cell scan on a patient with fever and abdominal pain. For several months, every patient with abdominal pain and low-grade fever had a white cell scan to rule out a subphrenic abscess. The patients all recovered uneventfully in a few days and wondered why they had to have an expensive test.

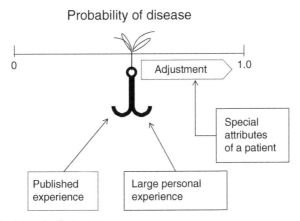

Figure 3.5 Schematic depiction of anchoring and adjustment.

The third heuristic is the mental process by which special characteristics of the patient are used to estimate probability. This heuristic is called **anchoring and adjustment**.

3.3.4 Heuristic III: anchoring and adjustment

Clinicians often assess probability starting from an initial probability and arriving at a final probability by *adjusting* to take account of the individual features of a patient. For example, they start with a probability based on the prevalence of the target condition and adjust upward or downward based on the individual patient's findings. This very important heuristic is often used incorrectly. According to experimental evidence, the usual mistake is to adjust too little after acquiring additional information. The bias toward the initial probability estimate is a failure of adjustment. The anchor depicted in Figure 3.5 represents the cognitive resistance to adjusting the starting probability. This heuristic for assessing probability is biased because people tend to place too much emphasis on the starting point (the first impression) and too little on new information.

There are several reasons why the anchoring and adjustment bias leads to incorrect adjustment of probability estimates.

- People tend to *overestimate* the probability of events that are defined by two or more features occurring at the same time. This type of event is called *conjunctive* because the events have an apparent connection with each other. The error in estimating probability may be due to overconfidence in redundant cues, one of the misuses of the representativeness heuristic.
- People tend to *underestimate* the probability of an event that is defined by one and only one of several features occurring. This type of event is called **disjunctive** because the events lack an apparent connection with each other.
- When asked to describe their uncertainty about a probability, people tend to over-state their certainty, as manifest by a narrower distribution of probabilities than is consistent with their stated level of certainty.
- People make a subjective judgment about how much to adjust a probability after getting new information. Research shows that their adjustment is closer to the starting point than it should be as determined by the post-test probability calculated with Bayes' theorem.

Bayes' theorem, which is the topic of the next chapter, is an unbiased approach to adjusting probabilities from a starting point. Bayes' theorem indicates exactly how much to adjust an initial probability when additional information becomes available.

Example

A patient with chest pain has atypical angina, and the clinician estimates the probability of coronary artery disease to be 0.70. The clinician orders an exercise electrocardiogram, which is very abnormal. Instead of diagnosing coronary artery disease, the clinician orders a costly cardiac CT angiogram.

Comment: When the probability of disease prior to the test is estimated to be 0.70 and the exercise electrocardiogram is very abnormal, the probability of coronary artery disease is at least 0.95. At this point, most clinicians would tell the patient that they had coronary artery disease and discuss the choice between medical treatment or revascularization. Relying on intuition rather than Bayes' theorem, this clinician underestimated the effect of a very abnormal exercise ECG on the probability of coronary artery disease and ordered an unnecessary confirmatory test.

3.3.5 Correctly using heuristics for estimating probability

Using personal experience to estimate probability is among the most important topics in this book because it happens many times in a day in the practice of medicine. The student of medicine must learn how to avoid the pitfalls of the methods that people use to estimate the probability, which requires a secure understanding of the heuristics for recalling the experience.

Making precise, unbiased probability assessments from personal experience is beyond the cognitive ability of almost everyone. Clinicians do their best, and their best is often astonishing. Nonetheless, the wisest among us seek guidance from published experience, which is our next topic.

3.4 The role of empirical evidence in quantifying uncertainty

Earlier in this chapter we defined probability as *a quantification of judgment about the likelihood of an event*. In the preceding section, we focused on the use of judgment to determine a patient's probability. We referred to patterns of clinical features that comprise a description of the disease. Other than the iterative process called indirect probability assessment, we said nothing about how to use judgment to quantify one's uncertainty. The processes to be described in this section will determine *a number that can inform the judgments that establish a probability*.

The italicized phrase may seem less obscure if you remember the anchoring and adjustment heuristic. A probability assessment often starts with a number that represents a broad population. Clinicians arrive at a final probability by *adjusting* the starting probability to take account of the individual features of a specific patient. Published experience is often the source of that starting number. The mortality rate from an operation, the probability of an adverse effect of therapy, and the prevalence of a severe form of coronary artery disease are examples of starting probabilities obtained from published studies. Published studies are useful for several reasons:

A published report usually reflects a much larger experience with a disease than most clinicians see in a lifetime in practice.
 A published report is the product of systematic study and unbiased reporting according to the fundamental principles of epidemiology.
 Statistical analyses in published studies often organize the findings in a form that is useful for determining a specific patient's probability.

Published studies often report *prevalence*, which is the proportion of a population that has a characteristic *at a specified instant in time* (e.g., the proportion of 23-year-old men in the population of a town on a certain date). The prevalence of a disease can be a starting point for determining its probability in a specific patient. Do not confuse prevalence with *incidence*, which is the number of occurrences during a specified *period of time* (e.g., the number of men in a defined population who had a stroke during one year).

Prevalence can also mean the proportion of a subgroup defined by a *formal process* for combining clinical findings (i.e., *a clinical prediction model*), which is our next topic.

In the next several pages, we describe three ways to form a group of patients in which to measure the prevalence of a disease. In each, the common feature is a diagnostic problem.

3.4.1 Determining probability from the prevalence of disease in patients with a symptom, physical finding, or test result

The prevalence of a disease in patients who have a symptom, physical finding, or diagnostic test result helps a clinician to diagnose the disease ("common diseases are common").

Example

A medical student evaluates a young man with abdominal pain. Their main concern is appendicitis. The pain is present throughout the abdomen and is associated with loose bowel movements. The patient does not have localized abdominal tenderness, fever, or an increased blood leukocyte count. The medical student presents the patient to the chief surgical resident who, to the student's surprise, discharges the patient from the emergency room.

Comment: The chief surgical resident knows that the prevalence of appendicitis among self-referred adult males with abdominal pain is only 1%. The student should use this information as a starting point as they use the patient's clinical findings to determine the probability of appendicitis. If they do not suggest appendicitis, the probability of appendicitis is very low since it was 1% in the average male with abdominal pain. If the examination does suggest appendicitis, the student's probability must reflect the low prevalence of appendicitis in all men with abdominal pain.

A published prevalence of disease may not apply to a specific clinical situation. The most common problem is systematic differences between the published article's study population and the specific clinical situation. For example, the prevalence of renovascular hypertension in a specialty clinic is higher than in a primary care practice. A second problem is a small sample size, which means imprecise prevalence estimates that would propagate through subsequent calculations of post-test probability.

3.4.2 Determining the probability of a disease from its prevalence in patients with a clinical syndrome

Definition

Syndrome: a collection of signs and symptoms that consistently occur together and are associated with one or more specific diseases.

After evaluating a patient, the clinician may identify a clinically defined syndrome (e.g., nephrotic syndrome) whose causes, and their prevalence, are known from published studies. This process sounds straightforward, but the prevalence of a disease in a syndrome may depend on how the researchers assembled the study population. For example, the prevalence of the diseases may be higher in hospital patients than in office-based practice. Therefore, deciding that the prevalence in a published study applies to an individual requires attention to the match between the study setting and the clinical setting in which the individual was seen.

Example

A resident is examining a 45-year-old man who came to the emergency room after experiencing retrosternal chest pain for the first time earlier in the day. The pain was pressure-like in quality and was confined to the chest. The pain came on after a hurried meal and lasted about ten minutes. He has felt fine since then.

The resident is trying to decide whether to test for coronary artery disease. They know that the decision about testing should depend on how well the patient's history fits the typical history for exertional angina pectoris, atypical angina, or non-anginal chest pain. The resident looks up an article which indicates the prevalence of coronary artery disease in each of these syndromes. After consulting with a cardiologist, they decide that the patient's history is most consistent with non-anginal chest pain, counsels the patient against eating too fast, and schedules a follow-up visit in two weeks.

Comment: This hypothetical study illustrates some of the problems of studies of disease prevalence in patients with a syndrome like chest pain. The study may lack standardized criteria for assigning a patient to one of the three chest pain syndromes. A related study design problem: the placement into one of the three syndromes depends on one clinician's diagnosis. A better study design would ask two clinicians to independently classify each study patient's chest pain syndrome. They may get the same history and differ in its interpretation or obtain different descriptions of the illness and classify the patient's history differently. A well-designed study would have the two clinicians compare their diagnoses and try to resolve any differences.

The opportunities for using the prevalence of disease in patients with a clinical syndrome are limited because of a dearth of published information on the prevalence of diseases in clinical syndromes.

3.4.3 Establishing a probability using a clinical prediction model

Clinical prediction models use clinical features and other information to estimate a patient's probability of the target condition. This probability is the starting point for using the anchoring and adjustment heuristic to determine the patient's probability of the target condition. Most clinical prediction models are empirical. A typical study uses the following process.

1. Researchers obtain each item on a list of prespecified clinical findings from many patients with the same clinical symptom, sign, or test result. The researchers then establish the final diagnosis by a method that is independent of the clinical findings (e.g., a coronary arteriogram).
2. The researchers identify the predictors of disease by statistical methods that assign to each predictor a weight that takes the influence of the other predictors into account so that its weighting does not depend on whether the other predictors are present or absent.
3. The prediction model uses an explicit method for assigning patients to diagnostic subgroups based on their findings. For example, each patient has a score that is the sum of the weights of the patient's findings; patients with similar scores are assigned to the same subgroup.
4. The prevalence of the target condition in a diagnostic subgroup is the number of patients in the subgroup with the target diagnosis divided by the total number of patients in the subgroup.
5. The prediction model must be tested on additional patients to verify the prevalence of disease in the subgroups.

The principal statistical methods for clinical prediction models are regression analysis and recursive partitioning.

Regression analysis

Regression analysis describes the relationship between predictors (the independent variables or predictor variables) and the predicted event (the dependent variable). Regression analysis shows how the dependent variable changes when the value of a predictor changes while holding constant the values of the other variables. Regression analysis tests the hypothesis that a predictor variable is related to the dependent variable. It addresses the following question: "Independently of the other potential predictors, is the association of this predictor with the dependent variable real or due only to chance." Typically, a regression analysis shows that when all other candidate predictors are taken into account, some predict and some do not.

Regression analysis assigns a numerical weight to each predictor. The weight is a measure of how well the predictor discriminates between different values of the dependent variable (i.e., does the patient have the target diagnosis, or not). The larger the weight assigned to a predictor, the better it discriminates and the greater the change in the dependent variable when the predictor is present.

The weights have practical value in diagnosis. To use a prediction model derived by regression analysis, the clinician determines whether a predictor is present (e.g., asks a patient whether exertion causes the patient's chest pain). The clinician adds the numerical weights corresponding to the predictors that are present. The sum of the weights is a score. We will use the term **discriminant score** to represent this sum. The discriminant scores for diseased and non-diseased patients are distributed differently, as shown in Figure 3.6 for a hypothetical example.

As seen in Figure 3.6, the discriminant scores of diseased patients overlap with the scores of non-diseased patients. The researchers may choose a cutoff score below which most patients are not diseased and another cutoff score above which most patients are diseased. Between these two cutoff scores, the prevalence of the disease is intermediate. The clinician uses a patient's discriminant score to put the patient into a group, as shown in Table 3.1. This partitioning of patients may be linked to different actions: do nothing, get more information, or start treatment. Chapter 13 takes up this topic in depth.

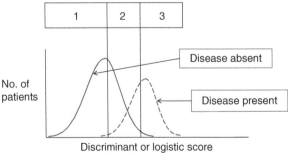

Figure 3.6 Hypothetical distribution of discriminant scores for diseased and non-diseased patients. The cutoff scores are represented by vertical lines. "Logistic score" refers to a regression analysis in which the dependent variable is binary (e.g. disease present or absent).

Table 3.1 Clinical prediction models scores and their meaning.

Score group	Range of scores	Probability of disease	Action
1	Low	Low	Do nothing
2	Intermediate	Intermediate	Do a diagnostic test
3	High	High	Start treatment

Alternatively, the researchers may divide the range of scores into equal-size segments (e.g., scores of 0–3, 4–6, 7–9, and so forth). The probability of disease assigned to a subgroup by a patient's discriminant score is the prevalence of disease in that discriminant score subgroup. As a reminder of our terminology, this prevalence is an *objective probability*; its basis is a study of a population of patients.

Example 1   Chest pain in referral practice

One of the authors asked 208 patients who had been admitted to the hospital for elective coronary arteriography to answer a set of questions about their chest pain and medical history. Seven findings in the history discriminated between patients with significant narrowing of at least one coronary artery and patients with no significant narrowing (Table 3.2).

Table 3.2 Empirical clinical prediction rule for coronary artery disease.

Attribute	Diagnostic weight
Age >60 years	+3
pain is brought on by exertion	+4
Patient must stop all activities when the pain occurs	+3
History of myocardial infarction	+4
pain relieved within 3 minutes after taking nitroglycerin	+2
At least 20 pack-years of cigarette smoking	+4
Male gender	+5

Adapted from Sox *et al.* (1990).

Example 2   Chest pain in primary care

The researchers from five studies of chest pain in primary care practice combined their study patients into one large data set from which they developed a clinical prediction model. They found seven independent predictors of a CAD diagnosis; because the weights were similar, they rounded them to +1 and −1 (Table 3.3). Note that one predictor has a negative weight; it reduces the probability of CAD.

Table 3.4 shows the number of patients with each chest pain score and the corresponding prevalence of CAD (see next page). Only 75 of the 644 patients (12%) had a CAD diagnosis.

Table 3.3 Chest pain predictors or coronary artery disease in primary care.

Clinical predictor	Weight of finding
Pain reproduced by palpating the chest wall	−1
Older age (male ≥ 55 years; female ≥ 65 years)	+1
Physician initially suspected a serious condition	+1
Chest discomfort feels like "pressure"	+1
Chest pain is related to physical effort	+1
History of CAD	+1
Chest pain score	range −1 to +5

Adapted from Aerts *et al.* (2017).

Table 3.4 Clinical prediction models scores and their meaning.

Chest pain score	−1	0	1	2	3	4	5
Patients with score and CAD/Patients with score	0/87	1/208	6/160	11/85	29/53	21/32	17/19
Probability of CAD (95% confidence interval)	0.00 (0.00–0.03)	0.00 (0.00–0.02)	0.04 (0.01–0.07)	0.13 (0.07–0.21)	0.55 (0.41–0.67)	0.66 (0.49–0.80)	0.89 (0.71–0.98)

Adapted from Sox *et al.* (2019).

Recursive partitioning

Recursive partitioning is a statistical process that leads to an **algorithm** for classifying patients.

Definition

ALGORITHM: Step-by-step instructions for solving a problem.

The first use of clinical algorithms was to display the logic of diagnosis for medical corpsmen in the military, physician assistants, and nurse practitioners. Their use to describe a diagnostic or treatment strategy has spread to standard textbooks of medicine and journal articles. A person can use an algorithm to describe their own logic in solving a problem. The first clinical algorithms were based on clinical judgment. Algorithms can be based on a study in which researchers obtain prespecified clinical findings from many patients and then use other means to establish the final diagnosis in each person.

In analyzing a dataset of such study patients using recursive partitioning, the diagnostic process is represented by a series of yes-no decision points. A finding that is associated with the final diagnosis places the patient in one group; if the finding is not present, the patient is placed in a second group. The patients in each of the two groups are asked a second yes-no question about another finding. This process continues until it reaches a predefined stopping point. The goal of the process is to place each patient into a group in which the prevalence of the disease is either very high or very low. Typically, the finding at each yes-no decision point best discriminates at that point in the partitioning process between those with the target condition and everyone else.

Evaluating the performance of clinical prediction models

Clinical prediction models are based on the systematic study of patients. They reflect the accuracy of clinical findings in the real world of patient care, which makes them a strong foundation for determining a patient's probability. However, clinical prediction models can lead to incorrect probabilities, which could lead to poor decision making and clinical outcomes. Prediction models must be tested before they are used in clinical practice.

The principal problem is over-fitting. The statistical techniques optimize discrimination in the patient population that was used to create the model (the **training set**). When the model is used in other populations (the **test sets**), it typically discriminates less well. This outcome is known as over-fitting. Too many candidate predictor variables and too few patients in the training set are related causes of over-fitting. A good general rule: the training set should contain at least 10 patients with the target condition for every candidate predictor variable. A study with 10 candidate predictors and 50 training set patients with the target condition would fail this rule; one with 200 such patients would pass. A likely explanation for over-fitting? Small samples of patients are likely to be atypical.

A good general rule: Do not use an untested clinical prediction model!

The best way to test a prediction model is to apply it to patients from a different setting than the training set patients, establish the final diagnosis, and calculate measures of **discrimination** and **calibration**. *Discrimination* is the ability of the model to distinguish patients with the target diagnosis from everyone else. The *c-statistic* gives the probability that a patient with the target diagnosis will have a higher discriminant score than a patient with other diagnoses. A c-statistic of 0.50 denotes no discrimination; a c-statistic of 1.0 indicates perfect discrimination. *Calibration* is a set of techniques and methods to ensure that the model and its inputs incorporate and are consistent with available evidence and the accompanying uncertainty. Go to *Chapter 14* (Advanced Decision Models) for further discussion of calibration and other methods for evaluating decision models.

The last topic in this section is quality standards for clinical prediction models. Several articles have addressed this topic (see articles 5, 6, and 7 in the References list). Studies should clearly define the outcome to be predicted and the predictors. If the outcome is a diagnosis, it should be established by means that does not use the patient characteristics being assessed as predictors. A study should present the characteristics of the study population, so that potential users may judge its applicability to their clinical setting. A prediction model should have *face validity*; it should make sense clinically. As noted in this section, the developers of a clinical prediction model should, at a minimum, divide the study population into a training set and a test set. Better still, the test set should be from another clinical setting with different patients, clinicians, and researchers. The best test of a clinical prediction model is its effect on patient care; it should be useful in practice. A randomized controlled clinical trial would be the best way to measure the effect of a prediction model on clinical outcomes.

3.5 Limitations of published studies of disease prevalence

*Pub*lished studies can mitigate the problem faced by the clinician with a limited personal experience. However, a clinician faces several potential pitfalls when applying a published prevalence of disease to their own patients.

When using a prevalence from a published study, the clinician must compare the study's clinical setting and inclusion criteria with their clinical practice. The concern is selection bias: systematic differences between the study setting and the clinician's own practice. Many published studies are performed on patients referred to academic medical centers. Patients are seen by specialists because a referring clinician suspects a disease in the specialist's sphere of expertise. Specialists less frequently see patients with clinical findings that imply a low probability of disease. Therefore, the prevalence of serious diseases in the specialist's practice will be higher than in the primary care clinician's practice. Moreover, clinical findings may be weaker predictors of disease in referral practice, if only because they are often a reason for referral and therefore common in referral practice regardless of the final diagnosis.

One of the authors addressed this point in a study of four different populations of patients with chest pain (see Bibliography). He and his colleagues applied a clinical prediction model developed in a training set consisting of patients referred for elective coronary arteriography (overall prevalence, 76%) to three different test populations. One test population had been admitted to the hospital for an elective coronary arteriogram, and two were primary care populations. In each test set, patients with similar chest pain scores – and therefore similar histories – were compared to the training set. In each group of similar chest pain scores, the probability of coronary artery disease (CAD) in test set patients undergoing a coronary arteriogram (overall CAD prevalence 72%) was the same in the referral test set with similar histories. However, compared with the training set, the prevalence of CAD in patients with similar chest pain scores was lower in one primary care test set (overall CAD prevalence, 33%) and still lower in another primary care test set (overall CAD prevalence, 8%). The authors concluded that the probability of CAD in patients with a similar history varied according to the overall disease prevalence. In other words, the interpretation of the history depended on the overall prevalence of disease in the population.

Clinical prediction models – few and far between 40 years ago – have become common: in 2021, a database of prediction models contained more than 1000 for cardiology problems alone. Fewer than half had been tested in a new population. The Bibliography contains an article addressing the problems involved in being sure that a probability determined from a prediction model applies to the patient in your office

3.5.1 Caution in using published reports to determine probability

The preceding examples show that primary care clinicians should be cautious when using the prevalence of disease from published reports to determine probabilities in their practice. The following examples illustrate the consequences of uncritically applying published studies to primary care practice.

Example 1

A primary care internist feels a nodule in the prostate gland. How likely is prostate cancer? The only pertinent reference is a classic paper from the practice of a renowned urologist; in this study, half of the patients with a prostate nodule had prostate cancer.

Comment: Does the internist's patient have a 50% chance of having prostate cancer. Probably not. After all, the patients who were seen by the urologist who wrote the paper were seen first by primary care clinicians. These clinicians probably referred only when the patient's nodule was suspicious for prostate cancer.

Example 2

A 40-year-old man has a blood pressure of 160/110 mm Hg. An internist who just completed training at a large referral center for hypertension orders a screening x-ray of the kidneys. A senior radiologist in the internist's practice calls with the following reminder:

Comment: Studies in specialty practice showed that about 5% of hypertensive patients had surgically curable causes of hypertension, such as pheochromocytoma and aldosterone-secreting adrenal tumors. When a study of secondary hypertension in primary care patients was finally performed, the prevalence of curable causes was only about 1%. After this study was published, primary care clinicians became much more selective about launching an expensive work-up for secondary causes of hypertension.

Clinicians in referral practice have less reason for concern about the effects of selection bias on the accuracy of disease prevalence in their practice. Their patients go through the same filtering process as the patients in most published studies.

3.6 Taking the special characteristics of the patient into account when determining probabilities

After this digression into ways to estimate disease prevalence, we return to the central problem of how to determine a probability. After using objective probability or personal experience to begin the process, we realize that patients often have special characteristics that affect their probability. A patient may have a clinical finding that seems important in the circumstances but does not appear in a published clinical prediction model because it is uncommon. Clinicians use subjective judgment to adjust the initial probability from the starting point provided by published studies and prior experience.

Example

A man in his mid-thirties has chest pain that has a few characteristics of anginal pain but is atypical. Clinical prediction models and other published studies indicate that the probability of disease should be approximately 0.20. However, the patient's two siblings and his father all had a fatal myocardial infarction before the age of 40. Because of these unusual findings, the patient's internist sharply increases the starting estimate of the probability of coronary artery disease and initiates a search that ends with a diagnosis of severe coronary artery disease.

Comment: Having several young siblings die of coronary artery disease happens so seldom that multivariate statistical methods are unlikely to identify the finding as a significant independent predictor of coronary artery disease. This alarming family history should influence the probability of disease. Common sense ruled in this case.

Summary

1. Clinicians often work in a state of uncertainty about the true state of the patient.
2. Clinical findings are imperfect indicators of disease. Almost invariably, negative results occur in patients with the target disease, and positive results occur in patients who do not have the disease.
3. We define probability as a **quantification of one's judgement about the likelihood of** a present state or a future event.
4. Several factors can influence an individual's probability: the clinicians' prior personal experience, published experience, the clinical setting of care, the presence of characteristic clinical features, and special or unusual attributes of the patient.

5. Probability assessment goes astray when people misuse cognitive methods to determine probability (heuristics). Errors in using these heuristics include the following:
   - Neglecting the influence of disease prevalence on probability when the patient's findings match up nicely with the features of the disease (Representativeness Heuristic).
   - Matching the patient's characteristics against poor predictors of the disease (Representativeness Heuristic).
   - Placing too much weight on a large number of predictors when some of them add little certainty (redundancy) (Representativeness Heuristic).
   - Overestimating the probability of an event that is easily recalled: it happened recently or was especially vivid (Availability Bias).
   - Failing to adjust probability adequately after learning about additional information (Anchoring and Adjustment).
6. Published disease prevalence estimates may be misleading if used in a clinical setting that differs from the study setting.
7. Clinical prediction models transform a large clinical experience into a form that enables clinicians to determine probabilities reliably and reproducibly.

Bibliography

Aerts, M. Minalu G.,Bösner S., *et al*. (2017) A clinical prediction rule for coronary artery disease in primary care derived from pooled individual patient data from five countries. *Journal of Clinical Epidemiology*, **81**, 120–8.

Bryant, G.D. and Norman, G.R. (1980) Expressions of probability: words and numbers (Letter). *New England Journal of Medicine*, **302**, 411.

A brief but influential article showing that each of the words used to express uncertainty corresponds to a range of probabilities that overlap one another. As an expression of uncertainty, words are no substitute for a probability.

Kahneman, D. (2011) *Thinking, Fast and Slow*, Farrar, Straus & Giroux, New York.

A book written for the general public about two systems of thinking, fast and slow, and how faulty reasoning and biases can send the former off the track.

Laupacis, A., Sekar, N., and Stiell, I.G. (1997) Clinical prediction rules: a review and suggested modifications of methodological standards. *Journal of the American Medical Association*, **277**, 488–94.

The authors review prediction models from a later era and propose modifications and additional standards for producing them.

McGinn, T.G, Guyatt, G.H., Wyer, P.C. *et al*. and The Evidence-Based Medicine Working Group (2000) Users' guides to the medical literature: XXII: how to use articles about clinical prediction rules. *Journal of the American Medical Association*, **284**, 79–84.

One of the JAMA series of articles on the critical use of clinical information.

Sox, H.C., Hickam, D.H., Marton, K.I. *et al*. (1990) Using the patient's history to estimate the probability of coronary artery disease: a comparison of primary care and referral practices. *American Journal of Medicine*, **89**, 7–14.

This article describes the development of a prediction model for chest pain and its testing in primary care and referral practice. The article shows that the interpretation of the patient's history can depend on the clinical setting.

Sox, H.C., Aerts, M., Hassenritter, J. (2019) Applying a clinical prediction rule for coronary artery disease in primary care to select a test and interpret the results *American Family Physician*, **99**, 584–6.

Spetzler, C.S. and Stael von Holstein, C.A.S. (1975) Probability encoding in decision analysis. *Management Science*, **25**, 340–57.

A classic paper on probability assessment.

Tversky, A. and Kahneman, D. (1974). Judgment under uncertainty: heuristics and biases. *Science*, **185**, 1124–31.

A classic, readable article on biased heuristics in subjective probability estimation. Kahneman won the Alfred Nobel Memorial Prize in Economics in 2002. Tversky, his partner in research, had died a few years earlier.

Wasson, J.H., Sox, H.C., Neff, R.K. *et al*. (1985) Clinical prediction rules: applications and methodological standards. *New England Journal of Medicine*, **313**, 793–99.

The authors evaluate published clinical prediction models and propose standards for developing and testing them.

Interpreting new information: Bayes' theorem

Clinicians often must take decisive action despite uncertainty about the patient's diagnosis or the outcome of treatment. **Chapter** 3 introduced probability as a language for expressing one's uncertainty. Using probability theory does not eliminate uncertainty about the patient. Rather, by providing tools to work with probability, it reduces *uncertainty about uncertainty*. This chapter builds upon the preceding chapter to show how to interpret new information in the language of probability.

4.1 Introduction

Why is it important to understand how new information affects uncertainty? Clinicians want to minimize their margin of error, in effect bringing probability estimates as close as possible to 1.0 or to zero. Without knowing how new information affects probability, the clinician may acquire too much or too little information.

How does a clinician monitor progress toward understanding the patient's true state? Let us represent the process of diagnosis by a straight line (Figure 4.1). Probability provides a ruler for measuring progress along this line. Subjective probability or a clinical prediction model (**Chapter** 3) tell us where to put the first mark on the line. When we obtain more information, Bayes' theorem tells us where to put the next mark.

The following examples illustrate the importance of modifying one's probability as new information becomes available.

Example 1: An intern on duty in the emergency department sees a man because of chest pain. The man has no health insurance.
The patient's history is 45 years old and has no cardiac risk factors. The pain began suddenly 4 days ago. The pain is in the left anterior chest; does not radiate to the arms, neck, or shoulders; has never occurred before; and is not accompanied by sweating. An electrocardiogram (ECG) does not show ST segment changes indicative of myocardial ischemia or Q waves indicative of myocardial damage. The serum troponin (a measure of cardiac muscle death) is normal. The intern in the emergency department admits the patient to cardiac intensive care. At the end of the first 24 hours, the patient is doing fine, the serum troponin is still normal, and the ECG is unchanged. After 2 days in cardiac care, the patient's cardiologist tells him that he did not have a myocardial infarction and discharges him from the hospital. Months later, he receives a $40 000 bill for this brief admission.

Medical Decision Making, Third Edition. Harold C. Sox, Michael C. Higgins, Douglas K. Owens, and Gillian Sanders Schmidler.
© 2024 John Wiley & Sons Ltd. Published 2024 by John Wiley & Sons Ltd.

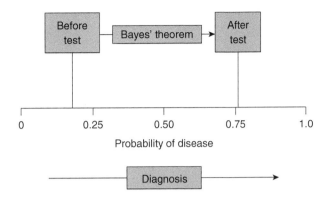

Figure 4.1 Role of Bayes' theorem.

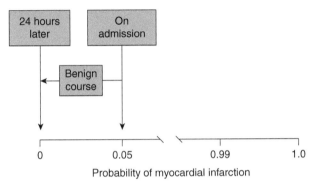

Figure 4.2 The effect of an uncomplicated hospital course on the probability of myocardial infarction.

Comment: The intern was uncertain about whether the patient was having an infarction and admitted him in order to be on the safe side. Once admitted, the clinicians were too cautious about interpreting what they had learned at the end of 24 hours. The complication-free course, the normal serum enzyme levels, and the unchanged ECG reduced still further the probability of infarction (Figure 4.2). They should have discharged him from the hospital, after the first 24 hours.

Example 2: The patient is a 60-year-old man with chest pain.
The pain began 6 months ago. It is a retrosternal sensation of pressure. When the pain is present, he cannot do anything. Exertion brings on the pain, and nitroglycerin relieves it within 3 minutes. The man has been a heavy cigarette smoker. The clinician interprets the history as "typical exertional angina pectoris" and obtains an exercise ECG to confirm their judgment. The patient is able to continue on the treadmill for 10 minutes, and there are no electrocardiographic indications of myocardial ischemia. The clinician tells the patient that the treadmill test indicates he probably does not have coronary heart disease. After six more months of chest pain with exertion, the patient obtains a second opinion. This physician tells him that, based on his history, he probably does have coronary artery disease despite the normal exercise ECG. To help the patient understand, he draws the diagram shown in Figure 4.3 (see next page).

Comment: The second clinician correctly interpreted the history as indicating a high probability of coronary artery disease. The probability of coronary disease in a 60-year-old man with typical angina is 0.89. The exercise ECG is often normal in patients with coronary artery disease. If the test is negative, as in this patient, the probability of coronary artery disease is 0.65.

These two examples involved estimating a probability before and after acquiring new information. The standard terminology for these two probabilities is:

Definition

PRIOR PROBABILITY: The probability of an event before acquiring new information. *Synonyms*: pre-test probability, pre-test risk.

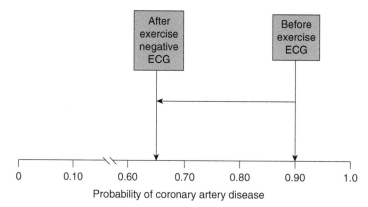

Figure 4.3 The effect of a normal exercise ECG on the probability of coronary artery disease in a man with typical exertional angina.

Definition

POSTERIOR PROBABILITY: The probability of an event after acquiring new information. *Synonyms*: post-test probability, post-test risk.

Explaining test results is part of the work of a clinician. Arguably, the explanation of a test result should include the post-test probability in addition to other aspects of the test and its meaning for the patient. Describing a test result as a probability may help patients to understand that the cause of their symptoms is not known for sure.

In this context, the key to test interpretation is calculating the probability of the disease that may be causing a clinical finding. Bayes' theorem is the key to making this important calculation. Bayes' theorem is one of the foundations of decision analysis. To understand the basis for Bayes' theorem requires a brief excursion into probability theory in order to learn a simple but helpful notation.

4.2   Conditional probability defined

The probability of a disease given that a clinical finding is present is an example of a **conditional probability**.

Definition

CONDITIONAL PROBABILITY: The probability that an event is true if another event is true (i.e., conditional upon the second event being true).

The notation of conditional probability is quite easy to understand. The conditional probability of **event A** given that **event B** is true is written:

$p[A \mid B]$, which means "the probability of event A *conditional upon* event B." The vertical line is read "conditional upon."

The formal definition of conditional probability is

$$p[A \mid B] = \frac{p[A \text{ and } B]}{p[B]}$$

This expression may be translated as "the conditional probability that *A* is true given that *B* is true is the ratio of the probability that both *A* and *B* are true divided by the probability that *B* is true."

A clinical example of a conditional probability is:

"What is the probability of coronary artery disease conditional upon an abnormal exercise ECG?"

To answer this question, the first step is to translate the formal definition of conditional probability into a form in which the conditional probabilities correspond to a measurable quantity. The Reverend Bayes found the way forward.

4.3 Bayes' theorem

Relatives of the Reverend Thomas Bayes (1702–61), an English clergyman, discovered his lasting contribution to knowledge when they were sorting his effects after his death. They discovered an unpublished manuscript that showed how, starting from the definition of conditional probability, to derive what came to be called Bayes' theorem. With Bayes' theorem, the clinician can calculate the posterior probability of a disease conditional on a test result using the following quantities:

- The prior probability of the disease
- The probability of a test result conditional upon the patient having the disease
- The probability of the test result conditional upon the patient not having the disease.

4.3.1 Derivation of Bayes' theorem

Notation: We generally use "target condition" instead of "disease" in this book because a clinician orders a test with a specific hypothesis in mind, the target condition. In writing equations, we prefer more compact notation and use "disease."

Suppose we are trying to calculate the probability of disease D given that a particular test result (R) occurred. Using the notation of conditional probability, we must calculate:

$$p[D|R]$$

where R represents a test result. This notation reads "probability of the disease conditional upon the test result." Here we adopt the convention of using $D+$ to indicate "target condition present" and $D-$ to indicate "target condition absent." "Target condition" refers to the suspected disease. For test result, we use R for "result" or $T+$ or $T-$ for "test positive" and "test negative"

We know from the definition of conditional probability that

$$p[D+|R] = \frac{p[R \text{ and } D+]}{p[R]}$$

$p[R]$, the probability of a test result, is simply the sum of the probability of the test result in patients with the target condition ($D+$) and its probability in patients who do not have the target condition ($D-$):

$$p[R] = p[R \text{ and } D+] + p[R \text{ and } D-]$$

Thus, we get:

$$p[D+|R] = \frac{p[D+ \text{ and } R]}{p[R \text{ and } D+] + p[R \text{ and } D-]}$$

By the definition of conditional probability

$$p[R|D+] = \frac{p[R \text{ and } D+]}{p[D+]}$$

and

$$p[R|D-] = \frac{p[R \text{ and } D-]}{p[D-]}$$

Rearranging these expressions, we get:

$$p[R \text{ and } D+] = p[D+] \times p[R \,|\, D+]$$

$$p[R \text{ and } D-] = p[D-] \times p[R \,|\, D-]$$

Substituting the left-hand side of these equations into the equation for $p[D+ \,|\, R]$, we obtain Bayes' theorem

$$p[D+\,|\,R] = \frac{p[D+] \times p[R\,|\,D+]}{\left(p[D+] \times p[R\,|\,D+] + p[D-] \times p[R\,|\,D-]\right)}$$

4.3.2 Clinically useful forms of Bayes' theorem
Bayes' theorem when a test result is positive

To translate Bayes' theorem into a clinically useful form, we will make several changes.

First, we express the test result (R), which could potentially have any biologically reasonable value, as a dichotomous variable (positive or negative). Many test results are expressed as a continuous variable (e.g., the concentration of an enzyme in the blood). The amount of information in a test result may vary depending on whether the result is a small number or a larger one. So, why give up that information by picking a single number to define the result of the test?

The purpose of a test result is to inform a decision to act. To act on a test result, we must choose a threshold value for taking action (e.g., the smallest lung mass that experts feel should be biopsied, rather than monitored to see if it grows). All values of the test result above the threshold we call "positive." All values below the threshold, we call "negative." Choosing the cut-point that defines "positive" and "negative" is a topic in Chapter 5.

Second, since the probability of all causes of a diagnostic problem must add to one, $p[D-]$ is equivalent to $1-p[D+]$.

Third, we will express $p[T+\,|\,D]$, the probability of a positive test result given that the patient is diseased, as the *sensitivity* of the test. Articles about the performance characteristics of tests use the term *sensitivity* rather than its equivalent in conditional probability notation.

$$\text{Sensitivity} = \frac{\text{number of diseased patients with positive test}}{\text{number of diseased patients}}$$

Fourth, we will rewrite $p[T+\,|\,D-]$, the probability of a positive test result given that the target condition is absent, in terms of the *specificity* of the test, which is the probability of a negative test if the hypothesized disease is absent: $p[T-\,|\,D-]$. The reason for this change is that studies of diagnostic test performance report their findings as test specificity. The probability of all test results in patients who do not have the target condition must add up to one. Therefore, $p[T+\,|\,D-]$ is equivalent to $(1-p[T-\,|\,D-])$ or $(1-\text{specificity})$.

$$\text{Specificity} = \frac{\text{number of non-diseased patients with negative test}}{\text{number of non-diseased patients}}$$

Combining these four changes, we have Bayes' theorem in a useful form:

$$p[D+\,|\,T+] = \frac{\left(p[D+] \times \text{sensitivity}\right)}{p[D+] \times \text{sensitivity} + \left(1-p[D+]\right) \times \left(1-\text{specificity}\right)}$$

Figure 4.4 shows the result of using Bayes' theorem to calculate the post-test probability after a positive test result ($p[D+\,|\,T+]$) for every value of the pre-test probability between 0 and 1.0. At very low pre-test probabilities, the post-test probability rises steeply above the pre-test probability, which is represented by the 45° line, as the pre-test probability increases. At very high pre-test probabilities, it rises slowly as the pre-test probability increases. The impact of a positive test result on the patient's pre-test probability of disease is largest at low pre-test probabilities and smallest at high pre-test probabilities.

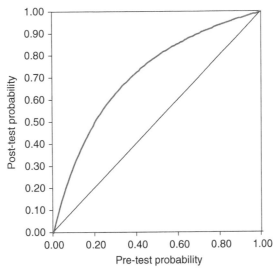

Figure 4.4 Post-test probability corresponding to a positive test result, calculated for all possible pre-test probabilities using Bayes' theorem. Test sensitivity set at 0.8. Specificity set at 0.8.

A note on navigating this book: Diagnostic tests and Bayes' theorem are closely related. So, it is difficult to describe one without describing the other. This book treats these two topics in separate chapters. In this chapter, we provide just enough information about sensitivity and specificity to support the presentation of Bayes' theorem. We present methods for measuring the sensitivity and specificity of a diagnostic test in **Chapter** 5. Some readers may prefer to read Chapter 5 before reading Chapter 4.

In applying Bayes' theorem to medicine, people often combine the potential causes of a diagnostic problem into two mutually exclusive states, just as they often combine test results into "positive" (above the threshold for taking action) and "negative" (below the action threshold). These two states are:

1. The disease whose probability we want to determine: the "target condition").
2. All other states that are known to cause the diagnostic problem (including the state in which no disease is demonstrable). This state means "the target condition is absent." Since the probability of all possible causes must add up to one, the probability that the target condition is absent is
   {1 – the probability of the target condition}

Later in the chapter, we will consider what to do when several diseases are under consideration, and a test can detect each of them.

Bayes' theorem when a test result is negative

To calculate the probability of the disease, if a test result is negative (i.e., the result lowers the probability of the target condition), we use Equation 4.5 after substituting minus signs (to denote a negative test result) for R in Equation 4.5. Thus, $p[D+ \mid T+]$ becomes $p[D+ \mid T-]$.

$$p[D+ \mid T-] = \frac{p[D+] \times p[T- \mid D+]}{\left(p[D+] \times p[T- \mid D+] + p[D-] \times p[T- \mid D-]\right)}$$

To translate this equation into a clinically useful form, note that:

$p[T- \mid D+]$ is the probability of a negative test result given that the patient is diseased, which is 1 – the probability that the test is positive when the patient is diseased = (1–sensitivity).

$p[T- \mid D-]$ is the probability of a negative test result given that the patient does not have the hypothesized disease, which is the *specificity* of the test.

$$p[D+ \mid T-] = \frac{p[D+] \times p(1-\text{sensitivity})}{\left(p[D+] \times p(1-\text{sensitivity}) + p[D-] \times \text{specificity}\right)}$$

Figure 4.5 shows the result of using Bayes' theorem to calculate the post-test probability after a negative test result ($p[D+ \mid T-]$) for every value of the pre-test probability between 0 and 1.0 (see next page). After a negative test, the post-test probability is lower than the pre-test probability, which is represented by the 45° line. At low pre-test probabilities, the post-test probability after a negative test rises slowly as the pre-test probability increases. At very high pre-test probabilities, it rises steeply. The impact of a negative test result on the patient's pre-test probability is smallest at low pre-test probabilities and largest at high pre-test probabilities.

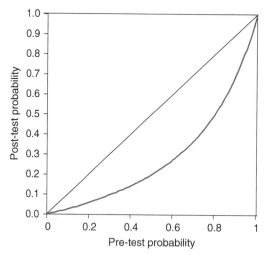

Figure 4.5 Post-test probability for a negative test result. Test sensitivity set at 0.8. Specificity set at 0.8.

Example: For illustration, imagine a 55-year-old man with hemoptysis (coughing blood) and a long history of smoking cigarettes. The clinician suspects lung cancer and estimates the pre-test probability of lung cancer to be 0.4. The interpretation of the chest x-ray is "mass lesion in the right upper lobe."

The sensitivity of the chest x-ray for detecting lung cancer is 0.60 and the specificity is 0.96:
How should the clinician interpret the finding of a "mass lesion in the right upper lobe?"

$$p[D+|T+] = \frac{p[D+] \times \text{sensitivity}}{\left(p[D+] \times \text{sensitivity} + (1-p[D+]) \times (1-\text{specificity})\right)}$$

$$= \frac{0.4 \times 0.60}{\left(0.4 \times 0.6 + (1-0.4) \times 0.04\right)} = 0.94$$

What if the chest x-ray had *not* shown a mass lesion?

$$p[D+|T-] = \frac{p[D+] \times (1-\text{sensitivity})}{\left(p[D+] \times (1-\text{sensitivity}) + (1-p[D+]) \times (\text{specificity})\right)}$$

$$= \frac{0.4 \times 0.4}{0.4 \times 0.4 + (1-0.4) \times 0.96} = 0.22$$

Explanation: Since the chest x-ray showed a mass lesion, the patient almost certainly has lung cancer. If the chest x-ray had shown no evidence of lung cancer, the clinician should still be suspicious, since the post-test probability of lung cancer was so high. Some patients with lung cancer do not have chest radiographic evidence at the time the disease is first detected.

This case is an example, among many, of a negative test result that reduces the probability of a disease but is not low enough to "rule it out." How low is low enough? What does "rule it out" mean in practice? Chapter 13 will address these important questions.

Probability of a test result

The probability of a test result can be a consideration in deciding to do a test. For example, suppose the patient's probability of a disease is 0.95. Although the next step appears to be to start treatment, a negative result on a test could reduce the probability to the point at which the clinicians should re-examine the decision to treat. Should they do the test? Knowing the probability of a negative test result would help them to decide.

As noted earlier, the probability of a positive test result ($p[T+]$) is the sum of its probability in diseased patients and its probability in nondiseased patients:

$$p[T+] = p[T+ \text{ and } D+] + p[T+ \text{ and } D-]$$

In the previous section, we rearranged the definition of conditional probability to show that

$$p[T+ \text{ and } D+] = p[D+] \times p[T+|D+]$$

$$p[T+ \text{ and } D-] = p[D-] \times p[T+|D-]$$

Since $p[T+|D+]$ = sensitivity and $p[T+|D-] = 1 -$ specificity

$$\boxed{\text{probability of a positive result} = p[D+] \times \text{sensitivity} + \left(1 - p[D+]\right) \times \left(1 - \text{specificity}\right)}$$

$$\boxed{\text{probability of a negative result} = p[D+] \times \left(1 - \text{sensitivity}\right) + \left(1 - p[D+]\right) \times \text{specificity}}$$

The following is another way to calculate the probability of a negative test.

$$\boxed{\text{probability of a negative test result} = \left[1 - \text{probability of a positive test result}\right]}$$

Figure 4.6 shows the relationship between the pre-test probability and the probability of a test result when the test has a sensitivity of 0.8 and a specificity of 0.8. The probability of a negative result is lowest when the pre-test probability of the target condition is nearly 1.0. **At that probability, the probability that the patient does not have the target condition is very low, and one should expect few negative test results.** Note that the probability of a positive test result is lowest when the pre-test probability is low.

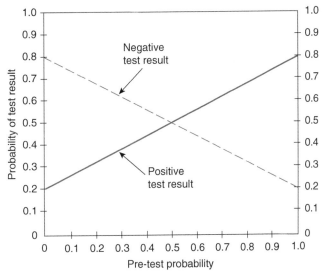

Figure 4.6 Probability of a test result for different pre-test probabilities. The sensitivity of the test is 0.8 and the specificity is 0.8.

4.4 The odds ratio form of Bayes' theorem

One disadvantage of Bayes' theorem is that most people need a calculator to do the math. A second disadvantage is that sensitivity and specificity alone do not convey their combined effect on probability. The solution to these problems is to rewrite Bayes' theorem to calculate the post-test odds, which is the same information as the post-test probability but expressed differently. The odds ratio form of Bayes' theorem is easy to remember and entails multiplying one number by another number.

Expressing the pre-test probability of the disease in terms of the *pre-test odds* of the disease simplifies Bayes' theorem. Using the odds ratio format of Bayes' theorem, anyone can easily update probabilities. Moreover, expressing Bayes' theorem in its odds ratio format leads directly to a simple, intuitive way to describe the effect of new diagnostic information on probability. It is the **likelihood ratio (LR)**, one of the most important ideas in this book.

4.4.1 The derivation of the odds ratio form of Bayes' theorem
Derivation:

To derive the odds ratio form of Bayes' theorem, start with Bayes' theorem in its familiar form (here we use R to denote any test result)

$$p[D+|R] = \frac{p[D+] \times p[R|D+]}{(p[D+] \times p[R|D+] + p[D-] \times p[R|D-])}$$

Now, convert $p[D+]$, a probability, to odds using the relationship learned in Chapter 3:

$$p[D+] = \frac{odds[D+]}{1 + odds[D+]}$$

Instead of Odds$[D+]$, we write $O[D+]$. Substituting $\frac{O[D+]}{1+O[D+]}$ where we see $p[D+]$ in Bayes' theorem, we get this expression:

$$p[D+|R] = \frac{\left(\frac{O[D+] \times p[R|D+]}{(1+O[D]]} \right)}{\frac{O[D+] \times p[R|D+]}{(1+O[D+]]} + \left(1 - \left(\frac{O[D+]}{1+O[D+]}\right) \times p[R|D-]\right)}$$

Using simple algebra, we obtain the odds ratio form of Bayes' theorem

$$O[D+|R] = O[D+] \times \frac{p[R|D+]}{p[R|D-]}$$

Look carefully at this equation. It's telling you that the post-test odds of disease D after test result R, ($O[D|R]$), is equal to the pre-test odds ($O[D]$) times a number. That number is the amount that the odds change after the test result, R. An expression that tells you how much the odds of disease change after new information is so useful that it ... $\frac{p[R|D]}{p[R|no\,D]}$ ... has a name: *the likelihood ratio*, also referred to as LR.

Definition: Likelihood Ratio = a number that shows how much the odds of disease change after getting a test result.
Another way to state the odds ratio form of Bayes' theorem is:

$$\text{Post-test odds} = \text{pre-test odds} \times \text{likelihood ratio}$$

The LR is convenient and powerful: a single number that shows how much one's uncertainty should change after a test result.

4.4.2 The likelihood ratio: a measure of test discrimination
We saw in the previous section that

$$\text{Likelihood ratio} = \frac{p[\text{result in diseased persons}]}{p[\text{result in non-diseased persons}]}$$

Any clinical finding may be characterized by its LR. Different amounts of ST segment depression during an exercise stress test indicate different likelihoods of coronary artery disease on an arteriogram, as shown in this example (Table 4.1).

In contrast to this example of a continuous variable having separate LRs for each of several results, the results can be combined, a single cut-point chosen, and a dichotomous test result formed, with its own LR. With a dichotomous result, a result that raises the odds of the target condition is "positive," and a result that lowers the odds is "negative." For example, physicians often treat the amount of ST segment depression on a stress ECG as a dichotomous variable. Less than 1 mm ST segment depression is a negative test; ST segment depression of ≥ 1 mm is a positive test, one that may require additional testing. Table 4.2 shows the LR for any amount of ST segment depression that is at least 1 mm.

Note that the data for Tables 4.1 and 4.2 are taken from different studies.

Table 4.1 Likelihood ratios for exercise ECG results.

Test result (mm ST segment depression)	Likelihood ratio for coronary artery disease
<1.0	0.40
1.0–1.49	2.09
1.5–1.99	4.50
2.0–2.49	10.80
≥2.5	38.00

Diamond and Forrester (1979).

Table 4.2 Likelihood ratios for exercise ECG results as a dichotomous test.

Test result (mm ST segment depression)	Test result label	Likelihood ratio for coronary artery disease
<1.0	Negative	0.40
≥1	Positive	7.45

Adapted from Rifkin et al. (1977).

Both of the results in Table 4.2 have a LR, one corresponding to ≥1 mm ST segment depression (abbreviated **LR+**) and another corresponding to <1 mm ST segment depression (abbreviated **LR−**):

$$LR+ = \frac{p[\text{finding present in } \textbf{diseased} \text{ persons}]}{p[\text{finding present in } \textbf{nondiseased} \text{ persons}]}$$

From the definitions of sensitivity and specificity, this definition takes the following form:

$$LR+ = \frac{\text{sensitivity}}{1-\text{specificity}}$$

$$LR- = \frac{p[\text{finding absent in } \textbf{diseased} \text{ persons}]}{p[\text{finding absent in } \textbf{nondiseased} \text{ persons}]}$$

From the definitions of sensitivity and specificity, this definition takes the following form:

$$LR- = \frac{1-\text{sensitivity}}{\text{specificity}}$$

The LR is especially useful for expressing the discriminatory power of a test result because the clinician needs to remember only one number (the LR) instead of two numbers (sensitivity and specificity).
- If the LR is 10.0, the odds increase 10-fold after a positive test.
- If the LR is close to 1, the odds change very little.
- If the LR is 0.1, the odds decrease a lot after a negative test.

4.4.3   Using the odds ratio form of Bayes' theorem
The LR is used in the odds ratio form of Bayes' theorem. To understand the odds ratio format, recall the following definitions from **Chapter** 3:

$$\text{Odds of event} = \frac{p[\text{the event will occur}]}{p[\text{the event will not occur}]}$$

$$\text{Odds of event} = \frac{p}{1-p}$$

Thus, if the probability of an event is 0.33, the odds that the event will occur are:

$$\text{Odds of event} = \frac{p}{1-p} = \frac{0.33}{1-0.33} = \frac{1}{2} \text{ or } 1:2$$

If a finding is present, the amount that the pre-test odds increases may be calculated with the odds ratio form of Bayes' theorem.

> Post-test odds = pre-test odds × likelihood ratio

The first example of the odds ratio form of Bayes' theorem shows how to calculate the post-test probability with a test result that is one point on a continuum of results. The test is a stress ECG, a test whose results can be expressed as a continuous variable, the amount of ST segment depression (Table 4.1).

Example 1: What is the post-test probability of coronary artery disease in a middle-aged man with a history of atypical angina pectoris? His exercise stress ECG showed 2.0 mm ST segment depression.

Step 1: Determine the LR for the patient's stress test result. From Table 4.1, we know that ≥2.0 mm ST segment depression has a LR of 10.8.

Step 2: Calculate the pre-test odds of coronary artery disease. From Table 4.1 in Chapter 3, we know that a male with a history of atypical angina pectoris has a pre-test probability of 0.70. To convert this probability to odds, we do the following:

$$\text{Odds of event} = \frac{p}{1-p} = \frac{0.7}{1-0.7} = \frac{0.7}{0.3} = 2.3:1$$

Step 3: The third step is to use the odds ratio form of Bayes' theorem to calculate the post-test odds:

> Post-test odds = pre-test odds × likelihood ratio

$$\text{Post-test odds} = \frac{0.7}{0.3} \times 10.8 = 25.2:1$$

In this case, the very positive stress test result has increased the probability of coronary artery disease to a virtual certainty.

In the second example, we repeat an early clinical scenario but now as an example of using the odds ratio form of Bayes' theorem. The test result is a dichotomous variable: a lung mass is either present on the chest x-ray (a positive test) or it is not (a negative test). In this example, the mass is present.

Example 2: How should a radiologist interpret a lung mass on a chest radiograph taken in a man whose pre-test probability of lung cancer is 0.4?

Step 1: The first step in answering this question is to calculate the LR for the radiographic finding of a lung mass.

$$\text{LR+} = \frac{p\left[\text{finding present in \textbf{diseased} persons}\right]}{p\left[\text{finding present in \textbf{nondiseased} persons}\right]}$$

The probability that a lung mass is present in persons with lung cancer is 0.6, which is the sensitivity of the chest radiograph for lung cancer.

The probability that a lung mass is present in persons who do not have lung cancer is 0.04, which is **1 – the specificity** of the chest radiograph. Thus, the specificity of the chest radiograph for lung cancer is 0.96.

Thus, *when a finding is present*, the LR is:

$$\text{LR+} = \frac{\text{sensitivity}}{1-\text{specificity}}$$

The LR+ for a lung mass on the chest x-ray is:

$$\text{LR+} = \frac{0.60}{0.04} = 15.0$$

Step 2: The second step in obtaining the post-test odds is to convert the pre-test probability to the pre-test odds:

$$\text{Odds of event} = \frac{p}{1-p} = \frac{0.4}{1-0.4} = \frac{0.4}{0.6} = 0.67:1$$

Step 3: The third step is to use the odds ratio form of Bayes' theorem to calculate the post-test odds:

> Post-test odds = pre-test odds × likelihood ratio

$$\text{Post-test odds} = \frac{0.4}{0.6} \times 15.0 = 10:1$$

Thus, the post-test odds are higher than the pre-test odds when the chest x-ray shows a mass. The expression "10:1" is read "10 to one." In words, "for every ten persons who have lung cancer, 1 person will not have lung cancer."

Thinking in terms of odds of events and LRs for tests simplifies computation. The odds of an event may be converted back to the probability of the event, if desired.

$$\text{Probability} = \frac{\text{odds}}{1+\text{odds}} = \frac{10:1}{1+10:1}$$

$$\text{Probability} = \frac{10}{11} = 0.91$$

In the third example of using the odds ratio form of Bayes' theorem, the test result is a dichotomous variable: a lung mass is either present (a positive test) or it is not (a negative test). In this example, the mass is absent despite a high pre-test probability of lung cancer.

Example 3: How should a radiologist interpret a normal chest radiograph taken because of concern about lung cancer? The patient had a pre-test probability of lung cancer equal to 0.4.

Step 1: The first step in answering this question is to calculate the LR for lung cancer when the chest radiograph does not show a lung mass.

$$\text{LR}- = \frac{p[\text{finding absent in } \textbf{diseased} \text{ persons}]}{p[\text{finding absent in } \textbf{nondiseased} \text{ persons}]}$$

The probability that a lung mass is present in persons with lung cancer is 0.6, which means that the probability that a lung mass is absent in persons with lung cancer is **1 − sensitivity**, (Explanation: since a lung mass is either present or absent, the sum of the two probabilities must add to 1.0).

The probability that a lung mass is absent in persons who do not have lung cancer is 0.96 is the **specificity** of the chest x-ray.

When a finding is absent, the LR is:

$$\text{LR}- = \frac{1-\text{sensitivity}}{\text{specificity}}$$

The LR− for a lung mass on the chest x-ray is:

$$\text{LR}- = \frac{0.40}{0.96} = 0.42$$

This LR tells us that a negative chest x-ray reduces the odds of lung cancer by a little more than half, which is not likely to be the end of the story given a pre-test probability of 0.4 in this man.

Step 2: The second step in obtaining the post-test odds is to convert the pre-test probability to the pre-test odds, as in the second example:

$$\text{Odds of event} = \frac{p}{1-p} = \frac{0.4}{1-0.4} = \frac{0.4}{0.6} = 0.67:1$$

Step 3: The third step is to use the odds ratio form of Bayes' theorem to calculate the post-test odds:

> Post-test odds = pre-test odds × likelihood ratio

$$\text{Post-test odds} = \left(\frac{0.4}{0.6}\right) \times 0.42 = 0.28:1 = 1:3.5$$

Thus, the post-test odds are lower than the pre-test odds when the chest x-ray does not show a mass. The expression "1:3.5" is read, "for every 1 person who has cancer, 3.5 people will not have cancer."

The post-test probability of lung cancer is quite high despite the normal chest radiograph. We will return to this point later in the chapter.

While thinking in terms of odds of events and LRs for tests simplifies computation, many people find probability an easier language of uncertainty. We can convert the odds of an event back to the probability of the event.

$$\text{Probability} = \frac{\text{odds}}{1+\text{odds}} = \frac{0.28:1}{1+0.28:1} = 0.22$$

4.5 Lessons to be learned from using Bayes' theorem

The following is a list of lessons that Bayes' theorem teaches us. The text lists the lessons in related groups, and the applicable evidence follows in the form of a plot of pre-test probability (horizontal axis) and post-test probability (vertical axis).

Lesson 1: The interpretation of new information depends on what you already knew.

Lesson 2: At low and high pre-test probabilities, the post-test probability is close to the pre-test probability. The test has the largest effect for intermediate range probabilities, where diagnostic uncertainty is greatest.

Lesson 3: Close to a probability of zero, the probability rises most steeply after a positive test result. Close to a probability of 1.0, the probability falls most steeply after a negative test result.

Lesson 4: A positive test is least likely when the pre-test probability is close to zero. A negative test is least likely when the pre-test probability is near 1.0.

Lesson 5: A test done to confirm that the probability is close to 0 or 1.0 is highly likely to confirm it and very unlikely to disconfirm it.

Lesson 6: The bottom-line: test results are least likely to occur when you need them the most.

4.5.1 Further thoughts

The last three lessons suggest that doing a test to confirm a probability that is close to 0 or to 1.0 is seldom warranted.

However, disconfirming a strong clinical suspicion is potentially quite useful. An unexpected negative test result when the pre-test probability is high, may lower the probability of disease enough to reverse a decision to start treatment. The same holds when the pre-test probability is very low: an unexpected positive result could change management.

Do these observations mean that one should order a test when the pre-test probability is very low or very high in the hope of a test result that could change treatment? The answer is "on occasion, but certainly not as a routine practice," for several reasons.

First, the probability of a surprising, disconfirmatory test result is lowest when the pre-test probability is at the extreme ends of the probability scale. As shown earlier in Figure 4.6, when the pre-test probability is above 0.95, the probability **of** a negative test result is as low as 20% for a test whose sensitivity and specificity are 0.8.

Second, a low-probability test result could be a false-positive or a false-negative, due to an error in the laboratory. Being skeptical of surprising test results is good clinical policy, as is confirming the unexpected finding by repeating the test.

Third, to change management, the post-test probability would have to cross a treatment threshold probability, which is the topic of Chapter 13. Treatment threshold probabilities are usually less than 0.50 and often considerably less.

By how much must the probability change to alter the next step in management? Discussions of the role of diagnostic tests should focus on this question. Before proceeding further, some readers may wish to learn more about how to use diagnostic tests in clinical practice. The first five pages of **Chapter** 13 provide a brief introduction.

4.5.2 The clinical significance of test specificity

The considerations when deciding about doing a test are its safety, cost, and suitability for the situation. If the patient's probability is relatively low, a test with high specificity (few false-positives) should be the prime consideration. This section will use Figure 4.7 to explain why.

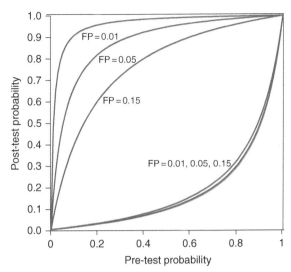

Figure 4.7 Effect of the specificity of a test on the post-test probability of the disease. The sensitivity of the test was set at 0.90. The post-test probability was calculated when the specificity was 0.99, 0.95, and 0.85 (in the figure, labeled FP = 0.01, FP = 0.05, and FP = 0.15, respectively, where FP stands for $p[T+|D-]$). The upper group of curves represent a positive test result. The lower group of curves represent a negative test result.

The role of test specificity in choosing between tests

When the pre-test probability is relatively low, the role of testing is to increase the probability of the target condition. High specificity is far more important than high sensitivity when the pre-test probability is relatively low. Figure 4.7 shows that the probability after a positive test (the upper group of curves) increases as the specificity of the test increases. Specificity is important when the pre-test probability is low. It is much less important when the pre-test probability is higher.

When the pre-test probability is high, the role of testing is to lower the probability of the target condition. Figure 4.7 shows that the probability after a negative test (the lower group of curves) is the same irrespective of the specificity.

4.5.3   The clinical significance of test sensitivity

The clinical significance of test sensitivity sharply contrasts with specificity (Figure 4.8). Test sensitivity is important when the pre-test probability is high, the important result is a negative test, and the main effect of a negative test is to lower the probability.

Figure 4.8 illustrates several concepts:
- The sensitivity of a test strongly affects the probability after a **negative** test result (lower family of curves in **Figure** 4.8). The higher the sensitivity of a test, the lower the post-test probability of the disease after a negative test result.
- The sensitivity of a test has a small effect on the post-test probability after a **positive** test result (upper family of curves in Figure 4.8).

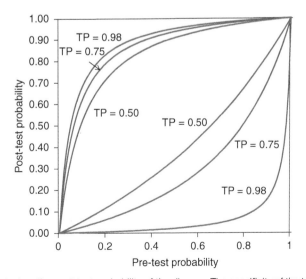

Figure 4.8 Effect of the sensitivity of a test on the post-test probability of the disease. The specificity of the test was set at 0.95. The post-test probability was calculated when the sensitivity of a test (where TP stands for p[T+|D+]) was set at 0.98, 0.75, and 0.50. The upper group of curves represent a positive test result. The lower group of curves represent a negative test result.

Table 4.3 Contrasting effects of test sensitivity and specificity.

	Sensitivity of test	Specificity of test
Preferred pre-test probability	High pre-test probability	Low pre-test probability
Test result that matters most for decision-making	Negative test	Positive test
Direction of the largest effect on probability	Lowers probability	Increases probability

Most tests have good sensitivity or specificity but seldom both. As a guide to choosing a test in specific situations, Table 4.3 summarizes the effects of sensitivity and specificity.

In choosing a test, strategies keyed to one test performance characteristic (sensitivity or specificity) and the patient's pre-test probability can be helpful. However, a diagnostic test has both characteristics, and the interplay between them is important in determining the post-test probability. The LR, discussed earlier in this chapter, reflects both sensitivity and specificity and determines the post-test odds.

$$LR+ = \frac{sensitivity}{1-specificity} \quad LR- = \frac{1-sensitivity}{specificity}$$

Post-test odds = pre-test odds × likelihood ratio

Using the LR to represent test performance has powerful advantages:
- *Test performance*: In one number the LR reflects two very different but inter-related characteristics of test performance: sensitivity (detection) and specificity (discrimination).
- *Ease of use*: The odds ratio form of Bayes' theorem requires the multiplication of two numbers. The conditional probability form of Bayes' theorem requires 3 multiplications, one addition, and one division. With a handy list of LRs, a clinician can use on-the-fly Bayesian reasoning to inform the choice of a diagnostic test.

Maintaining a list of commonly used tests and their LRs for common diseases should be on every clinician's to-do list. The bibliography for Chapter 5 includes a reliable source.

4.6 The assumptions of Bayes' theorem

Bayes' theorem is an oversimplification of real life. It requires us to make several assumptions. To understand them, we shall express Bayes' theorem in conditional probability notation:

$$p[D+|R] = \frac{p[D+] \times p[R|D+]}{(p[D+] \times p[R|D+] + p[D-] \times p[R|D-])}$$

where:
R = test result
$D+$ = disease present
$D-$ = disease absent

Assumption No. 1: *The probability of a test result conditional on the presence of the disease (i.e., sensitivity and specificity) is independent of the prior probability of the disease.*

We assume that this relationship is true whenever we calculate the post-test probability using the same sensitivity and specificity and different prior probabilities of the disease. The following example shows how this assumption can be wrong. Imagine a radionuclide scan of the liver that detects metastases from colon cancer. This scan detects all metastases that are larger than 2 cm. Now consider two patients with recently discovered colon cancer. Unbeknownst to anyone, both patients have metastases to the liver.
- One has lost weight. Their liver is considerably enlarged and has a stony hard consistency. This patient's prior probability of liver metastases is high. If a pathologist could examine this patient's liver, most of the metastases

would be larger than 2 cm, easily detectable by the liver scan. If similar patients were used to measure its sensitivity for liver metastases the result would be close to 1.0.
- The other patient feels and looks well, and their liver is not enlarged on physical examination. The patient's prior probability of liver metastases is low. If similar patients were used to measure the sensitivity of the scan for liver metastases, the result would be far from 1.0.'

In this hypothetical example, the sensitivity of the test depends on the prior probability of the disease, in violation of the assumption that the sensitivity and specificity are both constant. Few such examples exist, probably because few researchers determine the pre-test probability of the target disease when they measure sensitivity and specificity.

Table 4.4 shows a study in which a history of chest pain was obtained in patients along with an exercise ECG and a coronary arteriogram. In men and women, the sensitivity of the exercise ECG increased as the prior probability of coronary artery disease increased.

Table 4.4 Exercise ECG test performance in patients with different chest pain syndromes.

	Type of chest pain	No. patients	p[CAD]	Exercise ECG sensitivity	Exercise ECG specificity
Men	Definite angina	487	0.88	0.84	0.71
	Probable angina	443	0.67	0.72	0.80
	Nonischemic pain	203	0.22	0.46	0.79
Women	Typical angina	67	0.58	0.80	0.57
	Atypical angina	153	0.35	0.67	0.69
	Nonischemic pain	175	0.05	0.22	0.81

Adapted from Weiner *et al.* (1979).

Assumption No. 2: *The probability of a test result conditional on the presence of the disease (i.e., sensitivity and specificity) is independent of prior test results.*

To understand this assumption, imagine that two tests have been done in sequence (first test 1 with result $R1$ and then test 2 with result $R2$); now calculate the probability of the disease after the result of the second test.

$$p[D+\,|\,R1,R2] = \frac{p[D+]\times p[R2\,|\,D+,R1]}{\left(p[D+]\times p[R2\,|\,D+,R1] + p[D-]\times p[R2\,|\,D-,R1]\right)}$$

where:
$R1$ = result of test 1
$R2$ = result of test 2
$D+$ = disease present
$D-$ = disease absent

$p[D\,|\,R1,R2]$ = probability of the disease conditional upon the results of test one *and* test two
$p[R2\,|\,D+,R1]$ = probability of result on test 2 conditional upon the patient having the target condition *and* the result on test 1

To verify Assumption 2 would require the following study. First, divide patients with the target condition into two groups: one with a normal result on the first test and one with an abnormal result. Second, do the second test in both groups of patients with the target disease and a gold standard (reference) test on both groups. Then, calculate the sensitivity and specificity of the second test. Assumption 2 is verified (for that test) if they are the same. Since few investigators have studied two diagnostic tests done always in the same sequence, Assumption 2 of Bayes' theorem is seldom tested. *Therefore, clinicians must assume that the sensitivity of a second test in diseased patients is the same regardless of the results of the first test.*

The assumption of conditional independence also applies to test specificity. The specificity of the second test in a sequence is assumed to be the same regardless of the results of the first test in the sequence.

4.7 Using Bayes' theorem to interpret a sequence of tests

Diagnostic tests are often used in sequence. An abnormal finding on one test may raise concerns that only can be resolved by a second test. For example, when a screening test is performed on an asymptomatic person, an abnormal finding may raise concerns that a second test might resolve. What method should be used to interpret the results of the second test? The reader who has absorbed the lessons of this chapter will answer as follows:

> *"Use the post-test probability following the first test as the pre-test probability for the **second** test. Then, use the sensitivity and specificity of the second test and Bayes' theorem to calculate the post-test probability for the second test."*

We illustrate this concept for an exercise ECG performed on an asymptomatic 45-year-old man who is about to begin an exercise training program (Figure 4.9). The pre-test probability of coronary artery disease is 0.06 in asymptomatic men in the fifth decade of life. The sensitivity of the exercise ECG is 0.58 and its specificity is 0.88. The probability of coronary artery disease if the exercise test provokes ≥1 mm ST segment depression is 0.24, as calculated with Bayes' theorem. The odds of CAD corresponding to a probability of 0.24 are 1:3. Thus, following an unexpected abnormal stress test, the odds are one in four that the patient has significant coronary artery disease. Given the uncertainty about the diagnosis of CAD, the logical next step would be to perform a noninvasive test like coronary CT angiography.

Before using Bayes' theorem to calculate the post-test probability of coronary artery disease after coronary CT angiography, the clinician must answer two questions:

1. What should I use for the pre-test probability of coronary artery disease?
   This question is easy to answer. The probability of coronary artery disease after the positive exercise ECG *is* the probability of the disease prior to the second test.
2. What are the sensitivity and specificity of coronary CT angiography?
   The second question seems even more straightforward than the first. The apparently correct answer is its sensitivity and specificity, and therefore its LR, as measured in a large study of patients who had CT angiography and a definitive test, such as a coronary arteriogram.

This approach sounds logical, but it has a potential flaw. It assumes that the sensitivity and specificity of the CT angiogram, and therefore its LR+ and LR-, are the same in patients with a positive exercise ECG as it is in patients with a negative exercise ECG.

Recall Assumption 1 in the preceding section: The probability of a test result conditional on the presence of the disease (i.e., its sensitivity and specificity) is independent of the prior probability of the disease.

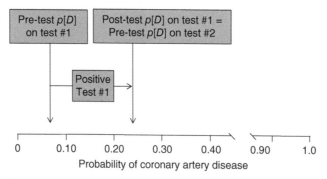

Figure 4.9 The post-test probability after the first test in a sequence is the pre-test probability for the second test. The pre-test probability for Test 1 is labeled as "Pre-test #1."

In contrast to the earlier case, here the post-test probability for the first test is the pre-test probability for the second test, the CT angiogram. In both cases, the question is whether the sensitivity and specificity of the second test are the same whether the first test is positive or negative. If the sensitivity and specificity of the CT angiogram are the same irrespective of the results of the exercise ECG, the post-test probability after the CT angiogram is *conditionally independent* of the exercise ECG results.

Definition

CONDITIONAL INDEPENDENCE: Two tests are conditionally independent if the sensitivity and specificity of one test do not depend upon the result of the other test.

Researchers typically measure the sensitivity and specificity of a test in the entire population of patients referred for the test irrespective of the results of earlier tests, such as an exercise ECG. When the results are used to interpret the scan in a patient with a positive exercise ECG, the clinician is assuming that the sensitivity and specificity of the scan are conditionally independent of the results of the exercise ECG.

In reality, clinicians assume conditional independence of the sensitivity and specificity of the tests in a sequence. Ideally, all study patients should have the first test in a sequence, the second test, and then a definitive test for the target condition. With this study design, it is possible to calculate the sensitivity and specificity of the second test in those with a positive result on the first test and in those with a negative result on the first test.

4.8 Using Bayes' theorem when many diseases are under consideration

This section contains advanced material and can be skipped without loss of continuity.

In this chapter, we have represented the denominator of Bayes' theorem by the sum of two quantities: ($p[D+] \times$ test sensitivity) and ($[1-p[D+] \times$ (1-test specificity), where $p[D+]$ is the probability of the target condition and ($1-p[D+]$) represents the probability of all other conditions. In effect, we are saying that the contribution of other diseases to the denominator of Bayes' theorem is a variable ($1-p[D+]$) times a constant (1-test specificity). As $p[D+]$ increases, the contribution of other diseases decreases.

Suppose that two diseases D_1 and D_2 are under serious consideration and that X is a symptom or test result associated with both diseases. Assuming that only one of them is actually present, Bayes' theorem would look like this:

$$p[D_1 \mid S] = \frac{p[X \mid D_1] \times p[D_1]}{p[X \mid D_1] \times p[D_1] + p[X \mid D_2] \times p[D_2] + p[X \mid \text{neither } D_1 \text{ nor } D_2] \times p[\text{neither } D_1 \text{ nor } D_2]}$$

More generally, assume that there are n possible diseases and that the patient has only one of these possibilities.

$$p[D_1 \mid S] = \frac{p[X \mid D_1] \times p[D_1]}{p[X \mid D_1] \times p[D_1] + \ldots + p[X \mid D_n] \times p[D_n]}$$

In this section, we derive Bayes' theorem in its most general form, one in which every "other disease" contributes to the denominator of Bayes' theorem individually (rather than being lumped under the term "no disease").

Suppose a clinician is considering three diseases (A, B, and C) as the possible cause of a patient's symptoms (the probability of other diseases is vanishingly small). The clinician's goal is to calculate the probability of disease A given the presence of a clinical finding.

In this instance, we know the prevalence of diseases A, B, and C, and we also know the frequency of finding X in these diseases (e.g. $p[X \mid A]$). Instead of representing two of the diseases (e.g., B and C) as "no disease," we can list them separately and perhaps gain additional precision in estimating the conditional probability that disease A is present.

The prior probabilities of these diseases are $p[A]$, $p[B]$, and $p[C]$, where $p[A]+p[B]+p[C] = 1$. The clinician makes observation X. The relationships between observation X and the three diseases are given by the following table (Table 4.5, see next page) of conditional probabilities.

Table 4.5 Probability of a symptom given three diseases.

Disease	Probability of finding X given disease A, B, or C
A	$p[X|A]$
B	$p[X|B]$
C	$p[X|C]$

The probability that finding X occurs in a patient with one of these diseases (e.g., $p[X$ and $A]$) arises from the definition of conditional probability:

$$p[X|A] = \frac{p[X \text{ and } A]}{p[A]}$$

$$p[X \text{ and } A] = p[A] \times p[X|A]$$

The probability of finding X occurring in all patients suspected of having diseases A, B, or C is the sum of the probability of its occurrence in each disease:

$$p[X] = p[A] \times p[X|A] + p[B] \times p[X|B] + p[C] \times p[X|C]$$

The probability of disease A given that finding X has occurred – $p[A|X]$—follows from the definition of conditional probability.

$$p[A|X] = \frac{p[X \text{ and } A]}{p[X]}$$

Substituting the expressions for $p[X$ and $A]$ and $p[X]$ into the expression for $p[A|X]$, we obtain the following equation, which is what the clinician is interested in:

$$p[A|X] = \frac{p[A] \times p[X|A]}{p[A] \times p[X|A] + p[B] \times p[X|B] + p[C] \times p[X|C]}$$

From this 3-disease case, it is a small step to express Bayes' theorem in its most general form, with n diseases and subject to the assumption that the patient has only one of the possible diseases. In this equation, X refers to a clinical finding, the subscript i refers to a specific disease and n refers to the total number of diseases under consideration.

$$p[D_1|X] = \frac{(p[D_1] \times p[X|D_1]}{\sum_{i=1}^{n} (p[D_i] \times p[X|D_i])}$$

Summary

1. A compelling reason to use probability to express uncertainty is to speak the language of Bayes' theorem, and thereby to calculate post-test probability.
2. Bayes' theorem takes two equivalent but different forms.
   - The algebraic form of Bayes' theorem is especially useful when several diseases are being considered. Downside: calculating a post-test probability requires a lot of facility with mental arithmetic. Most people need a calculator.
   - With the odds ratio form of Bayes' theorem, calculating the post-test odds requires multiplying two numbers: the pre-test odds and the LR of the test. Downside: moving back and forth between probability and odds requires some facility with mental arithmetic.
3. Perhaps the most important idea in this book: *the interpretation of a test result depends on the pre-test probability of the disease.*

4. Bayes' theorem provides other insights about interpreting test results and deciding when a test is likely to be useful.
   - Rare is the test that will *reduce the probability to near-zero* disease when the pre-test probability is quite high.
   - Still rarer is the test that will *raise the probability of the disease* to nearly 1.0 when the pre-test probability is quite low.
   - If you screen for occult disease, take particular care to avoid tests that have a low specificity.

Bibliography

Diamond, G.A. and Forrester, J.S. (1979) Analysis of probability as an aid in the clinical diagnosis of coronary-artery disease. *New England Journal of Medicine*, **300**, 1350–58.

   The authors estimated the pre-test probability of coronary artery disease using age, sex, and chest pain history and calculated post-test probabilities for 4 tests.

Gorry, G.A. and Barnett, G.O. (1968) Sequential diagnosis by computer. *Journal of the American Medical Association*, **205**, 849–54.

   A description of the sequential use of Bayes' theorem to interpret several clinical findings.

Gorry, G.A., Pauker, S.G., and Schwartz, W.B. (1978) The diagnostic importance of the normal finding. *The New England Journal of Medicine*, **298**, 486–9.

   A clear discussion of how a negative test result can be evidence against one disease and evidence for another.

Raiffa, H. (1968) *Decision Analysis: Introductory Lectures on Choices Under Uncertainty*, Addison-Wesley Publishing Co. Inc., Reading, MA.

   Chapter 2 of this classic book contains a derivation of Bayes' theorem.

Rifkin, R.O. and Hood, W.B. (1977) Bayesian analysis of electrocardiographic stress testing. *The New England Journal of Medicine*, **297**, 681–6.

   Probabilistic reasoning in test selection has become particularly well-accepted in cardiology practice. This article was very influential.

Weiner, D.A., Ryan, T.J., McCabe, C.H. *et al.* (1979) Exercise stress testing: correlation among history of angina, ST-segment response and prevalence of coronary artery disease in the Coronary Artery Surgery Study (CASS). *The New England Journal of Medicine*, **301**, 230–5.

   This study illustrates how measuring sensitivity and specificity in subgroups of patients can yield new insights. This study showed that in men the test performance of the exercise ECG depends on the patient's history.

CHAPTER 5

Measuring the accuracy of clinical findings

Clinicians must rely on imperfect knowledge to make decisions. Probability is a system for dealing with the uncertainty created by imperfect information, but it is only part of the story. The other part is the imperfect knowledge itself and how to measure it, which is the topic of this chapter.

When taking a patient's history, clinicians interpret the answer to a question as evidence for or against a diagnosis. They must decide if the answer favors the diagnosis or not and whether it is strong or weak evidence. Interpretive errors occur when:

- The clinician assumes that a negative response to a question is evidence that the hypothesized disease is absent. A *false-negative* result occurs when a patient has the target condition but answers no to the question.
- The clinician assumes that a positive response is evidence that the hypothesized disease is present. A *false-positive* result occurs when a patient has the finding but does not have the target condition.

In **Chapter** 4, we learned that the probability of a disease when a clinical finding is present depends on its sensitivity and specificity and the patient's pre-test probability. This chapter is about measuring sensitivity and specificity and evaluating published reports of diagnostic test performance.

5.1   A language for describing test results

This part of the chapter is about a language for describing test results. We first describe the distribution of test results in patients who have the target condition and patients who do not have the target condition. Building on this knowledge, we then consider several ways to describe test results.

Most test results are expressed as continuous variables. For example, the serum concentration of troponin I and troponin T (protein constituents of heart muscle cells) is a measure of heart muscle damage. The serum troponin level ranges from less than 100 units/ml to greater than 4000 units/ml, depending on the amount of damaged muscle. In a patient with a suspected myocardial infarction (MI), each point on this scale of troponin levels corresponds to a probability that the patient has had a recent MI. To understand this claim, first consider the results of a test in a

Medical Decision Making, Third Edition. Harold C. Sox, Michael C. Higgins, Douglas K. Owens, and Gillian Sanders Schmidler.
© 2024 John Wiley & Sons Ltd. Published 2024 by John Wiley & Sons Ltd.

population of healthy individuals. Figure 5.1 shows the distribution of values around the central value for a hypothetical test.

Figure 5.1 shows a symmetric distribution of values. The curve represents a *normal distribution*, which has many important statistical properties. The most important of these are the *mean* of the distribution, which is the unweighted average of all individuals' results, and the *standard deviation*, which is a measure of the degree of spread of the results around the mean of the distribution. The normal distribution has another important feature: the test results for 68% of the population fall within one standard deviation of the mean value. The test results for 95% of the population fall within two standard deviations of the mean (Figure 5.2).

The distribution of test results in patients with the target condition often overlaps the values in individuals who do not have the target condition (Figure 5.3).

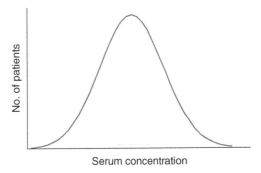

Figure 5.1 Results of a hypothetical test in a healthy population.

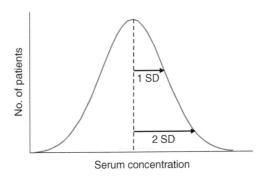

Figure 5.2 One and two standard deviations of a normal distribution.

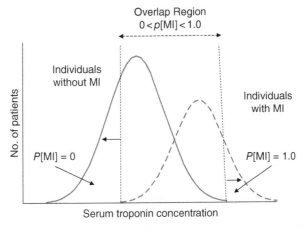

Figure 5.3 Distribution of test results in individuals with the target condition (dashed line) and individuals who do not have the target condition (solid line).

Notation: When describing the performance of a test (sensitivity, specificity, likelihood ratio), always specify the target condition to which these measures apply.

The interpretation of a test result depends on knowing the shape of the distribution curves in persons with and without the target condition and where the curves intersect. Very low test result values indicate "target condition absent," and very high values indicate "target condition present." Uncertainty is not a problem with these extreme values. Uncertainty is a problem for test result values in the range where the two distribution curves overlap because the patient could either have the target condition or not have it. Interpreting values in the overlap region requires Bayes' theorem.

5.1.1 Defining a test result
- A test result defined as a dichotomous variable
  - Below and above the upper limit of normal
  - Normal vs. abnormal
  - Positive vs. negative
- A test result defined as a continuous variable

A test result as a dichotomous variable: A test result is a gateway to taking an action. As discussed in Chapter 3, test results are typically expressed as a dichotomous variable: positive or negative. The reason for this practice is that these words connote action. To simplify, "positive test" implies "treat as if the patient has the target condition," and "negative test" implies "treat as if the patient does not have the target condition."

Imagine that the larger normal distribution curve in Figure 5.3 shows the distribution of serum troponin values in patients with chest pain who do not have an MI, and the smaller normal curve shows those who do have an MI. The horizontal axis is the concentration of serum troponin. Decision making is easy for very low or very high levels of troponin. The probability of an MI is zero in the lower of these two ranges of values and 1.0 in the upper range.

The diagnosis is more difficult in the region of troponin values where the two normal distribution curves overlap. As the troponin value increases, more and more patients do have an MI, and so the proportion of patients with an MI increases. Treatment for an MI benefits those with an MI and may harm those who do not have an MI. Therefore, each troponin value within the overlap region has a different ratio of benefits and harms from treating the patient as if they had an MI. Any value of serum troponin within the overlap region could be the cut point at which to treat the patient as if they had an MI. Picking the cut point value of serum troponin that maximizes net benefit – the treatment threshold value – is central to decision making and a recurring theme of this chapter.

The language commonly used to describe test performance uses terms that place test results into two categories. As described in Chapter 4, the terms are *sensitivity* and *specificity*, which are, respectively, the frequency of a "positive" test in patients with the target condition and the frequency of a "negative" test in someone who does not have the target condition. If the test result is expressed as a continuous variable (like serum troponin), we will take a different action depending on the troponin value at the cut point test result that separates a positive result from a negative result. Therefore, deciding on this cut point will require careful thinking about the consequences of treating or not treating the target condition. We discuss three possibilities for choosing the cut point:

Using the upper limit of normal as the cut point
Clinical laboratories usually report the patient's value and, as a guide to interpretation, the value that corresponds to the "upper limit of normal." The "upper limit of normal" is usually a value two standard deviations above the mean value. Is "above the upper limit of normal" a good way to describe a test result?

The words "upper limit of normal" sound as if they mean the highest result in someone without the target condition; this point would correspond to the right-hand end of the distribution labeled "individuals without disease" in Figure 5.3. While everyone with a serum troponin value above that point on the horizontal axis would have an MI, the serum troponin for many patients with an MI would be below the cut point value.

As described in the preceding section, the purpose of defining a cut point is to link the test result to action, such as "treat" or "do not treat." If the upper limit of normal is used as the cut point, many patients with the target condition would have results below the cut point and would not get treated for a MI. Lowering the cut point a little would result in treating more patients with a MI but also treating some who do not have a MI, which might cause more harm than the added benefit for those with a MI. In short, the placing of the cut point for starting treatment involves balancing benefit to the sick with harm to the well.

The "upper limit of normal" is a poor choice for the cut point for defining a test result as positive or negative. It accounts for the shape of the distribution of test results in normal people but not in patients who have an MI.

This is important because the intersection of the distributions for patients with and without an MI defines the overlap region, in which the balance of harms and benefits differs at each value of the test result.

Another reason for avoiding the "upper limit of normal:" the label encourages simplistic reasoning. The unwary might assume that a value above the upper limit of normal means the disease is present and a value below it means that the disease is absent. Figure 5.3 says otherwise.

The best cut point value for dividing "positive" from "negative" results will depend on the clinical situation. As we shall see at the end of this chapter, a higher cut point is best if the pre-test probability is low, and a lower cut point is best if the patient's pre-test probability is high.

Using normal and abnormal as the cut point

Clinicians often hear the following: "That chest radiograph is abnormal." Or, "this MRI scan is perfectly normal." Or, "that tuberculin skin test is abnormal." Here, the clinician has not categorized a test result in reference to a cut point along a continuous scale of test result values. Instead, the point of reference seems to be the normal condition. A central purpose of this book is to show how decision making can become more patient-centered by measuring uncertainty and personal preferences. This task is more difficult when the boundary that defines normal and abnormal – and thus action or no action – is ill-defined and personal. So, we will not use the terminology of normal and abnormal to help develop the ideas in this book.

Using the cut point to define positive and negative

In practice, most of the ideas that define the discipline of medical decision making depend on expressing numerical results as a dichotomous variable. Perhaps this usage reflects the nature of decision making: it is the act of choosing one action and not choosing another.

We follow the conventions of the scientists who conceived the ideas in this book and define the two categories of test results as "positive" and "negative." These terms are abstract and do not have a physical counterpart. The cut point, which divides the range of possible values into "positive" and "negative" regions, is a critical concept for deciding what a numerical test result means to the patient.

We define a "positive" test result as one that is more extreme than the cut point. It increases the probability that the patient has the target condition. A "negative" result is less extreme than the cut point, and it decreases the probability of the target condition.

A test result as a continuous variable

Dividing the range of values into positive and negative regions has an important shortcoming. It disregards the information contained in the magnitude of the numerical result. In general, a larger value of the serum troponin means a greater likelihood that the patient has an MI, and a very low value means a smaller likelihood. A result that moves the probability of the target condition closer to 1.0 – one that reduces uncertainty to a minimum – can be useful. However, as we will see in later chapters, crossing a threshold probability for taking action should be sufficient to take that action. When reducing uncertainty any further will not change management, the resources required are not well spent.

Referring to Figure 5.4 (see next page), within the range of test results that occur in both patients with the target condition and patients who do not have the target condition (the overlap region), a test result is consistent with either having the target condition or not having it. If the overlap region contains the cutoff value, it defines a positive and negative test result. Patients with the target condition can have a negative result (*false-negative*), and patients who do not have the target condition can have a positive result (*false-positive*) (Figure 5.4).

Definition

Cut point: The test result that divides the spectrum of test results into a test-positive region and a test-negative region.

In Figure 5.4 (see next page), we first introduced the problem of balancing harms and benefits of treatment versus no treatment when the diagnosis is uncertain.

Within the overlap region of the two distributions of individuals, the problem is distinguishing between persons who have the disease of concern and persons who do not. The cut point divides the diseased population into those with positive results, who are treated and benefit, and those with negative results, who are not treated and suffer harm. The cut point also divides the nondiseased population.

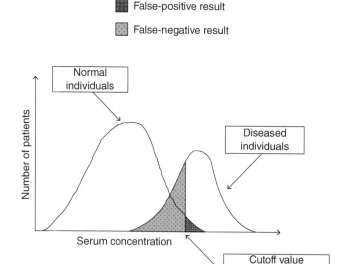

Figure 5.4 The figure shows the distribution of results in patients with and without the target condition. The cut point divides both distributions into regions that define false-negative results and false-positive results.

A small number of them are treated and suffer some harm, and most are not treated and do fine. The task is to find the cut point that best balances the potential benefits and harms of treatment for the individual patient, who may or may not have the disease of concern. We will revisit this problem in the appendix to this chapter and in Chapter 13.

In this part of the chapter, we have learned how the cut point test result leads to a language for describing misleading test results (e.g., false-positives and false-negatives and their truthful counterparts – true-positives and true-negatives). These terms apply to any information that might affect our certainty about the patient's true state: the history, physical examination, or a diagnostic test result. Using a cut point deprives us of the information conveyed by extreme test results, but it is in keeping with a focus on getting just the information we need to decide.

5.2 The measurement of diagnostic test performance

The key measure of any diagnostic information is its ability to discriminate between the target condition and all other conditions. What do we mean by "discriminate?" A test that perfectly discriminates between the target condition and all other conditions is positive in all patients with the target condition and negative in all patients who do not have it. Most tests fall far short of this ideal performance.

> **Definition**
>
> *TEST PERFORMANCE*: A test's ability to detect and discriminate.

5.2.1 How to measure test performance

Bayes' theorem defines the measures of test performance. The odds ratio form of Bayes' theorem (Chapter 4) states that:

$$\text{Post} - \text{test odds} = \text{pre} - \text{test odds} \times \text{likelihood ratio}$$

This form of Bayes' theorem reminds us that *the function of diagnostic information is to change the probability of disease.* The likelihood ratio is the most meaningful measure of diagnostic information because it directly shows the effect on the probability of disease. In other words,

To know the performance of a test, know its likelihood ratio.

Recall the definition of the likelihood ratio, as it emerges from the derivation of the odds ratio form of Bayes' theorem:

$$\text{Likelihood ratio} = \frac{p[R \mid D+]}{p[R \mid D-]}$$

where $p[R \mid D+]$ is the probability of a test result in patients with the target condition and $p[R \mid D-]$ is the probability of the result in people who do not have the target condition.

This line of argument leads us to the following method for measuring test performance:

1. To measure the performance of a test for a disease, first perform the test in patients who are known to have the target condition and in patients who are known to be free of it (but might have other diseases).
2. Then, calculate the frequency of a test result in patients with the disease and in patients who do not have the disease.

This simple prescription is hard to achieve to practice. Many studies of test performance have had serious flaws. These flaws can lead to inaccurate test performance measurements that can lead to incorrect interpretation of test results and potentially to mistakes in patient care.

We will first learn how to measure test performance. Then, we will learn how to evaluate articles about test performance and identify studies whose measurements of test performance we can rely upon.

Recall that the first step in measuring the performance of a test is to determine the frequency of a test result in patients with the target condition and in patients known to be free of it. Deciding if the patient has the disease requires doing another test, which is usually called the "gold standard" test (also "diagnostic reference standard").

Definition

"Gold Standard" Test: The procedure which defines the true state of the patient in a study of test performance (also known as "diagnostic reference standard").

Definition

Index Test: The test whose performance is being measured.

Definition

Source Population: The patients whose findings lead a clinician to order the index test. (Also known as the "clinically relevant population.")

Definition

Verified Sample: Patients who receive the gold standard test to *verify* their disease status (ideally, identical to the source population but too often, a *sample,* or subset, of the source population).

In the ideal study of a test, each patient in a source population containing N patients undergoes both the index test and the gold standard procedure. If the test results are expressed as a dichotomous variable (positive or negative), a 2 by 2 table is a convenient way to display the results of the study. The name "2 × 2" refers to the array of the four cells that contain the primary results, labeled TP, FP, FN, and TN in Table 5.1 (see next page).

Table 5.1 Test results defined.

	Results of the gold standard test		
Results of the index test	Positive	Negative	Totals
Positive	True-positive (TP)	False-positive (FP)	TP + FP
Negative	False-negative (FN)	True-negative (TN)	FN + TN
Totals	TP + FN	FP + TN	N = TP+FN+FP+TN

If the index test and the patient's true state were perfectly concordant, we would have that elusive animal, the perfect test, one with no false positive results and no false negative results. Misleading test results nearly always occur with most tests. Measures of the degree of concordance, such as the *sensitivity* and *specificity* of a test, are part of the basic vocabulary of medicine.

5.2.2 Measures of concordance between index test and disease state

Two types of test results reflect the true state of the patient: **true positive** results and **true negative results**. The relative proportions of these two types of results completely characterize the performance of a test.

The Sensitivity of a diagnostic test

Definition

Sensitivity: Probability of a positive test in a patient with the target condition.

In conditional probability notation, the sensitivity of a test result is:

p[positive test result | disease] or $p[+ | D+]$ which means "the probability of a positive test result if the patient has the target condition."

$$\text{Sensitivity} = \frac{\text{Number of diseased patients with positive test}}{\text{Number of diseased patients}}$$

To measure the sensitivity of a test, perform the index test and the gold standard test in a source population. In terms of the 2×2 table, the sensitivity of a test, is:

$$\text{Sensitivity} = \frac{\text{TP}}{\text{TP} + \text{FN}}$$

The specificity of a diagnostic test

Definition

Specificity: The probability that a patient who does not have the target condition has a negative test.

In conditional probability notation, the specificity of a test result is:

$p\left[\text{negative test result} | \text{disease is absent}\right]$ or $p\left[T- | D-\right]$

which means "the probability of a negative test result if the patient does not have the target condition."

$$\text{Specificity} = \frac{\text{Number of nondiseased patients with negative test}}{\text{Number of nondiseased patients}}$$

To measure the specificity of a test, perform the index test and the gold standard test in a source population. In terms of the 2×2 table (see Table 5.1), the specificity of a test is:

$$\text{Specificity} = \frac{\text{TN}}{\text{FP} + \text{TN}}$$

5.2.3 Measures of discordance between index test and disease state

Two types of test results that do not reflect the true state of the patient: *false negative* results and *false positive* results. Unlike sensitivity and specificity, these two quantities do not have their own names. Sometimes, "false-negative rate" and "false-positive rate" are used, but these names can be interpreted in several ways.

False-negative results

> **Definition**
>
> A negative test result in a patient who has the target condition.

The frequency of a false-negative result in conditional probability notation is the following:

$$p[\text{negative test result} \mid \text{disease}] \text{ or } p[T- \mid D+]$$

which means "the probability that a negative test result will occur if the patient has the target condition." Patients with the target condition can only experience a positive result or a negative result, so

$$p[T+ \mid D+] + p[T- \mid D+] = 1$$

Therefore, $p[T- \mid D+] = 1 - p[T+ \mid D+]$

$$1 - \text{sensitivity} = \frac{\text{No. of diseased patients with negative test}}{\text{No. of diseased patients}}$$

To obtain the value for $1 - \text{sensitivity}$, simply subtract the test sensitivity from 1. To measure it directly, perform the index test and the gold standard test in a source population. In terms of the 2×2 table

$$1 - \text{sensitivity} = \frac{\text{FN}}{\text{TP} + \text{FN}}$$

False-positive results

> **Definition**
>
> *False-positive*: A positive test result in a patient who does not have the target condition. The frequency of a false-positive result in conditional probability notation is the following:

$$p[\text{positive test result} \mid \text{no disease}] \text{ or } p[T+ \mid D-]$$

which means "the probability that a positive test result will occur if the patient does not have the target condition." Patients with the target condition can only experience a positive result or a negative result, so

$$p[T+ \mid D-] + p[T- \mid D-] = 1$$

Therefore, $p[T+ \mid D-] = 1 - p[T- \mid D-]$

$$1 - \text{specificity} = \frac{\text{No. of diseased patients with positive test}}{\text{No. of nondiseased patients}}$$

To measure $1 - \text{specificity}$, simply subtract the test specificity from 1. To measure it directly, perform the index test and the gold standard test in a source population. In terms of the 2×2 table:

$$1 - \text{specificity} = \frac{FP}{FP + TN}$$

5.2.4 Predictive value

Predictive value is another way to describe the results of performing the index test and the gold standard test in terms of the 2×2 table. Unlike the measures of test performance, for which the columns of the 2×2 table contain the key measures, the calculation of predictive value uses the rows. Predictive value is, in effect, a *post-test probability*. The two types of predictive value are **positive predictive value** and **negative predictive value**.

Positive predictive value

> **Definition**
>
> **Positive Predictive Value (PV+):** The fraction of patients with a positive test who also have the target condition.

$$PV+ = \frac{\text{Number of diseased patients with a positive test}}{\text{Number of patients with positive test}}$$

In terms of the 2 by 2 table,

$$PV+ = \frac{TP}{TP + FP}$$

Negative predictive value

> **Definition**
>
> **Negative Predictive Value (PV−):** The fraction of patients with a negative test result who do not have the target condition.

$$PV- = \frac{\text{Number of nondiseased patients with negative test}}{\text{Number of patients with negative test}}$$

In terms of the cells in the 2×2 table,

$$PV- = \frac{TN}{TN + FN}$$

Differences between predictive value and post-test probability

Predictive value and post-test probability appear to be very similar. Both answer this all-important question, *as a result of this test result, what is the likelihood that my patient has this disease?* However, posterior probability and predictive value are different in important ways. Posterior probability is far more useful than predictive value, but, unfortunately, authors of medical articles often use "predictive value" when the correct usage is "posterior probability."

Predictive value
- Defined as the proportion of patients with a test result who have the target condition.
- Calculated from a 2 by 2 table of results in a *specific* population of patients.
- Refers to a test as used in a particular population; strictly speaking, it does not apply to any other population because it depends on the prevalence of the target condition in the specified population. Applying a published predictive value for a disease to a population with a different prevalence of the target condition will cause error except when the prevalence of the disease is the same in both populations. The larger the difference in the prevalence of the target condition, the greater the error.
- There is no mathematical relationship with which to calculate the predictive value in another population.

Post-test probability
- Defined as the probability of the target condition after using Bayes' theorem to take new information, such as a test result, into account.
- A mathematical relationship (Bayes' theorem) makes it possible to calculate the post-test probability for *any* patient, regardless of the source population.
- According to Bayes' theorem, the post-test probability depends on the pre-test probability of the target condition, which is often a quantitative representation of a subjective *opinion* about the likelihood of an event.
- Uses sensitivity, specificity, and likelihood ratios obtained from published research. Assumes that the sensitivity and specificity applies to the patient at hand.

Thus, *the predictive value is an observable number obtained from a defined population. It usually will not apply to another population.*

An important caution: A reader might mistakenly believe that predictive value is a measure of test performance. It is not. Imagine a population consisting of patients who have undergone a diagnostic test. From this population, it is possible to calculate a predictive value, which will reflect the sensitivity and specificity of the test due to their influence on the number of true-positive and false-positive test results, which in turn affect the predictive value. The prevalence of the target condition also affects predictive value through its effect on the number of patients that can have a true-positive result (those with the target condition) or a false-positive result (those who do not have the target condition). Therefore, predictive value is a consequence of test performance and pre-test probability, not an independent measure of test performance.

The next several sections will illustrate the pitfalls of using predictive value as a surrogate for posterior probability.

5.3 How to measure diagnostic test performance: a hypothetical example

5.3.1 Description of the study

You must evaluate a new radionuclide scanning test for splenomegaly. The purpose of the test is to detect spleen enlargement that is too slight to be detected by palpating the abdomen. The scan uses radioactively labeled macroaggregated iron particles. When injected into the bloodstream, these particles attach preferentially to splenic macrophages, which ingest and then digest them. You decide to measure the accuracy of this test by comparing the size of the radionuclide scan image of the spleen to the weight of the spleen, which is a good gold standard test for splenomegaly. In order to weigh the spleen, someone must remove it. Therefore, you perform the spleen scan on all patients who are to undergo elective splenectomy.

A description of your study of the radionuclide spleen scan should contain the following information:
- *Index test*: Macroaggregated iron scan of the spleen.
- *Gold standard test*: Weighing the spleen after surgical removal.
- *Definition of abnormal index test*: Spleen silhouette as seen on the scan is more than 1.5 times normal size.
- *Definition of disease (splenomegaly)*: Splenic weight >250 grams.
- *Source populations*:
  - Patients whose clinicians cannot agree on the size of the spleen; some clinicians can feel it, but others cannot.
  - Patients whose spleen is not palpable, but they have a disease that is often accompanied by splenomegaly.
- *Verified sample*: Patients who are about to undergo splenectomy because their spleen is so large that it interferes with the survival of the formed elements of the blood.

A description of the flow of patients through the study appears in Figure 5.5 (see next page).

5.3.2 Description of results

The results of using the scan in 50 study patients appear in Table 5.2 (see next page).

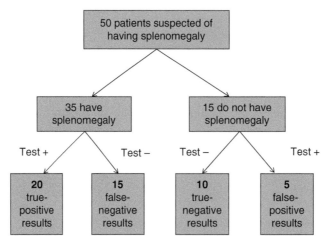

Figure 5.5 Flow of patients through an illustrative study of a hypothetical test for splenomegaly.

Table 5.2 Results of spleen scan study: verified sample consists of patients with palpable spleens.

	Number of patients		
Results of the spleen scan	*Spleen weighs >250 grams*	*Spleen weighs <250 grams*	*Totals*
Positive	True positive $N = 20$	False positive $N = 5$	$N = 25$
Negative	False negative $N = 15$	True negative $N = 10$	$N = 25$
Totals	$N = 35$	$N = 15$	$N = 50$

As shown in Table 5.2, 35 of the patients (70 percent) have splenomegaly. Of these 35 patients, 20 have a positive radioactive iron scan. Of the 15 patients with normal size spleens, 10 have a normal scan. Therefore,

$$\left(p[T+|D+]; \text{sensitivity}\right) = \frac{20}{35} = 0.57$$

$$\left(p[T-|D-]; \text{specificity}\right) = \frac{10}{15} = 0.67$$

Predictive value:

$$PV+ = \frac{\text{true positives}}{\text{total positives}} = \frac{20}{25} = 0.80$$

$$PV- = \frac{\text{true negatives}}{\text{total negatives}} = \frac{10}{25} = 0.40$$

5.3.3   An important limitation of the spleen scan study

The study of the spleen scan will be of little value to anyone because of a major error in design, one that occurs often and is the major reason why studies of test performance can mislead the unwary reader. Everyone who reads a study of test performance must be alert to its occurrence.

The error in the study design is the choice of the verified sample.

Recall these definitions:

Definition

Source Population: The patients whose findings lead the doctor to order the index test. (Also known as the "clinically relevant population.")

> **Definition**
>
> **Verified Sample:** Patients who receive the index test and the gold standard test (usually a subset of the source population).

When the verified sample and the source population are the same, the reader can be sure that the measurements of sensitivity and specificity apply to patients who receive the test in clinical practice. When, as in the spleen scan study, the verified sample differs from the source population, the reader cannot confidently use the findings in patient care.

Source population: Patients whose doctors cannot agree on the size of the spleen; some can feel it, but others cannot; patients whose spleen is not palpable, but they have a disease that is often accompanied by splenomegaly.

Verified sample: Patients who are about to undergo splenectomy because their spleen is so large that it interferes with the survival of the formed elements of the blood.

In fact, many patients in the verified sample have such large spleens that they do not need a spleen scan at all!

So far, in this section, we have learned this important paradox of technology assessment:

The patients in a study of test performance often differ from the patients who usually get the test.

The difference between the source population and the verified sample leads to two errors, which are easy to confuse with one another.

- *The predictive value of the spleen scan in the verified sample is not necessarily the same as the post-test probability in the source population.* The prevalence of an enlarged spleen was 70% in the verified sample, whose spleens were so large that they required surgery to remove them. The prevalence of splenomegaly would likely be considerably lower in the source population, patients who got a spleen scan because of uncertainty about the size of their spleens. Therefore, the predictive value in the verified sample is not necessarily the same as the post-test probability in the source population.
- *The measurements of test performance in the verified sample may not apply to the source population.* The large spleens in the verified sample would be easier to detect with the scan, increasing the sensitivity of the scan as measured in the verified sample. Many patients in the source population would have spleens that would be enlarged but not large enough to be detected by palpating the abdomen.

Both errors are important. We address the first in the next section, which is titled Pitfalls of Predictive Value. We focus on avoiding the second error in Section 5.6 of the chapter, which is about how to avoid biased estimates of test performance.

5.4   Pitfalls of predictive value

Applying the predictive value in one population to another risks error because differences in the prevalence of the disease in the two populations will affect the predictive value of a test. Here, we use the sensitivity (0.57) and specificity (0.67) of the spleen scan in the verified population to calculate the predictive value of the test in a primary care source population in which the prevalence of splenomegaly is only 20%. Figure 5.6 shows the results of using the scan in 1000 patients from this population (see next page).

Using the numbers from Figure 5.6, the predictive value of the test in the hypothetical source population is:

$$PV+ = \frac{114}{114+264} = 0.30$$

$$PV- = \frac{536}{536+86} = 0.86$$

The predictive value in the two populations differ, as seen in Table 5.3 (see next page).

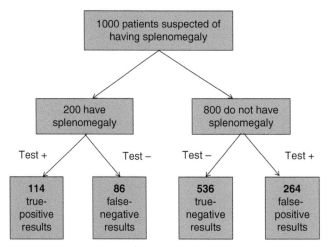

Figure 5.6 Results of applying the test for splenomegaly to a hypothetical population of primary care patients with a 20% pre-test probability of having splenomegaly.

Table 5.3 Predictive value in a verified sample population and the source population.

	Prevalence of splenomegaly in population	Positive predictive value	Negative predictive value
Verified sample population	0.70	0.80	0.40
Source population	0.20	0.30	0.86

The positive predictive value of the spleen scan is much lower (and the negative predictive value much higher) in the source population than in the verified sample. Therefore, *if two populations have a different prevalence of the target condition, their predictive values will differ.*

As discussed in Chapter 4, the predictive value is a number derived from a 2 × 2 table of results from a study of a test. The predictive value obtained in one population usually will not apply to another population unless the prevalence of the target condition in the two populations is the same.

A final point about using the term "predictive value:" the words "predictive value" do not precisely describe the meaning of the term. A person who is unsure of the meaning of "predictive value" would have to look it up. In contrast, consider the precision of the language of probability: "probability of the disease if the test is positive." More words are required, but their meaning is self-explanatory. In this book, we will not use predictive value when we mean post-test probability.

5.5   How to perform a high quality study of diagnostic test performance

We now return to a crucial question

Do measurements of the sensitivity and specificity of a test apply to the patients that I care for?

Readers of studies of test performance will find themselves asking this question many times and will often be disappointed. A skeptical frame of mind is the best way to read accounts of original research on diagnostic test performance. This section will itemize what to look for.

This book focuses on the use of a diagnostic test to help resolve diagnostic uncertainty. For that purpose, the clinician needs to know the state of the patient at the moment of diagnostic uncertainty. Therefore, the principal use of the index diagnostic test is to characterize the patient at a moment in time. The measurement of the sensitivity and specificity of a diagnostic test is an example of a *cross-sectional design*, in which the interval between the index test and gold standard test is as short as possible.

5.5.1   The features of a high-quality prospective study of a diagnostic test
Forming the study population
- Pre-specify the inclusion criteria. They should reflect the reasons that clinicians order the index test.
- Enroll study patients before they have the index test.

- Enroll enough patients to ensure reasonably precise measurements of sensitivity and specificity.
- When comparing two index tests, enroll enough patients to permit a statistically valid noninferiority interpretation of the measured difference in their sensitivity and specificity.

Study conduct
- Ensure that every patient who has the index test also has the gold standard test.
- Obtain a standard set of clinical features from each patient and use them, if necessary, to compare those who have the index test and the gold standard test with those who have only the index test.
- Record the time interval between having the index test and the gold standard test. Note any patient whose clinical status changes during the interval.

Interpreting the Index Test and Gold Standard Test
- Choose a gold standard test that accurately measures the patient's true state.
- Describe the criteria for labeling test results as positive or negative in the study protocol.
- If the test is a visual image, two clinicians must interpret the image independently, discuss any differences, and form a consensus interpretation.
- Conceal the clinical features of the patient from the study clinicians who interpret the index test or the gold standard test.
- Conceal the results of the index test from the study clinicians who interpret the gold standard.
- Conceal the results of the gold standard test from the study clinicians who interpret the index test.

The next parts of this section discuss the rationale underlying these rules of research conduct, focusing on (1) insuring that measurements of sensitivity and specificity apply to usual practice; and (2) assuring accurate, unbiased interpretation of images.

5.5.2   Study characteristics that help ensure that the results apply to usual practice
- **The criteria for including patients in the study should reflect test-ordering decisions in usual practice**

Recruitment and enrollment of study patients should maximize external validity by taking place in typical patient care settings. For example, the study of a test that is typically ordered by specialists should take place in a specialty clinic setting.

The setting of care can influence the study results. For example, many primary care physicians order a stress electrocardiogram (ECG) when they suspect coronary artery disease in a patient with chest pain. They refer some patients to cardiologists, often those with a test result that is alarming or confusing or because of a poor response to initial treatment. Study patients enrolled in primary care may differ from those drawn from a cardiologist's practice in ways that can influence the results of a test.

What to look for in a study: Read the description of the practice settings of the source population. Is it typical of your practice? How were patients identified for enrollment in the study? Who ordered the index test?

- **The study is prospective: Patients are enrolled before doing the index test.**

The ideal study enrolls patients in the clinical setting, not at the point of testing. Some patients may not show up for the index test, and it is important to know how they differ from those that do. In the ideal study, patients enroll early in the process of investigating their chief complaint. Data collection should occur according to a study protocol that enforces the discipline needed for good clinical research. A published report should include the criteria for excluding patients from the study cohort, as well as the criteria for including them.

Retrospective assembly of the study cohort is a much weaker research design. A retrospective study refers to a defined period in the past. Within this time frame, someone identifies all patients who had the index test and who among them also had the gold standard test. This approach invites biased results. First, a positive index test is often the reason for referring a patient for the gold standard test. Second, a positive index test is often sufficient to make a firm diagnosis. So, some patients do not get the gold standard test. Third, patients with a positive index test, whether referred or not, are not typical of the entire population who had the index test.

What to look for in a study: A description of the enrollment process. Were patients enrolled prospectively in the clinical setting where the test-ordering decisions occurred? Were inclusion and exclusion criteria stated clearly?

- **The study protocol describes a standard set of pertinent clinical features to obtain from each patient.**

A list of the frequency of clinical features in the source population helps clinicians to decide how well the measurements of test performance apply to patients in their practice. A full description of the source population should include race/ethnicity, gender, age, reasons for testing, duration and severity of the present illness, and past illnesses. By comparing the frequency of the items from the source population and the verified sample, the reader can identify possible selection biases that might limit the generalizability (external validity) of the study measurements of sensitivity and specificity.

What to look for in a study: A table listing key clinical features and their frequency in the source population and the verified sample. Reasons for failure to get the gold standard test.

- **Every patient who has the index test also has the gold standard test.**

The most important source of error in measuring test performance is due to differences between the verified sample and the source population that comprises the patients that undergo the test in usual practice. In the example of the hypothetical spleen scan, the source population was very different than the verified sample. This extreme example helps to understand the concept of *spectrum bias*, which we discuss in the next section.

What to look for in a study: A table comparing the clinical characteristics of those who had the gold standard test and those that did not have it.

5.5.3 Study characteristics that insure unbiased, reproducible interpretation of the index test and the gold standard test

Some index test results are expressed as numbers. The translation of a test result expressed as a number (e.g., the serum troponin level) into a positive or negative result requires knowing the cut point for the test as applied to a specific disease (e.g., acute MI).

In the study of the accuracy of diagnostic tests, imaging tests may be the index test (e.g., CT coronary arteriography) or the gold standard test (e.g., invasive coronary arteriography) or both, as in this sentence. With diagnostic imaging tests (e.g., a chest radiograph), the classification of the test result requires judgment about interpreting the image as positive (lung mass present) or negative (lung mass absent). This section addresses the interpretation of imaging tests. In a study of the sensitivity and specificity of an imaging test, at least two specialists interpret the images independently and adjudicate any disagreements.

- **If the test is a visual image, two clinicians should interpret the image independently, discuss any differences, and form a consensus interpretation.**

Many index tests and gold standard tests require someone to look at an image of a disease process, place the pattern into a category, and assign the correct label to the category. Many studies have shown that clinicians often disagree about the interpretation of a visual image. These interpretive errors can lead to incorrect numbers in the cells of the 2×2 table that describes the performance of a test.

The best way to avoid errors in interpretation is to have several people interpret the same image without knowing the others' interpretation. If they disagree, the usual procedure is to discuss the disagreement and come to a consensus interpretation or to ask a third person to participate in forming a consensus opinion.

What to look for in a study: With many tests (e.g., imaging tests), deciding what to call the result involves judgment (i.e., the result is not a number). When the index test, the gold standard test, or both is such a test, look for evidence that several people independently evaluated the test and settled any disagreement by consulting each other. The study should report how often two readers disagreed. The best measure is the kappa statistic, which accounts for agreement by chance alone (any kappa statistic above +0.5 is good agreement; kappa equal to zero signifies agreement due only to chance).

- **The study protocol describes the criteria for labeling test results as positive or negative.**

The raw data of a study of test performance are four numbers in a 2×2 table: the number of true-positive, false-positive, true-negative, and false-negative results. The source of these numbers are the results of the gold standard test and the index test. One essential step is being sure that the people who interpret the gold standard test and index test mean the same thing each time they classify a test result.

Suppose the index test is an imaging test, such as a chest radiograph. A radiologist looks at this image and sees a pattern (e.g., "patchy honeycomb appearance"). This pattern has certain characteristics that predict the underlying disease. The leaders of the study want to be sure that the radiologist looks for this pattern and uses the same name for it each time it is present and never when it is absent. They list the key features of a "positive" finding and provide criteria for using them to decide when the finding is present.

Studies of test performance try to maximize the internal validity of the judgments about whether a test result is positive or negative. Having two clinicians make the final decision independently is standard research procedure. They confer, and, if they disagree, ask a third individual to break the tie. Some studies assemble a group of expert radiologists, train them to read the imaging test according to the study protocol, and monitor for consistency in making the final interpretation. Some studies save the images and perform the final review at the end of the study.

What to look for in a study: do the authors define the criteria for deciding how to label a result, either with a name or by calling it "positive" or "negative?" Do they check for consistency in applying diagnostic criteria to images? Do their diagnostic criteria correspond to the system used in your hospital? Did at least two experts read each image independently?

- **The index test and gold standard test are both performed within a short time period.**

A cross-sectional study to measure the performance of a test describes the patient at one point in time. Its intent is to see how well the index test reflects the actual state of the patient at that time. Any change in the patient's condition between the index test and the gold standard test could bias the measures of sensitivity and specificity. The gold standard test must be performed before the patient's target condition has changed.

What do look for in a study: look for the average time elapsed between doing the index test and doing the gold standard test. Is it likely that the target condition may have improved or worsened since the index test?

- **The clinician should interpret the index test without knowing the clinical features of the patient. Likewise, the interpretation of the gold standard test should be concealed when interpreting the index text (and conversely for the interpretation of the gold standard test).**

Doing otherwise can result in two biases: Test-review bias and Diagnosis-review bias.

An example of Test-review bias. The physician interprets the index test: an exercise ECG result that is on the borderline between normal and abnormal. Whether to label the exercise ECG results as positive or negative is a close call. Knowing that the patient had an abnormal coronary arteriogram (the gold standard test) or had many risk factors for coronary artery disease may influence the clinician toward calling the difficult-to-interpret exercise ECG abnormal.

An example of diagnosis-review bias. The clinician is interpreting the gold standard test: a coronary arteriogram. The results must be classified as positive or negative, but it is not clear which interpretation to make. Knowing that the patient had very abnormal results on an exercise ECG or had many risk factors for coronary artery disease may influence the clinician toward calling the coronary arteriogram abnormal.

Test-review bias and diagnosis-review bias have similar effects on measured test performance: they increase the likelihood that the index test and the gold standard studies will agree, increasing the measured sensitivity and specificity of the index test.

What to look for in a study: Look at the study protocol. It should say that the clinicians who interpreted the index test were blinded to the results of the gold standard test and vice versa. Those who interpreted one of the tests should not have had any information about the other test or the clinical characteristics of the patient.

- **The number of enrolled patients, both with the target condition and free of the target condition, is sufficient for precise measurements of the sensitivity and specificity of the test.**

The 95% confidence interval for a proportion such as the sensitivity of a test is given by the following relationship:

$$95\% \text{ confidence interval} = \pm 1.96 \sqrt{\frac{p(1-p)}{N}}$$

where p is the proportion in question such as $p[T+ | D+]$, the sensitivity of a test. N is the number of patients with the target condition.

Figure 5.7 shows the relationship between the number of diseased patients used to calculate the sensitivity of a test and the half-width of the 95% confidence interval (see next page). In this example, above 100 patients with the target condition, the width of the confidence interval changes very little.

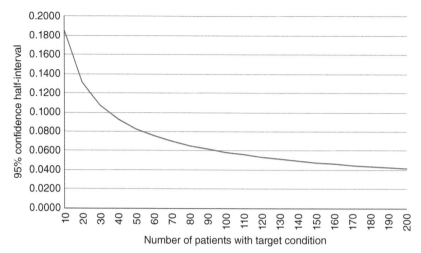

Figure 5.7 Relationship between 95% confidence interval for the sensitivity of a test and the number of patients used in a study to measure the sensitivity of a test. In this calculation, the sensitivity of the test is 0.90.

What to look for in a study: Evidence that, given the measured sensitivity in the study, the number of patients with the target condition is large enough for the half-width of the 95% confidence interval for the measured sensitivity of the test to be on the flat of the curve as depicted in Figure 5.7. The same applies for the number of study patients who do not have the target condition and the measured specificity of the test.

A well-reported study of the sensitivity and specificity of a test will address all of the key characteristics of a well-designed and carefully executed study. The STARD (Standards for Reporting of Diagnostic Accuracy) statement describes a 25-item checklist of the important features. QUADAS-2 is the corresponding statement for systematic reviews of diagnostic test performance (see Bibliography).

5.6   Spectrum bias in the measurement of test performance

> **Definition**
>
> **Spectrum bias:** The effect of differences in the spectrum of disease in different study populations on measurements of sensitivity and specificity.

Spectrum bias affects the measurement of test performance in two phases of the uptake of a test into day-to-day medical practice. In the first phase, the test is unproven, clinicians do not order the test, and it is difficult to find participants for a study of the test. In the second phase, clinicians have too much confidence in the test results and will not refer patients with a negative test result to undergo the gold standard test. The next section describes the mechanism of spectrum bias in studies of test performance. Later sections describe the effects of spectrum bias on test sensitivity and specificity.

5.6.1   The first phase of test evaluation: testing the "sickest of the sick" and the "wellest of the well"
The first studies of a diagnostic test are attempts to learn if the test is accurate enough to justify further study. The first concern is to be sure that the test will be positive for severe disease. A second concern is to be sure that the test is negative in most healthy people. The easiest way to accomplish these limited goals is to study the test in populations at the extreme ends of the spectrum of disease severity.

"The sickest of the sick:" One verified sample is the very sickest patients who, because they have advanced disease, are ideal for learning if the test can detect disease at all. Test sensitivity is apt to be high because advanced disease is typically extensive and easy to detect. In a broader spectrum of patients, sensitivity usually falls.

"The wellest of the well:" Healthy volunteers have advantages for measuring test specificity, which requires people who do not have the target condition. It is often reasonable to assume that healthy volunteers do not have the target condition because they are in excellent health. Therefore, performing a gold standard test is unnecessary. These advantages are outweighed by the disadvantages. The volunteers are often much younger than patients who undergo the test in practice, and they are also usually free of diseases that might cause a false-positive index test. When the test is evaluated with a broader spectrum of patients, the specificity of the test usually falls.

5.6.2   The second phase of test evaluation: reluctance to order the gold standard test because of over-confidence in a negative index test result

Using the index test result to decide whom to refer for the gold standard test is a special form of spectrum bias: *test-referral bias*. Because test-referral bias is a threat to the validity of studies of test performance, it is important to understand how it affects the measurement of sensitivity and specificity.

Why would a clinician be less likely to obtain the gold standard test on patients with a negative index test? Too often, a new diagnostic test becomes embedded in clinical practice before high-quality research has established its rightful role. In this phase, a clinician may gain confidence in a new test based on few if any high-quality studies of its performance and a small, and perhaps atypical, personal experience with it. Consequently, a negative index test increases their belief that the patient does not have the target condition, and so they are less likely to refer the patient for the gold standard test.

> **Definition**
>
> **Test-referral bias:** Systematic error in measuring test performance because the results of the index test influence the decision to refer a patient for the gold standard test.

The verified sample and the source population often differ. Would these differences affect patient care? When should spectrum bias change the interpretation of a test result? These effects of spectrum bias are the subject of the next two sections.

5.6.3   Effects of spectrum bias

Effects of spectrum bias on the sensitivity of a test

Spectrum bias causes the verified sample to have a different spectrum of disease than the source population.

To understand the effects of spectrum bias due to selective referral of patients for the gold standard test, imagine how a patient would become a member of the verified sample in our hypothetical study of the spleen scan to detect splenomegaly. The index test is the spleen scan and the gold standard test is the weight of the spleen after surgical removal.

Two forms of spectrum bias affect test **sensitivity**.

- *Disease severity bias*: Since the weight of the spleen is the gold standard for a study of the spleen scan, the source population is enriched with patients whose spleen is large enough to require surgery to remove it. The spleen scan can detect most of these very large spleens, so that the verification sample – those who undergo splenectomy – is enriched with patients with large spleens. This form of disease severity bias leads to a study that overestimates the sensitivity of the scan because larger spleens are easier to detect with a spleen scan.
- *Test referral bias*: Another reason for referral and enrollment in the verified sample is an enlarged spleen on the index test, the spleen scan. First, a positive index test is often the reason for referring a patient for the gold standard test. Second, a positive index test is often sufficient for the clinician to make a firm diagnosis without referring the patient for the gold standard test. Third, patients with a positive index test, whether referred or not, are not typical of the entire population who had the index test, many of whom had a negative spleen scan and were not referred. The net effect of these conflicting biases may be hard to predict.

These biases afflict retrospective studies, in which the physician decides whether to perform the gold standard based on the clinical need. They should not be a problem with prospective studies, which mandate doing both index test and gold standard test. However, prospective studies may be subject to referral bias because of failure to adhere to the study protocol which specifies that all patients who got the index test are to be referred to undergo the gold standard test. Failure to enroll all eligible patients will lead to a similar bias.

To see the effect of test-referral bias, first recall the study of the spleen scan, in which the verified sample were patients who had been referred for splenectomy because their spleens were very large on the spleen scan and needed surgical removal (Table 5.2).

Now, imagine doing the spleen scan in a hypothetical Source Sample of patients with suspected splenomegaly. This Source Sample contained 230 patients, of whom only the 50 shown in Table 5.2 were referred for splenectomy because of their large spleens. Now suppose—hypothetically—that we knew the true state of the spleen in the 180 patients who had a negative spleen scan and were not referred for splenectomy: 45 of them had an enlarged spleen, and 135 had a normal size spleen. Table 5.4 shows the results of the study in the Verified Sample (the same results as in Table 5.2) and as done in the Source Sample. In Table 5.4, the number of Source Sample patients who were not referred for the gold standard procedure appears in bold face type.

If it were possible to measure the sensitivity and specificity of the spleen scan in the Source Sample, the sensitivity would be lower (0.25 vs 0.57) and the specificity higher (0.97 vs. 0.67) than as measured in the Verified Sample (Table 5.5).

Figure 5.8 illustrates the effects of test-referral bias graphically. Focus first on the right half of the figure, which represents patients with the target condition, those needed to calculate test sensitivity. Source population patients with a positive index test (T+) all get referred for the gold standard test, while many with a negative test (T-) do not get referred (*test-referral bias*). In the verified population, the proportion of index test-positive patients is much higher than in the source population.

In other words, the sensitivity of the test as measured in the verified population is higher than it would be if it were possible to ascertain the true state of all of the patients in the source population.

As a general rule:

When test-referral bias is present, test sensitivity is higher in the verified sample than in the source population.

Table 5.4 Hypothetical results of doing the spleen scan in the source sample.

Study population	Results of the spleen scan	Number of patients		Totals
		Spleen weighs >250 g	Spleen weighs <250 g	
Verified Sample	Positive	True positive $N = 20$	False positive $N = 5$	$N = 25$
	Negative	False negative $N = 15$	True negative $N = 10$	$N = 25$
	Totals	$N = 35$	$N = 15$	$N = 50$
Source sample	Positive	True positive $N = 20$	False positive $N = 5$	$N = 25$
	Negative	False negative $N = 15$ **+45**	True negative $N = 10$ **+135**	$N = 205$
	Totals	$N = 80$	$N = 150$	$N = 230$

Note: The number of source population patients who were not referred for the gold standard procedure appears in bold face type.

Table 5.5 Comparison of sensitivity and specificity of the spleen scan as measured in the Verified Sample and the Source Sample.

	Sensitivity	Specificity
Verified sample	$p[T+ \mid D+]; = \dfrac{20}{35} = 0.57$	$p[T- \mid D-]; s = \dfrac{10}{15} = 0.67$
Source sample	$p[T+ \mid D+]; = \dfrac{20}{80} = 0.25$	$p[T- \mid D-]; = \dfrac{145}{150} = 0.97$

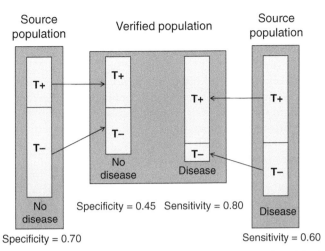

Figure 5.8 This representation of a retrospective study of test performance shows the effect of preferential referral of patients with positive tests on measurements of sensitivity and specificity. The heights of the T+ rectangles are the same in the source population and the verified population, reflecting the practice of referring all Test-positive patients to receive the gold standard test. The heights of the T- rectangles in the verified population are lower than in the source population, reflecting the practice of failing to refer every Test-negative patient to receive the gold standard test.

Effect of spectrum bias on the specificity of a test

Spectrum bias due to selective referral also affects the **specificity** of a test, causing it to be lower in the verified sample than it would be in the source population. Two forms of spectrum bias are at work:

Disease severity bias: When patients are very sick and the cause has not been identified, clinicians are likely to order the gold standard test after a negative index test. This practice enriches the verified sample with sick patients, relative to their proportion in the source population, which includes a broad spectrum of disease severity. Sicker patients have more severe, more easily detected forms of the target condition and other conditions that lead to referral for the gold standard test. They are therefore more likely to have positive gold standard test results, both true-positives but also false-positives due to other diseases. More false-positive results mean an index test with a lower measured specificity.

Test-referral bias: Physicians are less likely to refer a patient with a negative index test to have a gold standard test. Therefore, the verified sample has relatively few patients with a negative index test, which means relatively few true-negative test results and lower measured specificity. The left-hand side of Figure 5.8 depicts patients who do not have the target condition, those who are needed to calculate test specificity. Source population patients with a positive index test all get referred for the gold standard test, while many with a negative test do not get referred (*test-referral bias*). In the verified population, the proportion of index test-negative patients is lower than in the source population, which means that *test-referral bias underestimates specificity*, which is the probability of a negative test result in patients who do not have the target condition.

Thus, as a general rule: *test-referral bias causes test specificity to be lower in the verified sample than it would be in the source population*.

Table 5.5 uses the spleen scan study to illustrate the effect of test-referral bias on sensitivity and specificity. Sensitivity is higher and specificity is lower in the verified sample, a specific example of the general rule.

The spleen scan study does *not* reflect a general principle about the direction of the effect of test-referral bias on the *likelihood ratio*, which reflects the joint effects of sensitivity and specificity. Test referral bias affects the numerator and denominator of the likelihood ratio in the same direction. Therefore, the effect of bias on the ratio depends on the size of its effect on sensitivity relative to the size of its effect on specificity.

Because of referral biases, the verified sample may contain only a small fraction of the source population. Readers must scrutinize reports of test performance characteristics for evidence of these biases. One important clue is a retrospective study design in which the decision to order the gold standard test is up to the clinician rather than a prospective study, whose study protocol requires doing both the gold standard test and the index test.

The best clues to a trustworthy study are:

- Prospective design
- An accounting of how many patients dropped out before getting the gold standard test and why
- A comparison of the clinical characteristics of the source population and the verified sample.

Spectrum bias is a serious problem for *retrospective* studies, but remediation is possible. The next section contains advice about how to adjust sensitivity and specificity to reduce the effect of spectrum bias.

5.6.4 Adjusting for biased estimates of sensitivity and specificity

How should the clinician adjust published estimates of the sensitivity and specificity to improve their application to the source population? The following discussion, which outlines some general principles, pertains principally to retrospective studies of test performance.

General principles

Sensitivity and specificity are **conditional probabilities**.

Sensitivity is the probability of a positive test given that the patient has the target condition: $p[T+|D+]$.

Specificity is the probability of a negative test given that the patient does not have the target condition: $p[T-|D-]$.

In **Chapter** 3, we defined probability as a statement of opinion about the likelihood that a current state exists or a future event will occur. To arrive at a probability of the disease in a patient, we **anchor** on the prevalence of the disease in the subgroup to which our patient belongs and **adjust** to take account of the special characteristics of our patient. We can use the anchoring and adjustment heuristic to adjust a published sensitivity or specificity to take account of differences between the verified sample and the population to which the patient belongs.

5.6.5 Heuristics for adjusting published reports for disease severity bias

These heuristics assume that the target population for the test is the average patient in a primary care practice. Test performance measured in a prospective study in which everyone in the source population received the gold standard test would apply directly to the source population without any adjustment. Applying the same study to a very sick inpatient population might require adjustments in the opposite direction to that described here.

Sensitivity: The sicker the verified sample in comparison with the source population, the larger the downward adjustment of the sensitivity.

Specificity: If the verified sample consists of healthy volunteers, adjust the specificity downward. If the verified sample is mostly very sick patients, adjust the specificity upward.

These rules of thumb beg the question of *how much* to adjust the sensitivity and specificity estimates, which is the next topic.

Exact adjustment for spectrum bias

This material is advanced. The reader may want to skip to Section 5.7.

Exact correction for spectrum bias is possible in a retrospective study, subject to two related assumptions (Gray *et al.*, 1984).

- Selection for the gold standard test depends *only* on the index test result.
- Selection for the gold standard test depends on disease severity only through the correlation between the index test result and disease severity.

These assumptions are probably valid for screening tests, in which there are no clinical findings to influence selection for the gold standard test. The assumptions are less likely to be valid when the patient has symptoms and signs that might influence the clinician to refer the patient for the gold standard test even after a negative index test.

Begg and colleagues showed that, if these two assumptions are valid, the unbiased estimate of $p[R|D+]$ is

$$P[R|D+] = \frac{P[R] \times P[D+|R,S+]}{P[D+]}$$

where

$p[R|D+]$ is the probability of the index test result conditional upon the presence of the disease. If the result was a positive test, $p[R|D]$ would be $p[T+|D+]$, which is the sensitivity of the test.

$p[D+]$ is the disease prevalence in the verified sample
$p[R]$ is the probability of the test result in the source population
$p[D+|R,S+]$ is the post-test probability of the disease conditional upon R in the verified sample

Another approach to adjusting for test-referral bias is to focus on estimating the likelihood ratio in the source population.

If $L[R]$ is the likelihood ratio in the source population, and $L^*[R]$ is the likelihood ratio in the verified sample, $L[R] = c \times L^*R$, The correction factor, c, depends only on the odds of the disease in the verified sample and in the source population," and it is the same for all results of the test. (Gray *et al.*, 1984).

$$c = \frac{\text{Odds of target condition (verified sample)}}{\text{Odds of target condition (source population)}}$$

This research provides a pathway to measure the likelihood ratio of an index test in the source population of a retrospective study of test performance.

1. Measure the likelihood ratio in the verified population.
2. Determine the final diagnosis on all patients in both source and verified samples.
3. Calculate the odds of the target condition in both samples.
4. Calculate c, as noted earlier.
5. Calculate the likelihood ratio ($L^*[R\}$) in the source population using the formula listed earlier.

This source population likelihood ratio should give reliable estimates of post-test odds using the odds ratio form of Bayes' theorem.

5.7   When to be concerned about inaccurate measures of test performance

At this point in the chapter, the reader should be concerned about whether it is possible to measure test performance so that the results apply to the source population. The answer should be "yes" for well-conducted prospective studies and "maybe" for retrospective studies. Our focus on accurate measures of test performance should not obscure the real goal, which is making post-test probability estimates that guide decision making toward choices that maximize the probability of the outcomes that the patient values most. For this purpose, accurate measurements of test performance are sometimes important but not in all cases. Figures 5.9 and 5.10 illustrate this point by showing regions of pre-test probability in which the post-test probability changes very little as the sensitivity or specificity of a test changes quite a lot (see next page). These two figures are examples of *sensitivity analysis*, a powerful concept in the analysis of decision making.

When is accurate measurement of sensitivity important? Figure 5.9 shows the post-test probability for any value of the sensitivity, three values of the pre-test probability, and a specificity of 0.80. Remember that the sensitivity of most commonly used tests is usually larger than 0.75, which is the shaded area in Figure 5.9.

Figure 5.9 shows that accurate measurement of test sensitivity is not very important most of the time because the post-test probability changes very little as the sensitivity changes. Test sensitivity is important if your patient has an intermediate-to-high pre-test probability and a negative test result.

Figure 5.9 shows that test sensitivity in the range of 0.75–1.0 has little effect on the post-test probability for positive tests regardless of pre-test probability and for negative tests when the pre-test probability is low.

When is accurate measurement of test specificity important? Figure 5.10 shows the post-test probability for various values of the specificity, three values of the pre-test probability, and a sensitivity of 0.90. Remember that most tests have a specificity that is greater than 0.8, the shaded region to pay attention to in Figure 5.10.

Figure 5.10 shows that typical values of test specificity (shaded area) have little or no effect on the post-test probability for negative test results (dashed lines) in any patient. Test specificity strongly affects post-test probability for patients with positive test results if the pre-test probability is low and, to a lesser extent, intermediate.

Summary:
* *Worry about accurate measurements of test performance when your patient has an unexpected result:*
  * When the pre-test probability is high and the test is negative

- • When the pre-test probability is low and the test is positive.
- • Worry about test performance when your patient has an intermediate probability (i.e., when you are the most uncertain about the diagnosis).
- • Otherwise, do not worry.

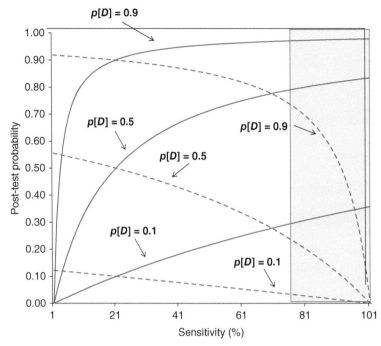

Figure 5.9 Change in post-test probability (vertical axis) because of changes in test sensitivity (horizontal axis). The specificity was 0.8 for all calculations. The pre-test probabilities (denoted by *p*[*D*]) were 0.1, 0.5, and 0.9 in successive calculations using Bayes' theorem and varying the sensitivity of the test from 0 to 1.0. The post-test probabilities after a positive test are denoted by solid lines. After a negative test, they are denoted by the dashed lines. The sensitivity of most tests in common practice is >0.75.

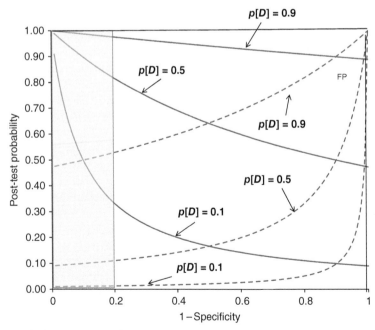

Figure 5.10 Change in post-test probability because of changes in test specificity. The sensitivity was 0.9 for all calculations. The pre-test probabilities (denoted by *p*[*D*]) were 0.1, 0.5, and 0.9 in successive calculations using Bayes' theorem and varying the 1 – specificity of the test from 0 to 1.0. The post-test probabilities after a positive test are denoted by solid lines. After a negative test, they are denoted by the dashed lines. The shaded section denotes the range of test specificity typically found in practice (0.8 to 1.0), so that 1 – specificity is low.

On reflection, accurate measurements of test performance are most important in all the situations in which a test result could have a big effect on probability.

5.8 Test results as a continuous variable: the ROC curve

In most of this chapter, we have described test results as "positive" and "negative." Often, we use these terms because the clinical laboratory provides only the "upper limit of normal" as information to guide test interpretation (by now, you should be feeling impatient with clinical laboratories that fail to provide sensitivity and specificity, and especially likelihood ratios, the information that you need to interpret test results!). This part of the chapter describes the advantages of expressing test results as a continuous variable (i.e., a number within a range) rather than as a dichotomous variable (positive or negative). The principal advantage is the freedom to choose the optimal cut point for the clinical situation.

5.8.1 The distribution of test results in diseased and well individuals

As discussed at the beginning of this chapter, the distribution of test results in patients with the target condition often overlaps the distribution of results in those who do not have it (Figure 5.11). That overlap region is where decision making requires tradeoffs between the benefits and harms of treating patients with a value on the horizontal axis that is above the cut point for the test.

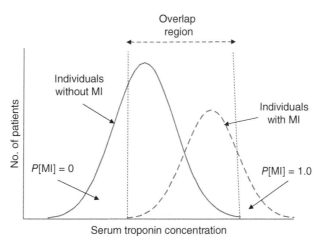

Figure 5.11 Distribution of test results in healthy and diseased individuals.

When published reports provide information about the distribution of test results in patients who have the target condition and those who do not have it, we can express the conditional probabilities of test result R ($p[R \mid D+]$ and $p[R \mid D-]$) in several ways.

- As the conditional probability of a result anywhere in a range of values of test results, here denoted by the distance between X_1 and X_2 on the horizontal axis (Figure 5.12, see next page). From $p[R \mid D+]$ and $p[R \mid D-]$, we can calculate the likelihood ratio of a test result that falls in this range.
- As the conditional probabilities of all test results above a cutoff value in the overlap region. $P[R \mid D+]$ would represent this result (Figure 5.13, see next page). From $p[R \mid D+]$ and $p[R \mid D-]$, we can calculate the likelihood ratio of a test result that falls above the cutoff value.

As discussed at the beginning of this chapter, test results should link to a decision for action. When the clinical laboratory reports a test result as a number (e.g., a serum troponin I value of 50 ng/dl), we must decide if that number exceeds the cut point for taking action.

The clinician who learns of a test result should always ask the question, "What do I do now?" The options are: do nothing, get more information, or start treatment. As we shall see in Chapter 13, these three options correspond to three ranges of probabilities: low probability: do nothing; intermediate probability: get more information; and high probability: start treatment. According to Bayes' theorem, the post-test odds of the disease depends on the likelihood ratio of the test, which in turn depends on the cut point for the test. In this section, we will lay the groundwork for determining the test result cut point that maximizes the patient's well-being.

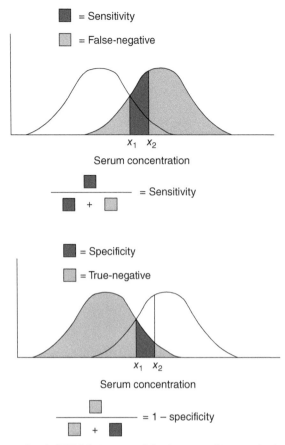

Figure 5.12 Calculation of $p[R|D+]$ (top panel) and $p[R|D-]$ (bottom panel) for the range of test results denoted by the distance between X_1 and X_2 on the horizontal axis.

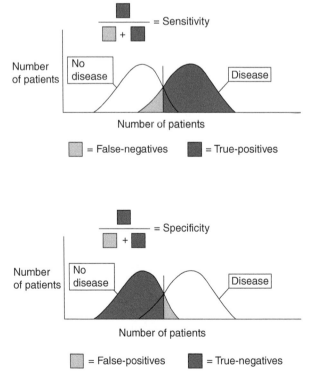

Figure 5.13 Calculation of $p[R|D+]$ (top panel) and $p[R+|D-]$ (bottom panel) for all test results above a cutoff value, which is denoted by the vertical line.

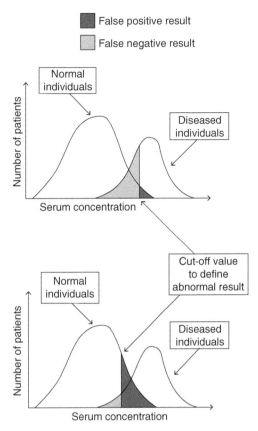

Figure 5.14 Effect of altering the cut point that defines a positive test result. See text for explanation.

Establishing a criterion for decisive action will require making a tradeoff. To understand the tradeoff, refer to Figure 5.14 and consider two cases. The only difference between the two panels is the position of the cut point (vertical line)

- *Upper panel*: Start at the right-hand end of the distribution of patients with the target condition. Move the cut point value of the test to the left until over half of the patients with the target condition have a test result above the cut point (a true-positive). In doing so, some patients who do not have the target condition will have results that are to the right of the cut point (a false-positive). Thus, to be sure of detecting more of the patients with the target condition, one must accept a cut point that will lead to treating patients who do not have the target condition.
- *Bottom panel*: Move the cut point still further to the left until nearly all patients with the target condition have a test result that is above the cut-point. False-negative results are few, but now many persons who do not have the target condition will have results above the cut point (false-positives). Thus, to be sure of detecting and treating more of the patients with the target condition, one must accept a cut point that will lead to treating more patients who do not have the target condition.

This example shows that changing the cut point changes the relative proportions of false-negative and false-positive results. Every cut point defines a different proportion of those that treatment will help relative to those whom treatment will not help and may harm. Recognizing this outcome as inevitable, we should choose a cut point that maximizes net benefit across everyone, which is the topic of the next section.

5.8.2 The receiver operating characteristic curve

The receiver operating characteristic (ROC) curve is a graphical method for depicting the tradeoff between the sensitivity and the specificity of a test at various cut points. To obtain an ROC curve, one does the index test and the gold standard test on patients suspected of having the target condition and calculates the conditional probability of a test result ($p[R \mid D+]$ and $p[R \mid D-]$) for each definition of the cut point that defines a positive test result. Figure 5.15 is an ROC curve (see next page). It shows the effect of several cut points for a test that detects different blood levels of a chemical. The ROC curve is a plot of $p[R \mid D+]$ on the vertical axis and $p[R \mid D-]$ on the horizontal axis. In Figure 5.15, each point corresponds to one of three definitions of a positive test result, as defined by three different cut points (shown on the inserts).

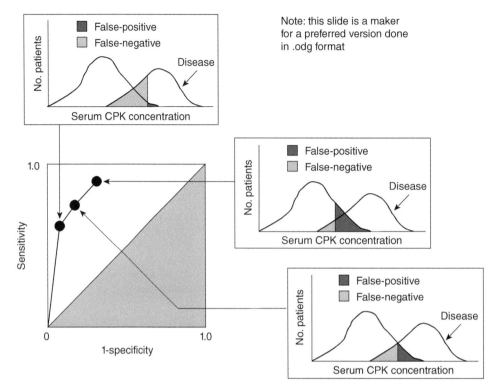

Figure 5.15 ROC curve for hypothetical test used to detect myocardial infarction.

The area of the ROC curve graph has three parts:

- *The 45-degree line*: Recalling that the likelihood ratio is $p[R\,|\,D+]/p[R\,|\,D-]$, the 45-degree line represents test results for which $p[R\,|\,D+]$ equals $p[R\,|\,D-]$, and, therefore, the likelihood ratio is 1.0. Since the post-test odds equals the pre-test odds times the likelihood ratio, points on the 45-degree line have no effect on the probability of the disease.
- *The area above the 45-degree line*: The likelihood ratio for test results that fall above the 45-degree line is greater than 1.0, indicating that the test result increases the probability of the disease.
- *The area below the 45-degree line*: The likelihood ratio for points below the 45-degree line is less than 1.0, indicating that the test result decreases the probability of the disease.

The three inserts in Figure 5.15 illustrate the effect of moving the cut point, this time from a higher serum concentration of creatine phosphokinase to a lower concentration. This figure reinforces the lesson learned from Figure 5.14.

Figure 5.16 displays the ROC curve for ST segment depression on an exercise ECG. One measure of an abnormal exercise ECG is how far the ST segment falls during exercise as compared with the baseline value prior to exercise. A cut point corresponding to deeper ST segment depression means a higher specificity but also a lower sensitivity.

This ROC curve illustrates the tradeoffs of choosing different cut points for defining a positive test. Suppose that the exercise ECG result determines whether a patient receives a coronary arteriogram. Setting the cut point at $\geq 2\,mm$ of ST segment depression would result in fewer false-positive results (and fewer negative coronary arteriograms). This cut point would lead to more false-negative exercise ECG results (and therefore more coronary artery disease patients who did not get a coronary arteriogram), and fewer coronary arteriograms (and lower costs). Setting the cut point at $1.0\,mm$ of ST segment depression would result in fewer false-negative results and more coronary arteriograms.

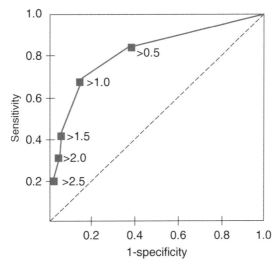

Figure 5.16 ROC curve for ST segment depression on an exercise electrocardiogram. Each point represents a different amount of ST segment depression, as indicated on the graph by the number of millimeters of ST depression. Adapted from Diamond and Forrester (1979).

5.8.3 Using the ROC curve to compare tests

The ROC curve is useful for comparing tests. The area under the ROC curve is a single measure of test performance that takes into account sensitivity and specificity. Of several tests for the same target condition, the test with the greatest area under its ROC curve best discriminates between people who have the target condition and those who do not have it. This method has become a widely used approach for comparing tests. A shortcoming is the requirement for knowing $p[R \mid D+]$ and $p[R \mid D-]$ for each definition of a test result. Two ROC curves could have different shapes and yet enclose the same area. As seen in the next section, the *shape* of the ROC curve is often the decisive factor in deciding when to use a test for a specific indication. Chapter 13 discusses another way to decide between two tests: given a pre-test probability, with which test would the post-test probability cross a treatment threshold probability and thereby alter the treatment plan?

5.8.4 Setting the cut point for a test

This chapter has prepared us to appreciate the importance of a method for setting the cut point for a test. This method takes into account two characteristics of the patient: the patient's pre-test probability of the target condition and the importance to the patient of avoiding false-negative and false-positive results. The principle is as follows:

The optimal cut point of a test is the test result corresponding to the point on the ROC curve at which the slope of the tangent to the ROC curve satisfies the following relationship.

$$\text{Slope of tangent to ROC curve} = \frac{H}{B} \times \frac{1 - p[D]}{p[D]}$$

where:

$p[D]$ = the pre-test probability of the target condition
H = the net harms of treating patients who do not have the target condition
B = the net benefit of treating patients with the target condition

The derivation of this relationship appears in the appendix to this chapter. To find the optimal point on the ROC curve, the derivation uses the principle that guides expected value decision making: choose the action that maximizes a person's expected utility. Thus, to maximize the patient's well-being, the cut point should be the test result corresponding to the point on the ROC curve where the tangent to the curve has a slope that satisfies this relationship. Maximizing the patient's well-being is a powerful foundation for a method to determine the optimal cut point of a test.

With a test whose results are expressed as a continuous variable, each point on its ROC curve corresponds to a different test result, each with its own sensitivity and specificity (Figure 5.15 illustrates this point) and a different ratio of Harms to Benefits, as shown in the equation for the slope of the tangent to the ROC curve (above). According to the equation for defining the optimal cut point:

- A test result corresponding to a point on the ROC curve where its slope is flatter than at the cut point reflects increased benefit relative to harm. Such results are classified as "positive" and should lead to action consistent with the target condition being present.
- A test result corresponding to a point on the ROC curve where its slope is steeper than at the cut point reflects increased harm relative to benefit. Such results are classified as "negative" and should lead to action consistent with the target condition being absent.

Chapter 13 contains a description of the method for determining the harms (H) and benefits (B) of treatment. In this chapter, we will use subjective judgment to estimate the ratio of H to B. Subjective estimates of this ratio often starts with a clinician imagining what it would feel like to make a mistake. An error of *commission* would be treating someone who does not have the target condition and thereby causing the harms of treatment (H) without corresponding benefit. An error of *omission* would be the failure to treat someone with the target condition and depriving the person of the benefit (B) of treatment.

Example

Consider a hypothetical antibody test to detect a form of cancer. The scale for the concentration of antibodies is divided into 10 equal-sized intervals. A reputable research group has measured the sensitivity and specificity of the serum concentration corresponding to each interval.

There are two target populations for this test: (1) those who have symptoms of active disease (*test done to confirm suspected disease*) and (2) those who have no symptoms but are worried that they may have it (*test done to screen for disease*). The net harms and benefits of treatment in the two populations may differ.

Cut point for disease confirmation: Imagine that a patient is suspected of having the disease that the index test is used to detect. Based on the patient's clinical findings, the probability of the target condition is 0.50. Patients with a positive test undergo a treatment that puts the patient at risk temporarily because of transient bone marrow toxicity. Patients with the disease derive considerable benefit from disease detection because treatment can prolong survival by several years. Patients who have similar symptoms but do not have the disease and have a positive test also receive the toxic treatment. They suffer transient bone marrow depression and no benefit from treatment. The clinician's ratio of harms to benefit for disease detection is 1 to 2.5, which reflects a judgment that it is worse to mistakenly withhold the treatment from someone who has the cancer and could benefit from treatment (an error of *omission*) than it is to give the treatment to someone with similar symptoms but who does not have the target condition and would suffer only transient bone marrow depression (an error of *commission*). In this population, the test result that divides "negative" from "positive" corresponds to the point on the ROC curve where the tangent has the following slope:

$$\text{Slope of ROC curve} = \frac{H}{B} \times \frac{1 - p[D]}{p[D]} = \frac{1}{2.5} \times \frac{1 - 0.5}{0.5} = 0.4$$

To find the cut point for the test, identify the point on the ROC curve where the tangent to the curve has a slope of 0.4, as shown in Figure 5.17. From differential calculus, the slope of the tangent to the ROC curve at any point is $\frac{dy}{dx}$, the instantaneous change along the vertical axis (sensitivity) for a given change along the horizontal axis ($1 - \text{specificity}$). With a relatively flat ROC curve at the cut point, Figure 5.17 shows that the sensitivity of the test will be high and the specificity of the test will be low, which means relatively few false-negative results that would lead to failure to treat those who have the target condition. The likelihood ratio (LR+) for the test at the optimal cut point is 1.51. The LR- is 0.32.

Cutoff value for screening: Candidates for screening for this cancer face a somewhat different situation. The prevalence of this disease in healthy people is only 0.001 (1 case in 1000 people). There is considerable benefit to disease detection because early detection and treatment could prolong life. The clinician's ratio of harms to benefits for treating the cancer in a screening population consisting of largely healthy people is 1 to 50, which reflects the judgment that it is worse to mistakenly give the treatment to an apparently healthy person who does not have the cancer and would suffer temporary harm from treatment than it is to withhold the treatment from an apparently healthy person who does have the cancer.

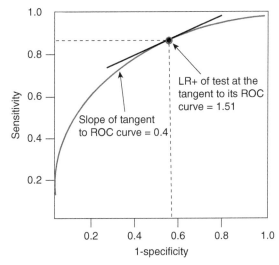

Figure 5.17 ROC curve for hypothetical test for antibodies to a form of cancer. The dotted lines denote the coordinates of the point on the curve at which the slope of the tangent to the curve is 2.5.

In the screening population, the test should be considered abnormal at the point on the ROC curve where its slope is:

$$\text{Slope of ROC curve} = \frac{H}{B} \times \frac{1-p[D]}{p[D]} = \frac{1}{50} \times \frac{1-0.001}{0.001}$$
$$= \frac{1}{50} \times \frac{0.999}{0.001} \cong 20$$

To find the cutoff value for the test, identify the point on the ROC curve where a tangent to the curve has a slope of 20. A test result corresponding to this point will occur in the lower left-hand corner of the ROC space plot. A slope of 20 means a large ratio of true-positive results to false-positive results and therefore a test result with a high likelihood ratio. A high likelihood ratio is fitting because the test result must produce a large increase in the probability of the cancer to justify screening asymptomatic persons. Therefore, the antibody level corresponding to the cut point should be much higher when testing asymptomatic persons in order to avoid false-positive results.

This example shows that choosing the definition of an abnormal test result requires attention to all facets of the clinical situation, including the clinical features of the patient and the consequences of managing a patient with a positive test.

5.9 Combining data from studies of test performance: the systematic review and meta-analysis

The sensitivity and specificity of commonly used tests have been measured in many studies. The results often differ, leaving the clinician to decide which study to believe. This problem has largely been solved by a systematic review. A **systematic review** summarizes the evidence from studies on the same topic. Systematic reviews have become a powerful force in shaping clinical practice, in part because clinical practice guideline panels rely on them to summarize the evidence that shapes their recommendation, which in turn influence insurance coverage decisions.

The systematic review starts with a systematic literature search to find and evaluate all studies, published and unpublished. The goal is to identify every study that fits the inclusion and exclusion criteria for the systematic review and evaluate and grade its study design characteristics. The risk of bias is a key measure of study quality. Factors to be assessed include (1) patient selection processes (prospective, consecutive patients); (2) blinding to index test results when assessing gold standard test results (and conversely); (3) adequacy of the gold standard test as a diagnostic benchmark; and (4) a short time interval between the index test and doing the gold standard test.

The second part of a systematic review is called a *meta-analysis*, which summarizes the results of high-quality studies. Studies of test performance are an excellent case example of the need for caution when trying to combine results from a group of studies. The same test could perform quite differently in different studies for the following reasons:

- Differing definitions of the cut point that defines an abnormal result.
- Different criteria for deciding that an image is a true-positive result.
- Different techniques for performing the test.
- The sample of studies includes several generations of the technology.

For these reasons, the first step in a systematic review of a group of studies of a diagnostic test is to do a qualitative analysis of the body of studies to decide if they are sufficiently alike to consider combining their results.

The product of a meta-analysis of studies of a diagnostic test is a summary estimate of sensitivity and specificity. Simply calculating an average sensitivity and, separately, an average specificity is not a valid approach because it ignores the correlation between sensitivity and specificity. To understand this correlation, imagine the cut point separating negative test results from positive test results. As this cut point increases, fewer patients with the target condition are classified as test-positive (decreasing sensitivity) while more patients who do not have the target condition are identified as test-negative (higher specificity and therefore fewer false-positives). Refer to Figure 5.14 to see the effect of raising the cut-point that divides positive from negative results. The opposite occurs when the cut point is lowered. A valid statistical approach to calculating a summary sensitivity and specificity must take account of the correlation between sensitivity and specificity: as one changes, so does the other. An approach that takes this dependency into account is the starting point for determining a valid average sensitivity and specificity.

A summary ROC curve is a robust approach to combining the results of diagnostic test accuracy studies. A summary ROC curve is the line that best fits the points defined by the sensitivity and specificity of individual studies as plotted in ROC space.

The first step in developing a summary ROC curve is to graph in ROC space the sensitivity (vertical axis) and 1 – specificity (horizontal axis) of the test as measured in each study. Each individual study of the test is one point in the space defined by the two axes (Figure 5.18, left-hand panel).

The next step is to define the line that best fits the points in ROC space. Two valid, equivalent methods are: (1) hierarchical SROC curve and (2) the bivariate random effects model. Using available statistical software, both methods give a valid estimate of the ROC curve that represents the individual studies in the ROC space. The methods also give the average sensitivity and specificity across all the included studies. The right-hand panel of Figure 5.18 represents these features.

These methods do not work for calculating a summary likelihood ratio. Instead, calculate a summary ROC curve and the average sensitivity and specificity. Use the latter to calculate a summary likelihood ratio-positive (sensitivity/ [1 – specificity]) and likelihood-negative ([1 – sensitivity]/specificity).

The right-hand panel shows a summary ROC curve and the point representing the average sensitivity and specificity with a 95% confidence interval. The article by Leeflang *et al.* (2008) discusses this topic in depth (see Bibliography). This illustration is a drawing, not a calculated plot. For an example with real-life data, see the article by Leeflang listed in the Bibliography.

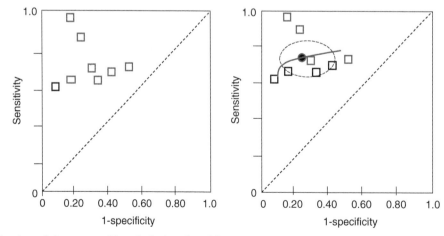

Figure 5.18 The left-hand panel shows several hypothetical studies of the accuracy of a diagnostic test plotted in the ROC. Each point represents a different study of test performance.

Summary

1. The following expressions completely characterize diagnostic information:
   - $p[R \mid D+]$: Likelihood of observing the finding in patients with the target condition (sensitivity)
   - $p[R \mid D-]$: Likelihood of the finding occurring in patients who do not have the target condition ($1-$specificity).
2. The predictive value-positive is the proportion of positive test results that are true positives in a study of diagnostic test performance. The predictive value applies to the population in which it was measured. Applying a predictive value to other populations will often lead to error.
3. Spectrum bias can occur when test performance is measured in one population (the verified sample) and applied to another population (the source sample). It occurs mostly in retrospective studies. In the source population, sensitivity is typically lower and specificity typically higher than in the verified population.
4. When the results of tests are expressed as a continuous variable, a result is defined by the value of the cut point, above which the test is positive. Each cut point defines a different test result. Each result has a $p[R \mid D+]$ and a $p[R \mid D-]$. The ROC curve is a plot of the $p[R \mid D+]$ (vertical axis) and $p[R \mid D-]$ (horizontal axis) of each possible test result.
5. A test has an optimum cut point value for defining a positive test result. Using that $p[R \mid D+]$ and $p[R \mid D-]$ to calculate a post-test probability will maximize the patient's expected utility. The optimum cut point is patient-specific. It depends on the patient's pre-test probability and the harms and benefits of treatment.

A.5.1 Appendix: derivation of the method for using an ROC curve to choose the definition of an abnormal test result

The topic of the last section of this chapter is a test that can have many results. The serum concentration of an enzyme released from damaged heart muscle, such as the serum troponin, can have any biologically reasonable value. When a test has many possible results, the clinician must pick a result that defines the threshold for acting as if the patient had the target condition. This appendix contains the derivation of the formula for identifying the point on the ROC curve that corresponds to the preferred definition of an abnormal result. The decision to give or withhold treatment to a patient depends on whether the patient's test result is above or below this cut point.

This derivation depends on concepts that first appear in the next several chapters. The reader should refer to these chapters as new concepts appear. The author has based this derivation on the one that appears in the Bibliography (Metz, 1978).

Our goal is to find the definition of an abnormal result that will minimize the net harm of doing the test. Since the true state of the patient is unknown, we express the net harm as an *expected value* (expected value decision making is introduced in Chapter 6). We will use the expected utility of the test (U[test]) as our measure of its worth. Refer to Chapter 8 to learn about utility.

$$U[\text{test}] = EU(\text{test}) - EU(\text{no test}) \tag{A.5.1}$$

To calculate the expected utility of doing the test, we use a decision tree (Figure A.5.1, see next page). See Chapter 6 for a description of decision trees. The first chance node on the tree represents the unknown true state of the patient ($D+$ = has the target condition; $D-$ = does not have the target condition). The second chance node (reading from left to right) represents the outcome of the test ($T+$ = test positive; $T-$ = test negative). The probability of disease is $p(D+)$. The probability of a positive test in a diseased patient is $p(T+ \mid D+)$, which is the sensitivity of the test.

Inspection of the tree shows four possible outcomes of the test (true-positive, false-negative, false-positive, and true-negative). If the patient's test result is above the optimum cut point that defines an abnormal test result, the patient will receive treatment ($A+$). If the result is below this value, the patient will not receive treatment ($A-$). Thus, depending on the patient's true state ($D+$ or $D-$) and the outcome of the test, a patient will be in one of four states:

True-positive result: $D+A+$
False-negative result: $D+A-$
False-positive result: $D-A+$
True-negative result: $D-A-$

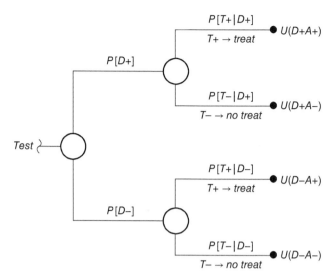

Figure A.5.1 Decision tree for calculating the expected utility of doing a test.

The patient's utility (or preference) for a true-positive result is $U(D+A+)$ or, in a more compact notation, U_{tp}. A true-positive result implies the treatment of a diseased patient, which presumably is a better outcome than a false-negative result, which implies not treating a diseased patient. Thus, one would expect U_{tp} to be greater than U_{fn}.

To obtain the expected utility of the test option, average out at the chance nodes in the tree shown in Figure A.5.1, as described in **Chapter** 6. To do so, multiply the utility of each outcome times the probability that it will occur, which is the product of the probabilities along the path to the outcome (the path probability).

$$U(\text{test}) = \left[p(D+)*p(T+|D+)*U_{tp} \right] + \left[p(D-)*p(T-|D-)*U_{tn} \right]$$
$$+ \left[p(D-)*p(T+|D-)*U_{fp} \right] + \left[p(D+)*p(T-|D+)*U_{fn} \right] \tag{A.5.2}$$

but

$$p(T-|D-) = 1 - p(T+|D-) \ and \ p(T-|D+) = 1 - p(T+|D+)$$

Substituting these relationships and rearranging terms, we get:

$$U(\text{test}) = \left[\left(U_{tp} - U_{fn} \right) \times p(D+) \times p(T+|D+) \right] + \left[\left(U_{fp} - U_{tn} \right) \times p(D-) \times p(T+|D-) \right]$$

The ROC curve describes the relationship between the sensitivity and $1-$ specificity for different cut points of a diagnostic test. Let the function $R[\ ]$ denote this relationship, which, plotted in ROC space, would describe the shape of the ROC curve. The relationship between the sensitivity and $1-$ specificity is given by this functional relationship:

$$p(T+|D+) = R\left[p(T+|D-) \right]$$

Substituting this relationship in Equation A.5.2,

$$U(\text{test}) = \left[\left(U_{tp} - U_{fn} \right) \times p(D+) \times R\left[p(T+|D-) \right] \right] + \left[\left(U_{fp} - U_{tn} \right) \times p(D-) \times p(T+|D-) \right]$$

The next step is from differential calculus. Differentiate $U(\text{test})$ with respect to $p(T+|D-)$ to find the point on the ROC curve where $U(\text{test})$, the patient's utility for testing, is a maximum. This step is an important reason to use this method for choosing the cut point because it maximizes the patient's best interests:

$$\frac{dU[\text{test}]}{d\left[p(T+|D-) \right]} = \left(U_{tp} - U_{fn} \right) \times p[D+] \times \frac{d\left[R\left[p(T+|D-) \right] \right]}{d\left[p(T+|D-) \right]} + \left(U_{fp} - U_{tn} \right) \times p(D-)$$

Now set the left-hand expression in the preceding equation equal to zero to find the point on the ROC curve where the utility of doing the test (U[test]) is a maximum.

$$0 = \left(U_{tp} - U_{fn}\right) \times p[D+] \times \frac{d\left[R\left[p\left(T+|D-\right)\right]\right]}{d\left[p\left(T+|D-\right)\right]} + \left(U_{fp} - U_{tn}\right) \times p(D-)$$

Solve this equation for $\dfrac{d\left[R\left[p\left(T+|\text{no }D\right)\right]\right]}{d\left[p\left(T+|\text{no }D\right)\right]}$, the slope of the ROC curve at the cut point that maximizes the value of testing,

$$\frac{d\left[R\left[p\left(T+|D-\right)\right]\right]}{d\left[p\left(T+|D-\right)\right]} = \frac{p[D-]}{p[D+]} \times \frac{\left(U_{fp} - U_{tn}\right)}{\left(U_{tp} - U_{fn}\right)} \tag{A.5.3}$$

In Chapter 13, we refer to $(U_{fp} - U_{tn})$ as the "harm" of treating a nondiseased person (denoted as H), and $(U_{tp} - U_{fn})$ as the "benefit" of treating a diseased person (denoted as B). Thus, Equation A.5.3 becomes

$$\frac{d[R\left[p\left(T+|D-\right)\right]]}{d\left[p\left(T+|D-\right)\right]} = \frac{p[D-]}{p[D+]} \times \frac{H}{B} \tag{A.5.4}$$

The left-hand side of Equation A.5.4 is the rate of change of the sensitivity with respect to 1 – the specificity of the test, which is the slope of the ROC curve.

With a test whose results are expressed as a continuous variable, each point on its ROC curve corresponds to a different test result and a different ratio of Harms to Benefits, as shown in Equation A.5.4.

- A test result corresponding to a point on the ROC curve where its slope is flatter than at the cut point reflects increased benefit relative to harm. Such results are classified as "positive" and should lead to action consistent with the target condition being present.
- A test result corresponding to a point on the ROC curve where its slope is steeper than at the cut point reflects increased harm relative to benefit. Such results are classified as "negative" and should lead to action consistent with the target condition being absent.

Equation A.5.4, which is the same expression that appears in the last section of Chapter 5, indicates that the cutoff value that maximizes the patient's utility is where the slope of the ROC curve equals the odds that the disease is absent times the ratio of harms to benefits of treatment.

Bibliography

Begg, C.B. and Greenes, R.A. (1984) Assessment of diagnostic tests when disease verification is subject to selection bias. *Biometrics*, **39**, 207–15.

  Information about correcting for disease verification bias in selecting participants in studies of diagnostic test performance.

Bossyut, P.M., Reitsma, J.B., Bruns, D.E. *et al.* (2003) Standards for reporting of diagnostic accuracy. Towards complete and accurate reporting of studies of diagnostic accuracy: the STARD Initiative. *Annals of Internal Medicine*, **138**, 40–4.

  A brief article describing the key elements of a study of diagnostic test accuracy and how to report them. An accompanying online-only article goes into much greater depth.

Diamond, G.A. and Forrester, J.S. (1979) Analysis of probability as an aid in the clinical diagnosis of coronary-artery disease. *New England Journal of Medicine*, **300**, 1350–8.

Gray, R., Begg, C.B., and Greenes, R.A. (1984) Construction of receiver operating characteristic curves when disease verification is subject to selection bias. *Medical Decision Making*, **4**, 151–64.

  If selection for the verified sample depends on the results of the index test, the method described in this article can be used to correct published sensitivity and specificity and obtain an improved estimate of these data in the source population.

Hanley, J.A. and McNeil, B.J. (1982) The meaning and use of the area under a receiver operating characteristic (ROC) curve. *Radiology*, **143**, 29–36.

  A good article for those who wish to learn more about ROC curves and how they may be used to compare diagnostic tests.

Irwig, L., Tosteson, A.N.A., Gatsonis, C. *et al.* (1994) Guidelines for meta-analyses evaluating diagnostic tests. *Annals of Internal Medicine*, **120**, 667–76.

An in-depth review of combining the results of different studies of test performance.

Leeflang, M.M.G., Deeks, J.J., Gatsonis, C.G., *et al.* (2008) Systematic review of diagnostic test accuracy. *Annals of Internal Medicine*, **149**, 889–97.

An up-to-date description of the key elements of a systematic review of diagnostic test accuracy, including reliable statistical methods for combining the results of studies.

McNeil, B.J., Keeler, E., and Adelstein, S.J. (1975) Primer on certain elements of medical decision making. *New England Journal of Medicine*, **293**, 211–5.

This classic article describes the use of ROC curves, including the method for selecting a definition of an positive result.

Metz, C.E. (1978) Basic principles of ROC Analysis. *Seminars in Nuclear Medicine*, **8**, 283–98.

This article contains a derivation of the method for choosing the optimum cut-off value for a diagnostic test.

Philbrick, J.T., Horwitz, R.I, Feinstein, A.R., *et al.* (1982) The limited spectrum of patients studied in exercise test research: analyzing the tip of the iceberg. *Journal of the American Medical Association*, **248**, 2467–70.

The authors show how selection factors limit the number of patients in the source population who can participate in studies of the sensitivity and specificity of a test.

Ransohoff, D.F. and Feinstein, A.R. (1978) Problems of spectrum and bias in evaluating the efficacy of diagnostic tests. *New England Journal of Medicine*, **299**, 926–30.

A description of the effect of biased patient selection on sensitivity and specificity.

Simel, D.L. and Rennie, D. (2008) *The Rational Clinical Examination: Evidence-based Clinical Diagnosis*, McGraw-Hill Medical, New York.

A source of trustworthy information about the performance of many different diagnostic tests. The following website has the information in the book as well as subsequent articles in JAMA: https://jamaevidence.mhmedical.com/content.aspx?bookid=845&sectionid=61357443. This site is proprietary. Access is through an institutional subscription or a personal subscription, Short-term access may also be available.

Weiner, D.A., Ryan, T.J., McCabe, C.H. *et al.* (1979) Exercise stress testing: correlation among history of angina, ST-segment response and prevalence of coronary artery disease in the Coronary Artery Surgery Study (CASS). *New England Journal of Medicine*, **301**, 230–5.

This study illustrates how measurement of the sensitivity and specificity in clinical and anatomic subgroups of patients can pay off in new insights. This study showed that the sensitivity of the exercise electrocardiogram depends on the patient's history.

Whiting PF, Rutjes AWS, Westwood ME *et al.* QUADAS-2: a revised tool for the quality assessment of diagnostic accuracy studies. *Annals of Internal Medicine* 2011;155:529–36.

A tool to assess the quality of studies of diagnostic accuracy. It covers patient selection, index test, reference standard, and flow of patients through the study.

CHAPTER 6

Decision trees – representing the structure of a decision problem

6.1 Introduction

This chapter begins the discussion of decision trees. These diagrams provide a foundation for many of the topics covered in later chapters. Chapters 3 and 4 discussed how uncertainty complicates medical decision making. A decision problem also involves choices. A test can be performed or skipped. A therapy can be started or delayed. The patient can be admitted or sent home. Moreover, choices and uncertainties can interact. Choosing a test can provide information that reduces uncertainty. That reduced uncertainty can alter the subsequent set of appropriate treatments. Decision analysis often uses the trees described in this chapter to represent these interactions.

The focus of this chapter is the structure of decision trees. We will see how decision trees can be organized to represent the relationships between the decision alternatives and uncertainties in a decision problem. Emphasis will be placed on how probabilities are used to quantify those uncertainties. We will see how the resulting probabilities can be combined to quantify the likelihood of the possible outcomes of a decision. Simple examples with a single decision will illustrate the discussion in this chapter. The simplicity of these examples will mean that a relatively simple calculation will identify the best decision alternative for the patient.

Ultimately, we will use decision trees in the analysis of complicated problems with multiple interdependent decisions. The analysis of those decision trees will be more complex. How to deal with complexity will be described in the next chapter.

6.2 Key concepts and terminology

A decision tree is a collection of nodes and branches showing the relationships between the alternatives and uncertainties in a decision problem. A choice between alternatives is represented by what is called a *decision node*. The uncertainty about something like the patient's condition, the results of tests, or the effect of treatments is represented by what is called a *chance node*.

The branches emanating from a decision node correspond to the alternatives available for the choice represented by the node. Each of the possible alternatives must be represented by exactly one of the branches. For example, suppose that a decision node represents a choice about the use of two possible drugs. The branches emanating from that decision node will include separate branches for each of the two drugs. In general, there will be a third branch

Medical Decision Making, Third Edition. Harold C. Sox, Michael C. Higgins, Douglas K. Owens, and Gillian Sanders Schmidler.
© 2024 John Wiley & Sons Ltd. Published 2024 by John Wiley & Sons Ltd.

representing the alternative of using neither drug. If medically appropriate, there also will be a fourth branch representing the combination of the two drugs.

The uncertainty represented by a chance node is what mathematicians call a *random variable*. The word "random" emphasizes what is known about the variable's actual value. That variable always has a value; however, the value is not known for certain within the timeframe of the decision problem. The branches emanating from a chance node correspond to the possible values for the corresponding patient condition, test result, or treatment effect. Each possible value must be represented by exactly one of the branches. Each of those branches corresponds to a possible chance node value.

For example, suppose that a chance node represents the uncertainty about two diseases as possible causes for a patient's symptoms. There will be separate branches for each of the two diseases representing the possibility that the corresponding disease is the sole cause of the symptoms. Often there will be a third branch representing the possibility that neither disease is causing the symptoms. If medically possible, there also will be a fourth branch representing the case where both diseases cause the symptoms. In the terminology we are using, the possible cause of the patient's symptoms is the random variable and the outcomes associated with the four branches are the possible values.

Definition: decision trees, decision nodes, and chance nodes

Decision tree: Collection of nodes and branches showing the relationships between the alternatives and uncertainties in a decision problem.

Decision node: Decision tree node representing a choice between alternatives. Branches emanating from a decision node correspond to the alternatives for the choice represented by the node.

Chance node: Decision tree node representing uncertainty about something like a patient characteristic, test result, or treatment effect. The branches emanating from a chance node correspond to the possible values for the corresponding patient condition, test result, or treatment effect.

6.2.1 Final outcomes

The starting point for a decision tree typically is a decision node. The branches leading from that initial node lead to other nodes, which in turn have branches leading to yet other nodes in the tree. A given sequence of nodes and branches, starting at the initial node, constitutes a path that includes the decision node alternatives and chance node values the patient might experience. Such a path ultimately ends with a *final outcome*, which summarizes that particular patient experience.

A key step in the analysis of a decision problem is the assignment of numerical values to the possible final outcomes. The methods discussed in this book are numerical in nature. In Chapter 3, we learned how to represent subjective beliefs by a number – a probability. The analysis of a decision also uses numerical values to quantify the desirability, or undesirability, of the possible outcomes.

The numerical values quantifying the desirability of outcomes are called *outcome values*. How best to determine the outcome value that is appropriate for the patient is a major challenge in decision analysis. Several later chapters will focus on this important topic. In the meantime, this chapter, and the one that follows, will use the length of the patient's life as the outcome value. Readers who question the use of the length of the patients as the sole measure of an outcome's desirability are right to do so. Patients usually are concerned about more than just how long they will live. However, a fuller discussion of this important topic will have to wait until those later chapters.

Definition: final outcomes and outcome values

Final outcome: The endpoint for a sequence of nodes and branches in a decision tree, starting at the initial node.

Outcome value: Numerical value quantifying the desirability of a final outcome.

6.2.2 Branch probabilities and outcome probabilities

Another key step in the analysis of a decision tree is calculating the probability for each of the possible outcomes of the decision. These are called the *outcome probabilities*. Methods for determining an outcome probability depend on knowing the probabilities for each of the branches encountered on the path leading to that outcome. These are called the *branch probabilities*.

Recall that a branch originating from a chance node corresponds to one of the possible values for the uncertainty represented by the node. Examples of chance node values include the presence of a disease, a test result, or the effect of a treatment. The branch probability for a chance node value is expressed as a conditional probability, which was first discussed back in Chapter 4. A conditional probability measures the likelihood of an event when another event is known or assumed to be true. For example, the test result sensitivity for a disease is the conditional probability measuring the likelihood of the result if the disease is present. In this case, the presence of the disease is called the conditioning event.

A branch probability measures the likelihood of the corresponding disease, test result, or treatment outcome, conditioned on the collection of decision node alternatives and chance node values encountered on the path leading to that branch. In other words, that collection of decision node alternatives and chance node values constitutes the conditioning event for the branch probability.

Because a branch probability depends on what happens earlier on the path leading to that branch, it is not surprising that the outcome probabilities share those same dependencies. Examples discussed later in this chapter demonstrate how an outcome probability is calculated. However, the defining property of an outcome probability is that it measures the likelihood of the outcome conditioned on what happens on the path leading to that outcome.

Definition: branch probabilities and outcome probabilities

Branch probability: The likelihood of the corresponding random variable value conditioned on all of the decision alternatives and chance node values encountered earlier in the decision tree.

Outcome probability: The likelihood of a final outcome conditioned on the decisions leading to that outcome.

6.2.3 Expected value calculations and life expectancy

The final step in any decision analysis is to compare what are called the *expected values* for each of the decision alternatives. The assumption behind this final step is that the best decision alternative will have the greatest expected value. The expected value is calculated for a decision alternative by multiplying the outcome probabilities and outcome values for each of the possible outcomes and summing the results.

Expected value calculations require a notation that identifies the numerous outcome values and probabilities. Suppose that a decision involves two alternatives, which will be denoted by A and B. Also, suppose that n possible outcomes can result from the choice between A or B. We will note these possible outcomes by the subscripted variables $x_1, \ldots, x_n$. The following notion will represent the outcome probabilities conditioned on which alternative is chosen:

Probability outcome is x_i if decision is $A = P[x_i \mid A]$
Probability outcome is x_i if decision is $B = P[x_i \mid B]$

In other words, the decision alternative becomes the conditioning event for the outcome probability.

The value associated with outcome x_i will be denoted by $V(x_i)$ and the expected value calculated for the two alternatives will be denoted by $EV(A)$ and $EV(B)$. The calculations used to determine the expected values can then be expressed as follows:

Expected value for $A = EV(A) = P[x_1 \mid A]V(x_1) + P[x_2 \mid A]V(x_2) + \cdots + P[x_n \mid A]V(x_n)$
Expected value for $B = EV(B) = P[x_1 \mid B]V(x_1) + P[x_2 \mid B]V(x_2) + \cdots + P[x_n \mid B]V(x_n)$

The final step for analyzing this decision is to compare $EV(A)$ and $EV(B)$. Decision alternative A is preferred to alternative B if and only if $EV(A)$ is greater than $EV(B)$.

Of course, the validity of this approach depends on how the values for the outcome values are determined. As noted earlier, in this chapter and the next, outcome is measured by the length of the patient's life. This is called *life expectancy analysis*. In later chapters, we will see an alternative outcome value called *utility*. Analysis based on utility is called *expected utility analysis*.

As already suggested, life expectancy analysis is problematic because length of life is not the only concern when making patient care decisions. However, life expectancy is commonly used for the outcome value, and it makes sense when the goal is to maximize the patient's life expectancy. Moreover, much of the mathematics used to analyze decisions does not care how outcomes are measured. Therefore, life expectancy will provide a suitable outcome value for the discussion in these two chapters.

Expected value calculations and life expectancy

Suppose the possible outcomes for alternative A are $x_1, \ldots, x_n$. Let $V(x_i)$ denote the outcome value for outcome x_i and denote the outcome probabilities as follows:

$P[x_i|A]$ = Probability outcome is x_i if the decision is A.

The expected value for alternative A, denoted $EV(A)$, is computed as follows:

$$EV(A) = P[x_1|A]V(x_1) + P[x_2|A]V(x_2) + \cdots + P[x_n|A]V(x_n)$$

When $V(x_i)$ is the length of the patient's life with outcome x_i, $EV(A)$ is called the *life expectancy*.

6.3 Constructing the decision tree for a hypothetical decision problem

This section uses a simple hypothetical decision problem to illustrate how the concepts described in the previous section are represented in a decision tree. This sample problem will be used again in the next chapter to demonstrate the analysis of decision trees. Therefore, we will give this problem a name – *Problem 1*. As mentioned in the previous section, the outcomes for this decision problem will be represented by the patient's corresponding length of life.

The initial decision in Problem 1 is whether to treat a patient suspected of having a possible disease. If the patient has that disease, treatment will increase the length of life from 4 to 12 years. Without the disease, the treatment will decrease the length of life from 20 to 16 years. Currently, the physician believes the probability of the disease is 0.40. A test is available that has a true-positive rate of 0.90 and a false-positive rate of 0.20. However, the test also has a risk, which reduces the patient's life by 1 year. Assume this reduction in the length of life is faced regardless of the test outcome and the presence or absence of disease.

In summary, Problem 1 has two decisions: (1) whether to test and (2) whether to treat. This problem also has three uncertainties: (1) the disease state, (2) the test result, and (3) the disease state after the test result is learned. This third uncertainty is an example of the interaction between decisions and uncertainties mentioned in the introduction to this chapter.

Definition: Problem 1

Decide whether to test and treat a patient who may have a disease
- Probability of disease is 0.40.
- With disease, treatment increases length of life from 4 to 12 years.
- Without disease, treatment decreases length of life from 20 to 16 years.
- Test has a true-positive rate of 0.90 and a false-positive rate of 0.20.
- Test reduces length of life by 1 year.

Figure 6.1 shows a decision tree for Problem 1. This book adopts the convention of drawing decision nodes as squares and chance nodes as circles. The nodes are organized so that the initial decision is placed on the left side of the diagram and the final outcomes are placed on the right. Often the other nodes are organized from left to right according to the temporal order in which the decisions are made, and the uncertainties are resolved. However, we will see that there is some flexibility in the ordering of the nodes.

Notice in Figure 6.1 that the nodes have been given labels, enclosed in parenthesis. For example, **A1** is the label for the initial decision node in the tree. These labels will simplify the following narrative.

Let us examine each of the nodes in the decision tree. Figure 6.2 focuses on the initial test decision. Node **A1** represents the decision of whether to use the test. This node can be thought of as the root for the decision tree since all other

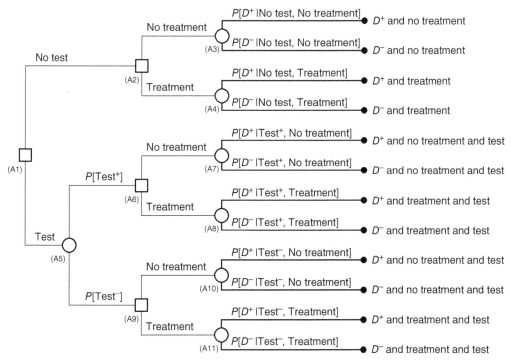

Figure 6.1 Decision tree for Problem 1, which has one treatment, one disease, and a test with two possible outcomes.

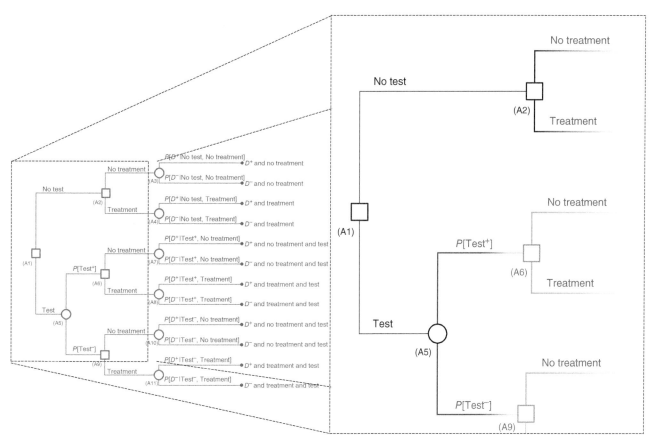

Figure 6.2 Portion of the decision tree in Figure 6.1 showing the initial test decision.

decisions and uncertainties follow this initial decision. There are two possibilities: (1) **No test** and (2) **Test**. These possibilities are represented by the two branches originating at node **A1**.

More complicated problems can have decision nodes with more than two possibilities, in which case additional branches would be used. However, recall that the essential feature of a decision node is that each of the emanating branches must represent exactly one of the possible alternatives. In other words, the alternatives represented by any two branches cannot overlap and all possible alternatives must each be represented by exactly one of the branches.

Figure 6.3 focuses on the portion of the decision tree immediately following the decision to forgo the test. In Figure 6.2, this is the portion of the decision tree starting with the branch from node **A1** to node **A2**. Node **A2** represents the treatment decision following the decision to forgo the test. Once again, Problem 1 has been designed so that there are only two possibilities: (1) **No treatment** and (2) **Treatment**. A more complicated treatment decision might require additional treatment alternatives. The only requirement is that each of the possible treatments must be represented by one and only one of the branches originating from the decision node.

Figure 6.4 focuses on the branch corresponding to the decision not to treat. Referring back to Figure 6.3, this branch connects the decision node **A2** with chance node **A3**. Node **A3** represents the uncertainty about the disease state. More precisely, node **A3** represents the uncertainty about the disease state if there is no treatment. There are two possibilities: (1) the disease can be present, denoted D^+, and (2) the disease can be absent, denoted D^-.

As before, this hypothetical problem has been designed with only two possible disease states, which are indicated by the pair of branches originating from node **A3**. As with decision nodes, the branches originating from a chance node

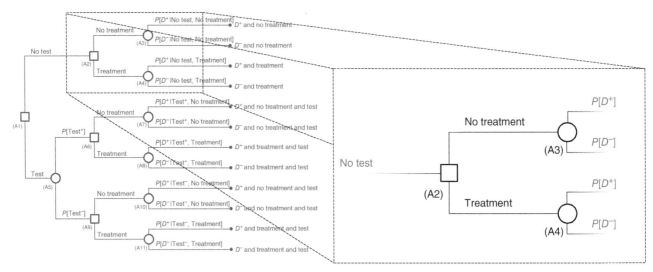

Figure 6.3 Portion of the decision tree in Figure 6.1 showing the treatment decision node following the decision to forgo testing.

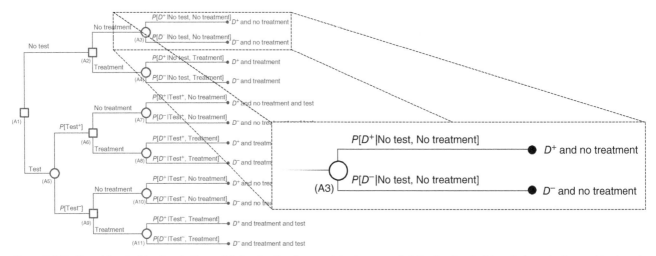

Figure 6.4 Portion of the decision tree in Figure 6.1 showing the disease state chance node following the decisions to forgo testing and treatment.

must correspond to a collection of mutually distinct and collectively exhaustive possibilities. The probabilities placed on the branches originating from a chance node – the branch probabilities – provide a test of this requirement. Each of these probabilities quantifies the likelihood that the possibility represented by the corresponding branch is true. Therefore, the probabilities for all branches originating from a chance node must sum to one. Not all possibilities have been represented if the sum is less than one. Conversely, more than one of the possibilities can be true, at the same time, if the sum is greater than one.

Determining the values for the branch probabilities often is the most challenging step in developing a decision tree. For this simple problem, the probability of disease is 0.40. That is

$$P\left[D^+\right]=0.40$$

Recall that the probabilities for the branches originating from a chance node are conditioned on the nodes and branches encountered earlier in the decision tree. Therefore, the probability for the upper branch shown in Figure 6.4 quantifies the possibility that disease is present if there is no treatment and the test has not been performed. This conditional probability is denoted $P\left[D^+\|\text{No test, No treatment}\right]$.

However, in Problem 1, treatment – or lack of treatment – does not affect the disease state that was present before the treatment decision is made. Nor does the decision to forgo the test. Once again, using the concept of independence introduced in Chapter 3, the disease state is independent of the test decision and the treatment decision. This means

$$P\left[D^+|\text{No test, No treatment}\right]=P\left[D^+\right]=0.40$$

Similarly

$$P\left[D^-|\text{No test, No treatment}\right]=P\left[D^-\right]=1-P\left[D^+\right]=0.60$$

Finally, notice that the branches originating from node **A3** each conclude with one of two final outcomes. Recall that node **A3** represents the uncertainty about the disease state if there is no treatment. Therefore, those two possible final outcomes are (1) disease present and no treatment and (2) disease absent and no treatment. From the definition of Problem 1, the corresponding lengths of life are 2 and 10 years, respectively.

Figure 6.5 focuses on the portion of the decision tree representing what happens if treatment is selected after deciding to forgo the test. Note that, the portion of the decision tree following chance node **A4** is almost identical to the structure after chance node **A3**, as shown in Figure 6.4. The only difference is how the treatment decision affects the lengths of life for the final outcomes. From the problem statement, the patient's life will last 6 years when disease is present, and the treatment is chosen. The patient's life will last 8 years when disease is absent, and the treatment is chosen.

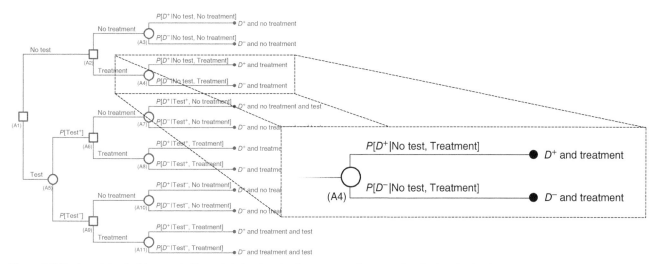

Figure 6.5 Portion of the decision tree in Figure 6.1 showing the disease state chance node following the decisions to treat after forgoing the test.

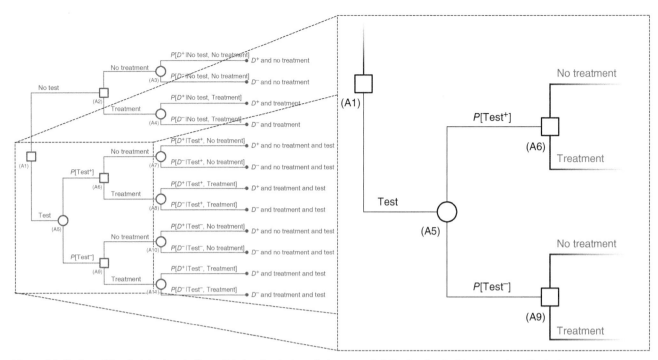

Figure 6.6 Portion of the decision tree in Figure 6.1 showing test result chance node following the decision to perform the test.

Figure 6.6 focuses on the portion of the decision representing what happens if the initial decision is to perform the test. This decision leads to node **A5**, which represents the uncertainty about the test result. In Problem 1, there are only two possibilities: (1) a positive test result, denoted Test⁺, and (2) a negative test result, denoted Test⁻.

Determining the corresponding branch probabilities requires some thought. Consider the probability that the test result is positive. This can happen in two ways. First, the test result can be positive when the disease is present – a true positive. Second, the test result can be positive when the disease is absent – a false positive. Together these two possibilities are the only way a test can be positive. Moreover, only one of these possibilities can occur at the same time. Therefore, as was explained back in Chapter 3,

$$P\left[\text{Test}^+\right] = P\left[\text{Test}^+ \text{ and } D^+\right] + P\left[\text{Test}^+ \text{ and } D^+\right]$$

Recall the definition of conditional probability

$$P\left[\text{Test}^+ \mid D^+\right] = \frac{P\left[\text{Test}^+ \text{ and } D^+\right]}{P\left[D^+\right]}$$

This expression can be rearranged as

$$P\left[\text{Test}^+ \text{ and } D^+\right] = P\left[\text{Test}^+ \mid D^+\right] \times P\left[D^+\right]$$

The term $P[\text{Test}^+ \mid D^+]$ is the true-positive rate, or sensitivity, for the test, which is given as 0.90. As stated in the definition of the problem, the term $P[D^+]$ is 0.40. So

$$P\left[\text{Test}^+ \text{ and } D^+\right] = 0.90 \times 0.40 = 0.36$$

Similarly,

$$P\left[\text{Test}^+ \text{ and } D^-\right] = P\left[\text{Test}^+ \mid D^-\right] \times P\left[D^-\right]$$

The term $P[\text{Test}^+ \mid D^-]$ is the false-positive rate, or one minus the specificity, which is given as 0.20. By definition, $P[D^-]$ is one minus $P[D^-]$. So

$$P\left[\text{Test}^+ \text{ and } D^-\right] = 0.20 \times 0.60 = 0.12$$

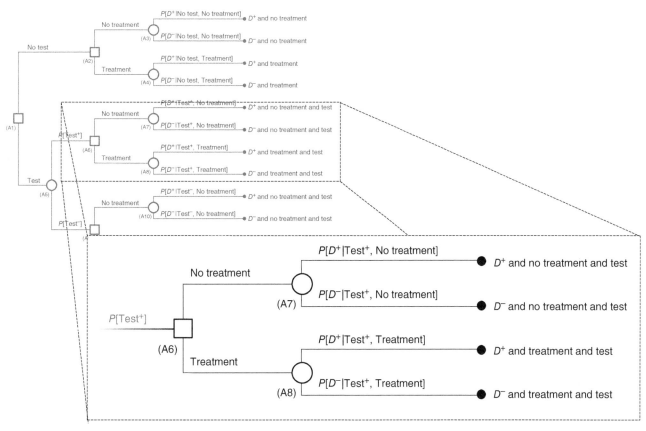

Figure 6.7 Portion of the decision tree in Figure 6.1 showing the treatment decision following a positive test result.

Combining these two results

$$P\left[\text{Test}^+\right] = 0.36 + 0.12 = 0.48$$

Since the test result must be either positive or negative

$$P\left[\text{Test}^-\right] = 1 - P\left[\text{Test}^+\right] = 0.52$$

Figure 6.7 focuses on the portion of the decision tree showing the treatment decision following a positive test result. Notice that the structure for this portion of the tree is the same as for the treatment decision when the test is not performed (see Figures 6.3, 6.4, and 6.5). The only differences are in the branch probabilities and the outcome values. First, the probability of disease is changed because of the positive test result. Second, the lengths of life for the final outcomes will be reduced by 1 year because of the risk associated with the test in this hypothetical problem.

As noted earlier, in Problem 1, the treatment does not affect the probability of disease. Therefore, the branch probabilities can be simplified by noting that

$$P\left[D^+ |\, \text{Test}^+ \text{ and No treatment}\right] = P\left[D^+ |\, \text{Test}^+\right]$$

and

$$P\left[D^- |\, \text{Test}^+ \text{ and No treatment}\right] = P\left[D^- |\, \text{Test}^+\right]$$

Similarly,

$$P\left[D^+ |\, \text{Test}^+ \text{ and Treatment}\right] = P\left[D^+ |\, \text{Test}^+\right]$$

and

$$P\left[D^- |\, \text{Test}^+ \text{ and Treatment}\right] = P\left[D^- |\, \text{Test}^+\right]$$

Bayes' theorem, which was described in Chapter 4, computes the new probability of disease after a positive test result.

$$P\left[D^{+}\mid \text{Test}^{+}\right]=\frac{P\left[\text{Test}^{+}\mid D^{+}\right]\times P\left[D^{+}\right]}{P\left[\text{Test}^{+}\mid D^{+}\right]\times P\left[D^{+}\right]+P\left[\text{Test}^{+}\mid D^{-}\right]\times P\left[D^{-}\right]}$$

$$=\frac{0.90\times 0.40}{0.90\times 0.40+0.20\times 0.60}=0.75$$

Since the disease must be either present (D^+) or absent (D^-)

$$P\left[D^{-}\mid \text{Test}^{+}\right]=1-P\left[D^{+}\mid \text{Test}^{+}\right]=1-0.75=0.25$$

Also, with Problem 1, the effect of the test on the length of life for the final outcomes is determined by subtracting 1 year from the length of life faced by the patient if the test was not performed. Therefore, without treatment, after testing the length of life with or without the disease is 1 year or 9 years, respectively. Similarly, with treatment, after testing the length of life with or without the disease is 5 or 7 years, respectively.

Almost the same analysis applies to the treatment decision following a negative test result – node **A9** in Figure 6.1. The lengths of life for the final outcomes are the same since, in this simple problem, the risk to the patient is assumed to be the same for both test results. The only difference is how the negative test result affects the probability of disease. Once again, Bayes' theorem can be used to determine the new probability of disease.

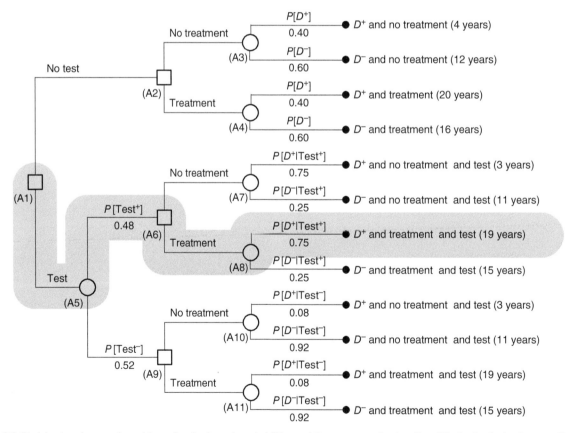

Figure 6.8 Decision tree for sample problem, showing branch probabilities and the corresponding lengths of life for the final outcomes. The path to the outcome *disease present*, *test performed*, and *treatment selected* has been highlighted for the decisions to perform the test and select the treatment if the test result is positive.

$$P\left[D^{+}\,|\,\text{Test}^{-}\right] = \frac{P\left[\text{Test}^{-}\,|\,D^{+}\right] \times P\left[D^{+}\right]}{P\left[\text{Test}^{-}\,|\,D^{+}\right] \times P\left[D^{+}\right] + P\left[\text{Test}^{-}\,|\,D^{-}\right] \times P\left[D^{-}\right]}$$

$$= \frac{\left(1 - P\left[\text{Test}^{+}\,|\,D^{+}\right]\right) \times P\left[D^{+}\right]}{\left(1 - P\left[\text{Test}^{+}\,|\,D^{+}\right]\right) \times P\left[D^{+}\right] + \left(1 - P\left[\text{Test}^{+}\,|\,D^{-}\right]\right) \times P\left[D^{-}\right]}$$

$$= \frac{\left(1 - 0.90\right) \times 0.40}{\left(1 - 0.90\right) \times 0.40 + \left(1 - 0.20\right) \times 0.60} = 0.08$$

In summary, Figure 6.8 shows the decision tree for the sample problem with the branch probabilities and the length of life for the final outcomes. The decision tree in Figure 6.8 fully describes this simple problem.

Notice that the decision tree in Figure 6.8 can be used to determine the outcome probabilities for a given set of decisions. For example, suppose that decisions are to (1) perform the test and (2) start treatment if the test result is positive. Assuming these two decisions, what is the probability that a patient with the disease will be both tested and treated?

The pathway through the tree for this outcome has been highlighted in Figure 6.8. Since the patient will be tested and treatment always follows a positive result, the probability of both being tested and treated is just the probability of a positive result. However, the outcome in question also includes having the disease. Therefore, with this set of decisions, the probability of the outcome in question is the probability of both a positive test result and the presence of disease. From the definition of conditional probability

$$P\left[\text{Test}^{+}\text{ and }D^{+}\right] = P\left[\text{Test}^{+}\right] \times P\left[D^{+}\,|\,\text{Test}^{+}\right]$$

Note that $P[\text{Test}^{+}]$ is the probability for the branch from chance node **A5** to decision node **A6**. Similarly, $P[D^{+}\,|\,\text{Test}^{+}]$ is the probability for the branch from chance node **A8** to the outcome in question. In short, the probability of the path from the initial decision node to a final outcome is the product of the branch probabilities encountered along the path.

This demonstration of how an outcome probability can be computed illustrates the fundamental requirement for assigning probabilities to the branches comprising a path. Each of the successive branch probabilities is conditioned on the uncertainties and decisions that precede the branch on a path from the initial decision to a final outcome. Often an uncertainty is independent of some of those preceding uncertainties and decisions. These independencies can simplify the branch probabilities. For example, the probability of disease is independent of treatment. So $P\left[D^{+}\,|\,\text{Test}^{+}\text{ and Treatment}\right]$ becomes $P\left[D^{+}\,|\,\text{Test}^{+}\right]$.

6.4 Constructing the decision tree for a medical decision problem

By using hypothetical tests, treatments, and diseases, Problem 1 has avoided much of the challenge involved in developing the decision tree for a real clinical decision. The probabilities and life expectancies were simply stated without any attempt at empirical justification. The discussion now turns to a more realistic clinical problem involving the management of coronary artery disease.

Coronary artery disease was selected for this first medical example because of the extensive body of published data that will simplify the determination of the decision tree parameters. The introduction of decision analysis to the medical community coincided with important advancements in the diagnosis and treatment of coronary artery disease in the 1960s and 1970s. Because of this coincidence, a large amount of data about test performance and patient outcomes for coronary artery disease appeared in the medical literature. The discussion that follows uses that empirical foundation to describe an analysis of an important medical problem. Some of the data that will be used is out of date. However, the important principle that complex medical decisions can be analyzed will be illustrated by these examples.

In addition, some simplifying assumptions will be used to reduce the complexity of the example that will be discussed. This means that what follows will not be a complete exploration of current coronary artery disease management. However, the simplified decisions described for the treatment of this important disease will illustrate the process of going from published results to decision tree parameters.

6.4.1 Management of coronary artery disease overview

Many of the model parameters used in this discussion will be taken from the Coronary Artery Surgery Study (CASS) (Taylor *et al.*, 1989). This large multicenter study conducted a randomized clinical trial of the effects of surgery-based therapies and drug-based therapies on the survival of patients with coronary artery disease.

The ACC/AHA Coronary Arteriography Guidelines (Scalon *et al.*, 1999) list the evaluation of stable angina as a reason for using arteriography. Management of stable coronary artery disease typically starts with drug-based therapies. Arteriography can show the anatomical findings needed for more aggressive treatment alternatives.[1] These include coronary artery bypass graft surgery (CABG). Other alternatives, known collectively as *percutaneous coronary intervention* (PCI), involve the placement of stents in partially blocked arteries that have been opened using angioplasty. The development of drug-eluting stents has resulted in types of PCI that approach the effectiveness of CABG while avoiding the risks of open-heart surgery.

Studies show that the effectiveness of the treatment alternatives varies with the location and extent of the narrowing in the coronary arteries. The patient's survival resulting from the choice of treatment also depends on other factors, such as the presence of arrhythmias, conduction defects, and other damage to the heart. However, the examples in this chapter condense this complex array of diagnostic endpoints into a pair of health states, denoted *CAD* and *NO CAD*. Similarly, the treatment alternatives will be grouped (1) as drug-based therapies (*MED*), (2) more aggressive arteriography-based treatments (*PCI/CABG*), and (3) no treatment (*NONE*).

The specific patient used in this example is a hypothetical 65-year-old woman, who will be called Ms. Maple. Suppose that both a beta-blocker and a statin drug have been prescribed for Ms. Maple. However, she dislikes the side effects of these drugs and has not adhered well to this typical medical regimen. Moreover, her older sister recently died from a heart attack. This raises Ms. Maple's concerns about her diagnosis and increases the likelihood that she may face a similar outcome. Therefore, Ms. Maple's physician is considering coronary arteriography as a first step toward a more aggressive therapy.

The outcomes in Problem 1 were specific lengths of life, such as the patient will live 3 years. The example discussed in this section will use a slightly more sophisticated view of how long the patient will live with a given outcome. In most cases a medical decision results in a prognosis that can only make a probabilistic statement about how long the patient will live. Chapter 11 provides a more detailed discussion of what a probabilistic statement about a patient's survival means. For now, we will use a life expectancy to represent the uncertainty about how long a patient will live. The goal will still be to find the decision that maximizes Ms. Maple's life expectancy.

For example, based on actuarial data published by the US Social Security Administration, a 65-year-old woman has a life expectancy of 24.2 years. What does this mean? It does not mean that the woman will live exactly 24.2 years. The woman could step off the curb in front of a car and die tomorrow. She also could get lucky, live for another 35 years, and become a centenarian. Each possible length of life has a probability. As we saw in the previous section, the woman's life expectancy is the sum of each possible life length weighted by the corresponding probability.

In general, denoting life expectancy by *LE*, someone's life expectancy, in years, is computed by the following summation:

$$LE = \left(P[\text{Die now}] \times 0 \text{ years}\right) + \left(P[\text{Die in 1 year}] \times 1 \text{ years}\right) + \left(P[\text{Die in 2 years}] \times 2 \text{ years}\right) + \left(P[\text{Die in 3 years}] \times 3 \text{ years}\right)$$
$$+ \left(P[\text{Die in 4 years}] \times 4 \text{ years}\right) + \left(P[\text{Die in 5 years}] \times 5 \text{ years}\right) + \dots$$

In theory, the summation should be extended forever. However, since no one appears to live longer than about 120 years, for a 65-year-old woman, like Ms. Maples, the sum only needs to consider the next 55 terms. The probabilities for the remaining terms are essentially zero.

When computing someone's actuarial life expectancy, the probabilities are determined using the life tables published by the Social Security Administration. Chapter 11 will describe how to make those calculations. The result is an age-specific life expectancy for a member of the general population.

Of course, Ms. Maple is not necessarily a "typical" member of the general population. She has a chest pain that her physician believes is caused by coronary artery disease. She certainly has a clinical presentation that would justify the risk and expense of arteriography. The CASS study reported the survival rates for patients found to not have coronary artery disease based on the results of arteriography (Meyer *et al.*, 1985). These published survival rates can be adjusted according to age and sex to estimate a life expectancy of 19.2 years for a 65-year-old woman with a clinical presentation that justifies arteriography (Fisher *et al.*, 1982).

Therefore, the Social Security Administration life tables and the CASS imply different life expectancies for Ms. Maple. How to proceed with this difference partly depends on how the analysis will be used. Suppose the goal is

---

[1] The examples in this chapter ignore important alternatives to arteriography that would be considered for the evaluation of an actual patient. Computerized tomography coronary arteriography can visualize blockages with the use of peripherally injected radiopaque dye, thereby avoiding the need for catheterization.

Table 6.1 Life expectancy for Ms. Maple derived from the CASS data.

Treatment	Disease state	
	NO CAD	CAD
No treatment (NONE)	19.2–24.2 years	<11.4 years
Drug-based therapy (MED)	<19.2 years	11.4 years
Aggressive treatment (PCI/CABG)	N.A.	15.2 years

to establish a clinical policy that will be applied to any 65-year-old woman with stable angina. In this case, the life expectancy of the patient with a normal arteriography finding probably should be estimated by 19.2 years, the life expectancy derived from studies of patient survival with treatments for coronary artery disease. The life expectancy of 19.2 years is a value that could be defended by objective evidence from these studies.

On the other hand, suppose the goal of the analysis is to determine the best decision for the specific individual represented by Ms. Maple in this example. Ms. Maple might differ significantly from that "typical" stable angina patient being considered for an invasive and expensive diagnostic procedure. Her physician might consider Ms. Maple to be truly disease free, except for the possibility of blockages in her coronary arteries. In this case, her physician might choose to assume Ms. Maple's life expectancy will be close to 24.2 years if the arteriography findings are negative. The discussion of sensitivity analysis in the next chapter will show how to address these discrepancies.

In either case, recall that the focus of this chapter, and the next chapter, is to find the choice that maximizes her life expectancy. Table 6.1 shows the values for Ms. Maple's life expectancies that will be used in this discussion. These life expectancies are sex and age-adjusted from the life expectancies published by CASS.

Notice that most of the life expectancies in Table 6.1 can only be determined to be within a range. For example, as we just saw, there is uncertainty about how long Ms. Maple will live if she does not have coronary artery disease and has no treatment. Her life expectancy if she has coronary artery disease and is untreated is even less certain. Based on published data, all we can say is that, almost certainly, her life expectancy will be less than the 11.4 years reported by studies of patients with coronary artery disease who are treated with drug-based therapy (Mock *et al.*, 1982). Similarly, unnecessary drug therapy, if Ms. Maple does not have coronary artery disease, will not increase her life expectancy over what she could expect without treatment. Therefore, Ms. Maple's life expectancy with unnecessary drug therapy can only be bounded above by the 19.2 years found in published data for untreated patients without disease. Once again, the discussion of sensitivity analysis later in the next chapter shows how to manage these problematic parameter values.

The entry in Table 6.1 for unnecessary aggressive treatment is "Not Applicable" (NA). This entry follows from one of the assumptions that will be made. Arteriography surely is not a perfect test of coronary artery disease. There is some evidence that this test can produce both false-positive and false-negative results. However, most likely those misleading results are extremely rare. Therefore, this analysis will assume that arteriography is a perfect test. The procedure also is the necessary first step for the more aggressive treatments. Therefore, assuming that arteriography is a perfect test is equivalent to assuming that Ms. Maple has PCI or CABG if and only if she has coronary artery disease.

We also must consider the risks to Ms. Maple's survival because of the procedures she might undergo. Since we assume that arteriography is a perfect diagnostic test and PCI or CABG will not be considered without a positive arteriography finding, the risk of these treatments for nondiseased patients is not a consideration. On the other hand, fatal complications do result from the more aggressive therapies. The risk from PCI is very low, probably causing approximately one death per 1000 cases (Peterson *et al.*, 2010). However, some patients subjected to more aggressive treatment for coronary artery disease must undergo CABG because of the location of the coronary obstructions and other considerations. Therefore, this example will assume a risk of death equal to 0.0295 for patients undergoing PCI/CABG.

Large studies of arteriography have reported fatal complications (Bourassa and Nobel, 1976). However, those deaths invariably occur in patients with coronary artery disease. This means the possibility of fatal arrhythmias or significant vascular trauma during catheterization does not appear to be a significant risk for patients without coronary artery disease. Therefore, the risk of death because of arteriography will be set at 0.0010 for patients with coronary artery disease. This risk of death will be set at 0.0001 for patients without coronary artery disease who undergo arteriography.

6.4.2 Simple decision in the management of coronary artery disease
The next chapter will analyze a coronary artery disease management decision that includes an additional diagnostic test. However, the coronary artery disease management decision – called *Problem 2* – discussed in this chapter will focus only on the decision of whether Ms. Maple should have coronary arteriography.

This decision assumes that Ms. Maple faces a perioperative risk of 0.0295 if she has coronary artery disease. As stated earlier, we also will assume that she will not undergo one of the more aggressive treatments if she does not have coronary artery disease. Ms. Maple's risk of death from arteriography is assumed to be 0.0010 or 0.0001 depending on whether she does or does not have coronary artery disease. We also assume that her life expectancies, depending on her treatment and actual disease state, are what are shown in Table 6.1. Finally, we assume that this decision is made with the opinion that the probability Ms. Maple actually has coronary disease is 0.7000. This probability matches the prevalence of positive arteriograms in the CASS study.

Definition: Problem 2

Decide whether to order coronary arteriography for a 65-year-old woman with stable angina and who is considering PCI or CABG because of dissatisfaction with drug-based therapy. Assume:

	NO CAD	CAD
Probability of disease state	0.3000	0.7000
Probability of death during arteriography	**0.0001***	0.0010
Probability of death during PCI/CABG	N.A.	0.0295
Life expectancy with no treatment	**19.2 years***	**5.7 years***
Life expectancy with drug-based therapy	**19.2 years***	11.4 years
Life expectancy with PCI/CABG	N.A.	15.2 years

* Low-confidence parameter values.

Figure 6.9 shows a decision tree for Problem 2. The branch labeled *NO ART* represents the decision to forgo the procedure. That branch leads to a chance node, labeled **B2**, which represents the uncertainty about Ms. Maple's disease state. Node **B2** has two branches, corresponding to the two possible disease states. Those two branches lead to the outcomes representing the continuation of drug-based therapy for the corresponding disease states. Notice that the outcomes are shown in Figure 6.2 with the corresponding values assumed for Ms. Maple's life expectancy. For example, Problem 2 assumes the life expectancies reported by studies of survival for medically treated coronary artery disease, adjusted to a 65-year-old woman (11.4 years).

The other branch from node **B1**, labeled *ART*, leads to the portion of the decision tree representing how undergoing arteriography will affect Ms. Maple's life expectancy. This begins with the chance node labeled **B3**, which represents the uncertainty about surviving the procedure.

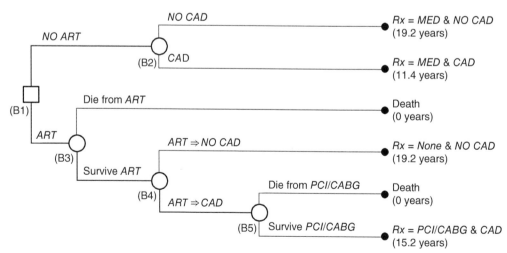

Figure 6.9 Decision tree for Problem 2. Chance nodes are ordered according to how the corresponding uncertainties in the problem typically resolve over time.

Two branches originate from node **B3**. The branch labeled "Die from *ART*" represents the possibility of a fatal complication from arteriography. This branch leads to the outcome labeled "Death," which has a life expectancy of 0 years. The other branch, labeled "Survive *ART*," represents what happens if Ms. Maple survives the procedure. This branch leads to node **A4**, representing the uncertainty about what arteriography will reveal if it does not cause Ms. Maple's death.

Problem 2 divides the range of arteriography findings into two groups represented by the abbreviations:

NO CAD   No significant coronary artery narrowing was found
CAD   Significant narrowing was found

The decision tree in Figure 6.9 labels the corresponding branches $ART \Rightarrow NO\ CAD$ and $ART \Rightarrow CAD$, respectively.

Because Problem 2 assumes arteriography to be a perfect test for coronary artery disease, the findings on the arteriogram will define Ms. Maple's final treatment. A negative finding means that she does not have coronary artery disease. So the drug-based therapy would be discontinued. A positive finding means that Ms. Maple faces the risk involved with the more aggressive treatment indicated by the arteriogram, as presented by the chance node **B5**.

So far, the Problem 2 decision tree has ordered the nodes according to how the corresponding uncertainties typically would resolve over time. For example, once the arteriography procedure has been ordered, the uncertainty about the patient's survival would be resolved first. Next, the uncertainty about the procedure findings would be resolved. Typically, the last uncertainty resolved would be Ms. Maple's actual disease state.

This temporal ordering of the chance nodes seems natural. Often this ordering helps assure that the tree represents all considerations in a decision problem. However, in a problem with only one decision node, there are no firm rules about the ordering of the nodes except that the primary decision is placed first and the final outcomes are placed last. The math used to analyze the tree does not care about the order of the nodes. On the other hand, other orderings of the nodes can reduce the work in determining the branch probabilities. These alternate orders are discussed later in this section.

6.4.3 Determining the branch probabilities

Figure 6.10 labels the branch probabilities for the decision tree in Figure 6.9. Note that some of these probabilities can be determined directly from the problem definition. For example, the probabilities on the branches starting at node **B2** are the probabilities that Ms. Maple has, or does not have, coronary artery disease. Therefore, from the definition of Problem 2:

$$P[NO\ CAD] = 0.3000$$
$$P[CAD] \quad = 0.7000$$

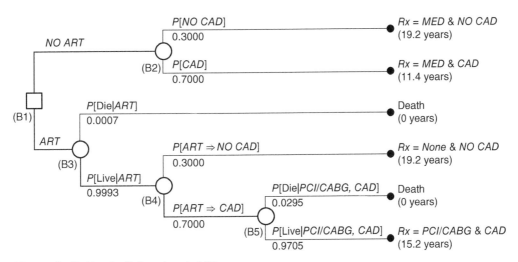

Figure 6.10 Decision tree for Problem 2 with branch probabilities.

Notice that because arteriography is assumed to be a perfect test for coronary artery disease, the branch probabilities for the possible arteriography findings equal the probabilities for the corresponding disease states. That is

$$P[ART \Rightarrow NOCAD] = P[NOCAD] = 0.30$$

and

$$P[ART \Rightarrow CAD] = P[CAD] = 0.70$$

Other branch probabilities require more thought. For example, what is the probability that Ms. Maple will survive coronary arteriography? This uncertainty corresponds to the branch probability labeled "$P[Live|ART]$" in Figure 6.10. The same method used to determine the probability of a positive test result in Problem 1 is used.

The probability of surviving arteriography depends on Ms. Maple's disease state. If her disease state is *NO CAD*, Ms. Maple's chance of surviving is 0.9999. Using the notation of conditional probability, this can be written:

$$P[\text{Live} | ART \text{ and } NO\ CAD] = 0.9999$$

or

$$P[\text{Die} | ART \text{ and } NO\ CAD] = 0.0001$$

This mathematical expression reads as "the probability of surviving conditioned on undergoing arteriography and not having coronary artery disease equals 0.0001." Similarly, if her disease state is *CAD*, her chance of surviving arteriography is

$$P[\text{Live} | ART \text{ and } CAD] = 0.9990$$

or

$$P[\text{Die} | ART \text{ and } CAD] = 0.0010$$

Before arteriography, the presence or absence of coronary artery disease is unknown. Therefore, combining the probabilities for each disease state with the corresponding probabilities of dying during arteriography yields:

$$P[\text{Live} | ART] = (0.3000 \times 0.9999) + (0.7000 \times 0.9990) = 0.9993$$

In short, $P[\text{Live}|ART]$ is the sum of the probabilities of living for each of the disease states, weighted by the corresponding probabilities for those health states.

The complication requiring this calculation is that Ms. Maple's disease state affects her chances of surviving the procedure. In the terminology of probability theory, Ms. Maple's disease state and her survival are not independent events. Knowing one event changes the probability of the other event. Put another way, not knowing the disease state means that the value for the arteriography risk must account for each possible value for the disease state random variable.

6.4.4 Alternate chance node ordering

Let us consider one of the alternate orderings of the nodes mentioned earlier. Figure 6.11 shows an alternate decision tree that simplifies how the branch probabilities are determined for Problem 2. The important change is the placement of the nodes representing the uncertainty about Ms. Maple's disease state. The first decision tree placed those nodes just before the final outcomes. These are nodes **B2** and **B4** in Figure 6.10. Notice that these nodes are located late in the tree. The decision tree shown in Figure 6.11 places the chance nodes for the disease state uncertainty just after the primary decision node. These chance nodes are **C2** and **C3** in Figure 6.11. Otherwise, the trees shown in Figures 6.10 and 6.11 are the same.

The significance of changing the order of the nodes becomes apparent when determining the branch probabilities. Consider the probability of the branch from node **C4** to Death. This branch now is on a path that includes knowing that Ms. Maple does not have coronary artery disease. Therefore, the branch probability measures the likelihood that Ms. Maple will die from the arteriography if there are no significant blockages in her coronary arteries. According to the definition for Problem 2, this probability equals 0.0001. Similarly, the probability for the branch from node **C5** to Death is 0.0010. Because the disease state chance node has been moved closer to the decision node, values for these

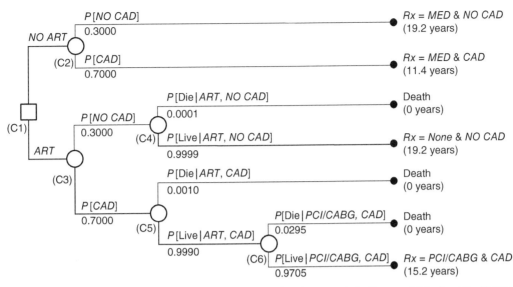

Figure 6.11 Alternate Decision Tree for Problem 2, with branch probabilities. The chance node for the uncertainty about the disease state has been moved forward.

branch probabilities can be taken directly from the problem definition. If Ms. Maple survives arteriography and has coronary artery disease, the same simplifications hold for the probabilities on the branches originating from node **C5** in Figure 6.11.

In general, for the purposes of determining the branch probabilities, the optimal ordering of the nodes depends on how the uncertainty in the problem is defined. In the case of Problem 2, the uncertainties about the outcome of the arteriography and surviving the procedures are conditioned on Ms. Maple's actual disease state. Therefore, placing the chance node for her disease state first in the tree means that many of the branch probabilities can be taken directly from the problem statement.

6.4.5 Computing the life expectancy for the decision alternatives

Recall that our goal is to determine the life expectancies for the two treatment alternatives. Since our focus in this example is the patient's life expectancy, the alternative with the greater life expectancy will be the preferred alternative.

Once the branch probabilities are known, straightforward arithmetic determines the life expectancies. Recall that life expectancy for an alternative is calculated by multiplying the outcome probability by the outcome life expectancy for each outcome. This calculation is simple for the *NO ART* decision because there are only two possible outcomes:

$$LE[NO\,ART] = (0.3000 \times 19.2\,\text{years}) + (0.7000 \times 11.4\,\text{years})$$
$$= 13.7\,\text{years}$$

Calculating the life expectancy for the ART decision involves more terms but still is just arithmetic:

$$LE[ART] = (0.3000 \times 0.0001 \times 0\,\text{years}) + (0.3000 \times 0.9999 \times 19.2\,\text{years}) + (0.7000 \times 0.0010 \times 0\,\text{years})$$
$$+ (0.7000 \times 0.9990 \times 0.0295 \times 0\,\text{years}) + (0.7000 \times 0.9990 \times 0.9705 \times 15.2\,\text{years})$$
$$= 16.1\,\text{years}$$

Note in both calculations that each of the branch probabilities on a path from the initial decision to a final outcome is conditioned on the branch probabilities that have been encountered earlier in the path.

For example, consider the path that starts with the decision *ART*, passes through chance node **C5** and chance node **C6**, and ends with the outcome labeled *CAD Rx = PCI/CABG*. Figure 6.12 focuses on this single path and the corresponding terms in the summation for *LE[ART]*. The first branch probability on this path is *P[CAD]*, which equals 0.7000. Nothing else is known at this point on the path so the probability is not conditioned by any prior information. The next branch probability is *P[Live|ART, CAD]*, the probability of surviving arteriography if Ms. Maple has coronary

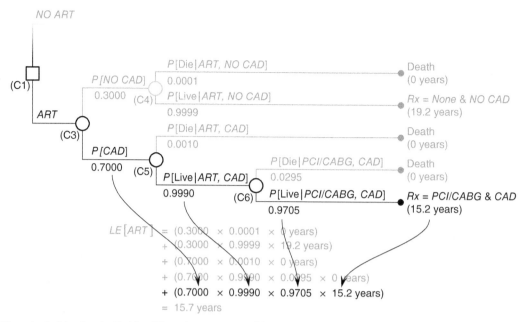

Figure 6.12 Alternate decision tree for Problem 2 focusing on one possible outcome resulting from the decision to order arteriography and the corresponding term in the expression for Ms. Maple's life expectancy with arteriography.

artery disease. This term comes after setting the disease state to *NO CAD*. Therefore, this branch probability is the probability Ms. Maple survives arteriography if she has coronary artery disease. From the definition of Problem 2,

$$P[\text{Live} \mid ART, CAD] = 0.9990$$

The third branch probability on the selected path measures the likelihood that Ms. Maple survives the treatment if she actually has coronary artery disease. According to the definition of Problem 2, this third and final branch probability is

$$P[\text{Live} \mid PCI / CABG, CAD] = 0.9705$$

The value for the last branch probability in the selected path is Ms. Maple's life expectancy with coronary artery disease if she has the aggressive therapy indicated for her disease. From the definition of Problem 2,

$$LE(Rx = PCI / CABG \,\&\, CAD) = 15.2 \text{ years}$$

Note that moving the chance node for the disease state forward only delays the arithmetic needed to compute some of the branch probabilities. With Problem 2, moving the node for the uncertainty about Ms. Maple's disease state simplified computing the probability that she would survive arteriography. With the original decision tree for Problem 2 (see Figure 6.10) the probability that Ms. Maple survives arteriography had to be computed.

The alternate design for the tree was drawn with the chance node for Ms. Maple's disease state placed before the other chance nodes in Problem 2. This allowed for the probability of surviving arteriography to be taken directly from the problem statement.

Figure 6.13 focuses on the two paths in the alternate decision tree that lead to the outcomes in which Ms. Maple survives arteriography. Figure 6.13 also highlights the corresponding terms in the summation for *LE[ART]*. Notice that these two terms contain the same multiplication steps that were used to compute the branch probability *P[Live|ART]* in the expression:

$$P[\text{Live} \mid ART] = (0.3000 \times 0.9999) + (0.7000 \times 0.9990) = 0.9993$$

In other words, the alternate design for the decision tree may have simplified the determination of some of the branch probabilities; however, the computation that is avoided is simply moved to the life expectancy calculation.

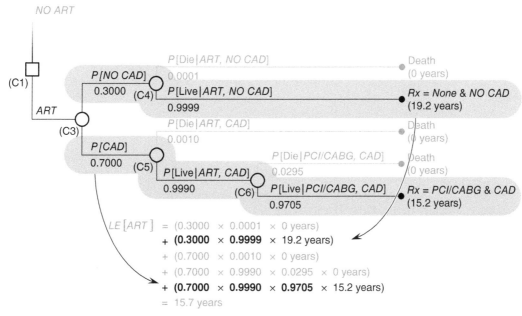

Figure 6.13 Alternate decision tree for Problem 2 focusing on the two outcomes with Ms. Maple surviving arteriography. The corresponding terms in the expression for Ms. Maple's life expectancy with arteriography also are highlighted.

In theory, calculating the life expectancies for the two decision alternatives completes the analysis. The life expectancy for ordering the arteriography is 16.1 years. The life expectancy for forgoing arteriography is 13.7 years. Therefore, the decision tree analysis concludes with the recommendation that Ms. Maple has arteriography because this decision would maximize her life expectancy.

In reality, this first calculation of the life expectancies would be where the real work begins in the analysis of a decision tree. The definition of Problem 2 assumes several problematic values that should be examined more carefully. This is done with sensitivity analysis, a topic discussed in the next chapter.

Summary

- A decision tree is used in decision analysis to depict the structure of a decision problem.
- The decision tree diagram is drawn using square-shaped nodes to represent choices or *decisions* and circular-shaped nodes to represent uncertainties or *chances*. Typically, an initial decision node provides the root for a decision tree. Sequences of decision node and chance node branches ultimately lead to each of the possible outcomes faced by the patient.
- Each branch originating from a *decision node* represents the options available for the corresponding decision in the problem. The options represented by the decision node branches are organized so that exactly one option can be chosen. Collectively, the options represented by the branches from a decision node represent all possible choices for that decision.
- Each branch originating from a *chance node* represents the possibilities for the corresponding uncertainty in the problem. The possibilities represented by the chance node branches are organized so that exactly one possibility can be true. Collectively, the possibilities represented by the branches from a chance node represent all possibilities for that uncertainty.
- The definition of a chance node branch includes a branch probability that measures the likelihood of the corresponding possibility, conditioned on the choices and possibilities that must occur to reach that branch.
- Multiplying the branch probabilities encountered on the path to a final outcome determines the probability that the outcome will occur.

Epilogue

This chapter described the organization of tree diagrams that represent the interactions between the decisions and uncertainties in a decision problem. The examples used to illustrate the process were simple. This meant we could easily compute life expectancies for the decision alternatives. Our focus was finding the decision alternative that would result in the greatest life expectancy for the patient. Therefore, a simple calculation found a solution to the decision problem.

For example, with our hypothetical patient named Ms. Maple, we calculated that her life expectancy would be 16.1 years if she underwent arteriography. We also calculated that her life expectancy would be 13.7 years if she did not undergo arteriography. Therefore, we concluded that undergoing arteriography would be the best decision for Ms. Maple because it would maximize her life expectancy.

This conclusion was based on straightforward calculations that determined the outcome probabilities by simply multiplying the branch probabilities encounter on each path to an outcome. That simple calculation was possible because of the simple structure of the decision tree.

The next chapter will expand on the concepts described in this chapter to show the analysis of more complicated decision problems.

Bibliography

Bourassa, M.G. and Nobel, J. (1976) Complication rate of coronary arteriography. A review of 5250 cases studied by a percutaneous femoral technique. *Circulation*, **53**, 106–14.

Fisher, L.D., Kennedy, J.W., Davis, K.B. *et al.* and The Participating CASS Clinics (1982) Association of sex, physical size, and operative mortality after coronary artery bypass in the coronary artery surgery study (CASS). *Journal of Cardiovascular Surgery*, **84**, 334–41.

Mock, M.B., Ringqvist, I., Fisher, L.D. *et al.* and Participants in the Coronary Artery Surgery Study (1982) Survival of medically treated patients in the coronary artery surgery study (CASS) registry. *Circulation*, **66**, 562–8.

Myers, W.O., Davis, K., Foster, E.D. *et al.* (1985) Surgical survival in the coronary artery surgery study (CASS) registry. *The Annals of Thoracic Surgery*, **40**, 245–60.

Peterson, E.D., Dai, D., DeLong, E.R. *et al.* (2010) Contemporary mortality risk prediction for percutaneous coronary intervention: results from 588,398 procedures in the national cardiovascular data registry. *Journal of the American College of Cardiology*, **55**, 1923–32.

Scanlon, P.J., Faxon, D.P., Audet, A.M. *et al.* (1999) ACC/AHA guidelines for coronary angiography: a report of the American College of Cardiology/American Heart Association task force on practice guidelines (Committee on Coronary Angiography). *Journal of the American College of Cardiology*, **33**, 1756–824.

Taylor, H.A., Deumite, N.J., Chaitman, B.R. *et al.* (1989) Asymptomatic left main coronary artery disease in the coronary artery surgery study (CASS) registry. *Circulation*, **79**, 1171–9.

CHAPTER 7

Decision tree analysis

7.1 Introduction

This chapter demonstrates how to analyze a decision tree. In particular, this chapter describes the analysis of complicated decision trees that include multiple decision nodes. The previous chapter used a decision tree example that had only a single decision node. The final step in analysis of that simple decision tree was the comparison of the expected values calculated for the decision alternatives. Recall that expected value was calculated by combining the outcome probabilities with outcome values that quantify how much one outcome is preferred relative to another. The fundamental assumption of decision tree analysis is that the alternative with the greatest expected value is the best choice.

This basic approach of comparing alternatives based on their expected values is common to all of the methods discussed in this book. However, the method described in this chapter – based on what is called the *folding-back operation*[1] – calculates an expected value using an approach that differs from what was demonstrated for the simple example in the previous chapter.

That example was simple because there was only one decision node. This meant the expected value for an alternative could be determined directly by calculating the probabilities for each of the possible outcomes. Those were called the *outcome probabilities*. Because the initial node represented the only decision in the tree, the probability for an outcome could be calculated by simply multiplying the branch probabilities encountered on the path leading to that outcome. Branch probabilities are expressed as conditional probabilities that accounted for how one chance node value depended on another chance node value. This meant multiplying the branch probabilities produced a valid outcome probability.

This direct approach to calculating the outcome probabilities becomes difficult to use when a decision tree represents multiple interdependent decisions. The multiplication of the branch probabilities on the path to an outcome must account for each of the decisions on the path that leads to those branches. With a medical decision involving multiple tests and multiple treatment options, tracking how those decisions interact can be complicated. The folding back operation manages that complexity by shifting the focus from outcome probabilities to the expected values computed from those outcome probabilities. The folding back operation that will be described still computes the outcome probabilities; however, it does so in the background while computing the expected value.

The previous chapter stressed the importance of how values are determined for outcomes. These two chapters use the patient's length of life as the value for an outcome. If Outcome A means the patient will live twice as long as the

---

[1] The folding-back operation also is called "averaging out" the decision alternatives.

Medical Decision Making, Third Edition. Harold C. Sox, Michael C. Higgins, Douglas K. Owens, and Gillian Sanders Schmidler.
© 2024 John Wiley & Sons Ltd. Published 2024 by John Wiley & Sons Ltd.

patient would live with Outcome B, then Outcome A is preferred twice as much as Outcome B. We called this approach *life expectancy analysis* since it identifies the alternative that maximizes how long the patient will live on average.

Later chapters will discuss alternate outcome values that provide a more complete representation of what is important in a decision. Those preference measures will have different numerical values; however, the same folding back operation will still determine an expected value that can be used to compare the alternatives in a decision.

Finally, this chapter also will demonstrate a process called *sensitivity analysis*. Recall the medical example called Problem 2 in the previous chapter. Constructing the decision tree for this problem depended on several problematic decision tree parameters. These parameters were problematic because there was limited or conflicting empirical evidence for their values. The sensitivity analysis described in this chapter will demonstrate a systematic examination of these low-confidence values.

7.2 Folding-back operation

The decision tree for Problem 2, first described in Chapter 6, is easy to evaluate because there is only one decision – whether to order coronary arteriography. The branch probabilities on the paths to the various outcomes fully describe the outcome uncertainties for this problem. Simple arithmetic computes the corresponding life expectancies for the patient. However, what if additional decision nodes are encountered on those paths to the final outcome? How do we compute life expectancy for a more complicated decision problem involving multiple decisions?

One answer is what we call the *folding-back* operation.

7.2.1 Folding-back operation applied to hypothetical problem

Problem 1, first described in Chapter 6, will be used to introduce the folding-back operation. The decision tree in Figure 7.1 is the same decision tree shown in Figure 6.8 for Problem 1. Recall that this decision problem concerns the management of a hypothetical disease that may be present (D^+) or absent (D^-). Initial assessment establishes a probability of 0.40 for the disease. Management of the disease requires a choice between two alternatives: **Treatment** and **No treatment**, which will lead to different life expectancies, depending on the disease state. In Problem 1, there is a test that can be used to change the probability of the disease. The treatment decision can be based on the result of this test. However, undergoing the test also affects the patient's length of life. Figure 7.1 shows a decision tree for this problem, including the various branch probabilities that were derived in the previous chapter. The outcome values are expressed as lengths of life for the patient.

> **Definition: Problem 1**
>
> Decide whether to test and treat a patient who may have a disease
> - Probability of disease is 0.40.
> - With disease, treatment increases survival from 4 to 12 years.
> - Without disease, treatment decreases survival from 20 to 16 years.
> - Test has a true-positive rate of 0.90 and a false-positive rate of 0.20.
> - Undergoing the test reduces survival by 1 year.

The folding-back operation involves a series of steps that sequentially eliminate nodes without changing the expected values for alternatives represented by the initial decision node. The process ends when that initial decision node is reached. The resulting tree is equivalent to the original tree, only reduced to a simple choice between alternatives with known expected values. For example, suppose that the decision tree shown in Figure 7.1 could be reduced to the following simple decision tree:

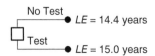

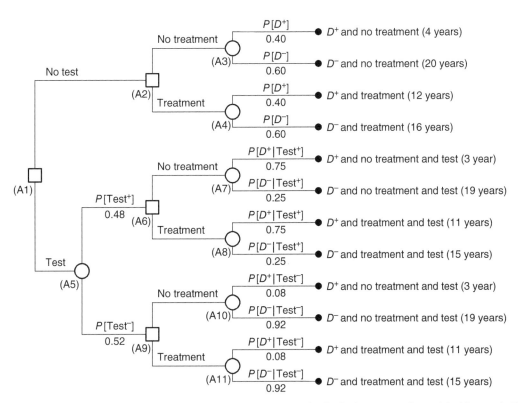

Figure 7.1 Decision tree Problem 1, showing branch probabilities and life expectancies for final outcomes. Copy of decision tree in Figure 6.8.

Clearly, **Test** is the best alternative because 15.0 years is longer than 14.4 years. As long as the expected values are unchanged by the operation, the obvious choice made for this reduced decision tree is the correct choice for the original decision tree.

Therefore, the key to the folding-back operation is how to replace a chance node or a decision node by a single outcome with an equivalent expected value. How this is done depends on the type of node.

Consider the following generic chance node:

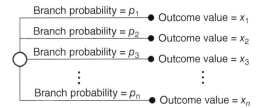

This generic chance node represents an uncertainty that has n possibilities. Each possibility corresponds to a branch probability denoted by $p_1, \ldots, p_n$. In turn, each of the branches leads to outcomes that have the values denoted by $x_1, \ldots, x_n$.

We are only interested in expected values so facing the uncertainty represented by this node would be equivalent to facing a single outcome that has the same expected value. As we saw in the previous chapter, the expected value for a chance node is computed by multiplying each branch probability by the corresponding outcome value and summing the results. That is

$$\text{Expected value} = p_1 \times x_1 + p_2 \times x_2 + \cdots + p_n \times x_n$$

Of course, the expected value for a single outcome is just the value for that outcome. Therefore, we can replace the generic chance node shown earlier by an outcome that has a value equal to the chance node's expected value. Moreover, the replacement will not change the expected value for any decision alternative that leads to this chance node.

Decision nodes are replaced using a similar operation. Consider the following generic decision node:

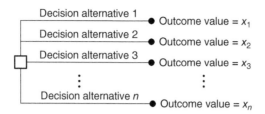

This generic decision node represents a choice between n alternatives. Each alternative is represented by a branch leading to an outcome. The values for those outcomes are denoted by $x_1, \ldots, x_n$.

The goal is to make choices that maximize expected value. Therefore, if faced with the decision represented by this node, the choice would be the outcome with the greatest value. This means a decision node can be replaced the possible outcomes for the node that has the greatest value. As with the chance node, this replacement will not change the expected value computed for any path that leads to this decision node.

The following demonstrates how the folding-back operation uses these two replacement steps to reduce the decision tree shown in Figure 7.1 for Problem 1. Keep in mind that the goal is to determine the life expectancies that would result from choosing either **Test** or **No Test**. Those life expectancies will determine the best alternative for the decision represented by node **A1**.

The folding-back operation starts with the nodes encountered just before the final outcomes. In the case of the decision tree shown in Figure 7.1, these are the chance nodes corresponding to the uncertainty about the disease (chance nodes **A3**, **A4**, **A7**, **A8**, **A10**, and **A11**).

Consider chance node **A3**. This node represents an uncertainty that can result in a life expectancy of 4.0 or 20.0 years. The corresponding branch probabilities are 0.40 and 0.60, respectively. Therefore, the life expectancy for chance node **A3** is:

$$LE = (0.40 \times 4.0 \, \text{years}) + (0.60 \times 20.0 \, \text{years}) = 13.6 \, \text{years}$$

Using the logic described earlier, chance node **A3** can be replaced by an outcome that has a life expectancy of 13.6 years without changing the life expectancies that will be calculated for decision node **A1**.

Figure 7.2 shows the result of repeating this replacement operation for each of the chance nodes representing the disease uncertainty. The result is a simpler decision tree with six fewer nodes. However, this simpler decision tree will still lead to the same life expectancy calculations for decision node **A1**. Therefore, this first step in the folding-back operation has reduced the original decision tree to an equivalent decision tree with six fewer nodes.

At first glance, it may appear that the folding-back operation has eliminated the uncertainty about the disease. That uncertainty originally complicated the treatment decision represented by the tree. In reality, the folding-back operation has incorporated the disease uncertainty into the revised life expectancies for the new final outcomes.

Continuing the folding-back operation, now consider the nodes encountered just before the final outcomes in the reduced decision tree shown in Figure 7.2. These are the decision nodes representing the choice between **Treatment** or **No treatment** (decision nodes **A2**, **A6** and **A9**).

Consider decision node **A2**. This node represents the choice between a life expectancy of 13.6 years and a life expectancy of 14.4 years. Once again, the goal is to maximize life expectancy. Therefore, the decision at node **A2** would be to choose 14.4 years, which corresponds to the **Treatment** alternative. This means that facing the decision represented by

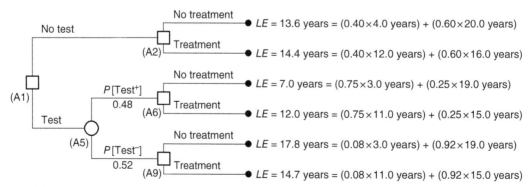

Figure 7.2 Reduced decision tree after step 1 of the folding-back operation is applied to the decision tree in Figure 7.1. The chance nodes for disease uncertainty in Figure 7.1 have been replaced with life expectancies computed for the eliminated chance nodes.

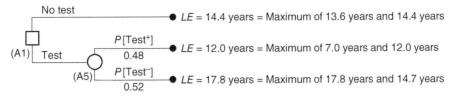

Figure 7.3 Reduced decision tree after step 2 of the folding-back operation is applied to the decision tree in Figure 7.2. The decision nodes for the choice of treatment in Figure 7.2 have been replaced with life expectancies for the best alternative for the eliminated decision nodes.

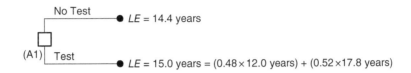

Figure 7.4 Reduced decision tree after step 3 of the folding-back operation is applied to the decision tree in Figure 7.3. The chance nodes for the test result uncertainty in Figure 7.3 have been replaced with life expectancies computed for that chance node.

node **A2** would be equivalent to facing an outcome that has a life expectancy of 14.4 years. Therefore, node **A2** can be replaced with an outcome with a life expectancy of 14.4 years without changing the life expectancies that will be calculated for decision node **A1**.

The decision tree shown in Figure 7.3 has used this logic to replace each of the treatment decision nodes in Figure 7.2. The resulting decision tree is equivalent to the original decision tree but with nine fewer nodes.

Finally, consider chance node **A5** in Figure 7.3. This node represents an uncertainty that can result in a life expectancy of 12.0 or 17.8 years. The corresponding branch probabilities are 0.48 and 0.52, respectively. This means the life expectancy for chance node **A5** is:

$$LE = (0.48 \times 12.0 \text{ years}) + (0.52 \times 17.8 \text{ years}) = 15.0 \text{ years}$$

Therefore, as shown in Figure 7.4, the third step in the folding-back operation results in an equivalent decision tree with a single decision node (**A1**). One of the alternatives for node **A1** is to forgo the test, which has a life expectancy of 14.4 years. The other alternative for node **A1** is to perform the test, which has a life expectancy of 15.0 years. Because 15.0 years is greater than 14.4 years, it follows that the life-expectancy maximizing decision is to have the test.

In summary, the folding-back operation reduces the original decision tree for the problem to an equivalent decision tree with a single decision node. The reduction follows a step-by-step process that replaces each node based on one of the following two operations:

Chance node: Replaced by an outcome with life expectancy equal to the life expectancy computed for the possible outcomes that can follow the node.

Decision node: Replaced by an outcome with life expectancy equal to the maximum life expectancy for the possible alternatives that can be chosen at the node.

In effect, the folding-back operation determines the life expectancy faced at each of the nodes in the decision tree.

Folding-back operation

1. Locate the nodes encountered just prior to a final outcomes in the decision tree. Replace each of those penultimate nodes as follows:
   - In the case of a chance node, replace the node by an outcome with an outcome value that equals the expected value for that node, computed by multiplying the probabilities for the branches emanating from the node by the values for the corresponding final outcomes.
   - In the case of a decision node, replace the node with an outcome that has a value equal to maximum outcome value for all of the final outcomes reachable from the node.
2. If the resulting decision tree consists of a single decision node, the best decision alternative is the alternative corresponding to the greatest outcome value.
3. Otherwise, repeat starting at Step 1.

7.2.2 Chance node ordering revisited

Before applying the folding-back operation to a clinical problem, we will return to the topic of how nodes are ordered in a decision tree. The ordering of nodes in a decision tree often matches the temporal order in which the corresponding uncertainty would be resolved or a decision would be made. Section 6.4.4 described an alternate ordering of the nodes in the arteriography decision tree discussed in Chapter 6. Determining some of the branch probabilities was simpler if the chance node representing the uncertainty about the presence of coronary artery disease was repositioned in the tree. How much flexibility is there in the positioning of a chance node in a decision problem like Problem 1, which involves more than one decision?

For example, Figure 7.1 shows a decision tree for Problem 1 that positions the disease state chance nodes just before the final outcomes. This placement makes sense conceptually because the patient's actual disease state often does not become apparent until the effects of treatment are observed. However, this ordering of the nodes required calculations, both for the test result branch probabilities as well as the branch probabilities for the possible disease state after the test result is known.

Figure 7.5 shows an alternate decision tree for Problem 1. This revised decision tree places the chance node representing the disease state uncertainty chance nodes that would appear to avoid those branch probability calculations. However, the resulting decision tree is called "problematic" for reasons that will become apparent.

Figure 7.6 shows the so-called problematic decision tree after the first step of the folding back operation. For this decision tree, the process starts with the treatment decision nodes since these are positioned just before the final outcomes (decision nodes **D3**, **D4**, **D7**, **D8**, **D10**, and **D11**). In Figure 7.6, each of these decision nodes has been replaced by outcomes with the corresponding maximum life expectancies. For example, decision node **D3** is a choice between a life expectancy of 4.0 and 12.0 years. Therefore, this decision node has been replaced by an outcome with a life expectancy of 12.0 years. Similarly, replacements were made for the other five decision nodes.

Figure 7.7 shows the continuation of the folding back operation. As shown in Figure 7.6, the first step concluded with a decision tree that placed the chance nodes for the test result as the nodes leading to the final outcomes (chance nodes **D6** and **D9**). These two chance nodes are replaced by outcomes with the corresponding life expectancies.

The remaining chance nodes in resulting decision tree (see Figure 7.8) represent the uncertainty about the disease (chance nodes **D2** and **D5**). Once again, these chance nodes are replaced by outcomes with the life expectancies computed for the corresponding node.

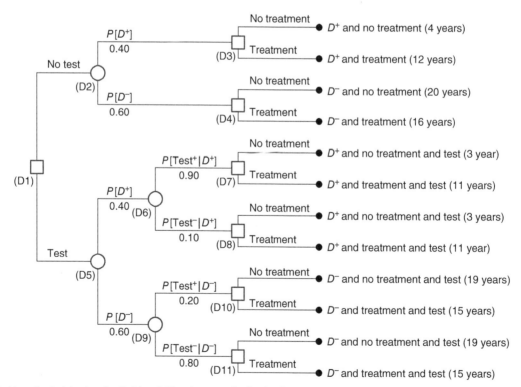

Figure 7.5 Problematic decision tree for Problem 1. The chance nodes for the disease state have been moved to before the treatment decision node.

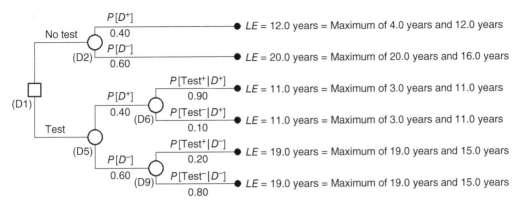

Figure 7.6 Reduced decision tree after step 1 of the folding-back operation is applied to the problematic decision tree shown in Figure 7.5. The decision nodes for the choice of treatment in Figure 7.5 have been replaced with life expectancies for the best alternative for the eliminated decision nodes.

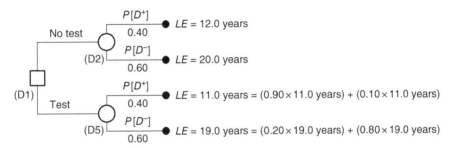

Figure 7.7 Reduced decision tree after step 2 of the folding-back operation is applied to the decision tree in Figure 7.6. The chance nodes for the test result uncertainty in Figure 7.6 have been replaced with life expectancies computed for these chance nodes.

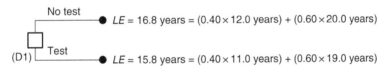

Figure 7.8 Reduced decision tree after step 3 of the folding-back operation is applied to the decision tree in Figure 7.7. The chance nodes for the disease uncertainty in Figure 7.7 have been replaced with life expectancies computed for those chance nodes.

Figure 7.8 shows the problematic decision tree after the third and final step in the folding-back operation. The life expectancies for the chance nodes representing the uncertainty about the disease (nodes **D2** and **D5**) have been computed. The result is a simple choice decision between an option that would lead to a life expectancy of 16.8 years and an option that would lead to a life expectancy of 15.8 years.

The preferred option for the decision posed in Figure 7.8 is clear – the **No test** alternative has a higher life expectancy than the **Test** alternative. However, this result is the opposite of the result determined by folding back the original decision tree for Problem 1. That is why the problematic decision tree is problematic. Moving the disease state chance node to a position before the treatment decision node resulted in a tree that no longer accurately represents the actual decision problem.

In hindsight, the mistake with the problematic decision tree was apparent back in Figure 7.6. This figure showed the decision tree after the first step of the folding back operation. The reduction step determined the optimal treatment decision based on the test result. However, for a given disease state, the same treatment decision is optimal for either test result. In other words, the test result no longer matters. Of course, this makes no sense. Why perform the test if the disease is already known, as implied by the revised decision tree?

The example provided by the problematic decision tree may now seem obvious; however, it illustrates the one rule that must be followed when ordering the nodes in a decision tree. A chance node represents an uncertainty.

The branches originating from the node represent how that uncertainty might be resolved. Therefore, a chance node cannot be placed before a decision node representing a choice that would not be made before that uncertainty would be resolved in the actual decision problem.

Node-ordering rule

When ordering the chance nodes in a decision tree, the relative position of one chance node relative to another chance node is arbitrary. However, the position of chance node A relative to a decision node B must be such that if node A is placed before node B then, in the actual decision problem, the uncertainty represented by node A must be fully resolved before the decision represented by node B would be made.

7.2.3 Two-stage decision in the management of coronary artery disease

We now will use the folding-back operation to analyze a more detailed example involving the management of coronary artery disease. The problem we will analyze extends the arteriography decision example (Problem 2) discussed in the previous chapter.

Definition: Problem 2

Decide whether to order coronary arteriography for a 65-year-old woman with stable angina and who is considering PCI or CABG because of dissatisfaction with drug-based therapy. Assume:

	NO CAD	CAD
Probability of disease state	0.3000	0.7000
Probability of death during arteriography	**0.0001***	0.0010
Probability of death during PCI/CABG	N.A.	0.0295
Life expectancy with no treatment	**19.2 years***	**5.7 years***
Life expectancy with drug-based therapy	**19.2 years***	11.4 years
Life expectancy with PCI/CABG	N.A.	15.2 years

*Low-confidence parameter values.

The extension to Problem 2 analyzed in this chapter adds the optional use of an exercise stress test (EST). We will consider only a small part of what can be learned from this multifaceted test. The results of an exercise stress test will be classified as either "positive" or "negative." A positive result supports a diagnosis of coronary artery disease whereas a negative result contradicts a diagnosis of coronary artery disease. The example also will include the possibility of an indeterminate exercise stress test result. This result occurs when the patient is unable to achieve the necessary exercise level. Table 7.1 shows the probabilities for positive, negative, and indeterminate exercise stress test

Table 7.1 Probability of positive, negative, and indeterminate exercise stress test results conditioned on the patient's disease state.

	Disease state	
Assumption	NO CAD	CAD
Probability exercise stress test result is indeterminate	0.3317	0.2720
Probability exercise stress test result is negative	0.6154	0.3523
Probability exercise stress test result is positive	0.0529	0.3757

Adapted from Bartel et al. (1974).

results, conditioned on the patient's disease state from one of the many published studies of exercise stress testing (Bartel *et al.*, 1974). These measures of the test's diagnostic accuracy will be used in our example.

There is a small chance an exercise stress test will cause the patient's death. In 1980 a national survey of facilities conducting exercise stress tests reported approximately one death per 10 000 tests (Stuart and Ellestad, 1980). As was the case with coronary arteriography, all of the fatal complications with exercise stress testing occurred in patients with confirmed coronary artery disease.

In summary, we will consider the case of the 65-year-old woman, we called Ms. Maple in the preceding chapter. She is thought to have coronary artery disease, although the diagnosis is not certain. This patient's condition currently is managed by a drug-based therapy. Because of poor compliance with this therapy, more aggressive treatment is being considered. Depending on further assessment of Ms. Maple's heart, the more aggressive treatment will either be percutaneous coronary intervention or coronary artery bypass graft surgery. These more aggressive treatments require coronary arteriography. Before proceeding with coronary arteriography, Ms. Maple could first undergo an exercise stress test. This less invasive test could provide information that affects the probability of coronary artery disease for Ms. Maple. We will call this example *Problem 3*.

Definition: Problem 3

Decide whether to order coronary arteriography for a 65-year-old woman with stable angina and who is considering PCI or CABG because of dissatisfaction with drug-based therapy. An exercise stress test also can be ordered and the result used to make the arteriography decision. Assume:

	NO CAD	CAD
Probability of disease state	0.3000	0.7000
Probability of death during arteriography	**0.0001***	0.0010
Probability of death during PCI/CABG	N.A.	0.0295
Life expectancy with no treatment	**19.17 years***	**5.70 years***
Life expectancy with drug-based treatment	**19.17 years***	11.39 years
Life expectancy with PCI/CABG treatment	N.A.	15.21 years
Probability for indeterminate EST result	0.3317	0.2720
Probability negative EST result	0.6154	0.3523
Probability positive EST result	0.0529	0.3757
Probability of death during EST	0.0000	**0.0001***

*Low-confidence parameter values.

7.2.4   Decision tree for two-stage coronary artery disease management decision

Figure 7.9a and b shows a decision tree for Problem 3. This problem requires a more complicated decision tree that no longer fits on a single page. However, portions of the tree have the same structure as the decision tree for Problem 2 discussed in the previous chapter.

Figure 7.10 shows the alternate decision tree that was developed for Problem 2 in the previous chapter. Recall that this version of the tree for Problem 2 placed the chance node representing the uncertainty about Ms. Maple's disease immediately after the arteriography decision node. Referring to Figures 7.9a and 7.9b, which show a portion of the decision tree for Problem 3, notice that after the decision to forgo the exercise stress test, the portion of the tree starting with decision node **E2** is identical to the decision tree for Problem 2 shown in Figure 7.10.

The changes to the decision tree, required by the addition of the exercise stress test decision, start with chance node **E8** in Figure 7.9a. This node represents the uncertainty about Ms. Maple's survival if she undergoes the exercise stress test. Problem 3 assumes this test is not life-threatening if Ms. Maple does not have coronary artery disease. However, there is a small probability (0.0001) that Ms. Maple will die during an exercise stress test if she does have coronary artery disease. Since the probability of coronary artery disease is 0.70 for Ms. Maple, it follows that

$$P\left[\text{Die} \mid EST\right] = P[CAD] \times P\left[\text{Die} \mid EST, CAD\right] = 0.70 \times 0.0001 = 0.00007 \approx 0.0001$$

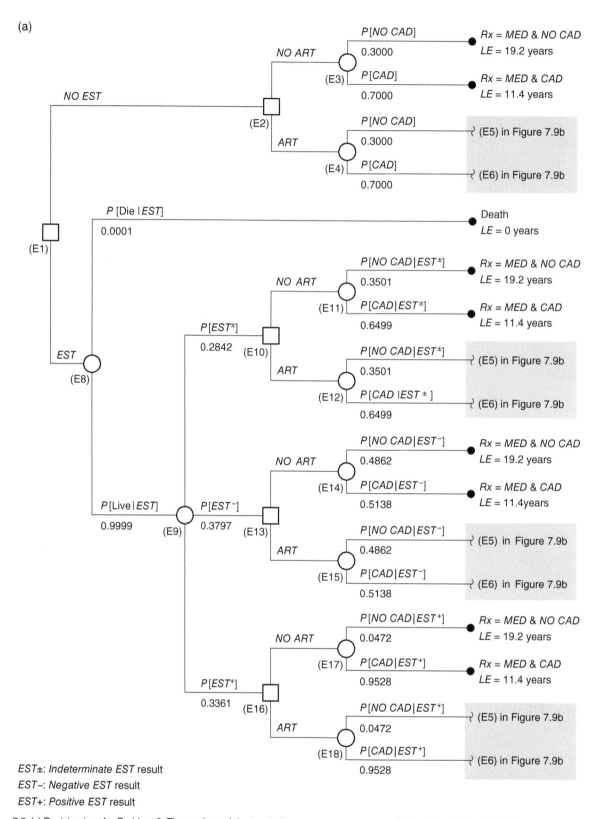

(a)

EST±: *Indeterminate EST result*
EST−: *Negative EST result*
EST+: *Positive EST result*

Figure 7.9 (a) Decision tree for Problem 3. The portions of the tree in the grey regions are expanded in Figure 7.9b. (b) Portions of the decision tree for Problem 3 are not expanded in Figure 7.9a. These expansions are for the portions of the decision tree shown in the grey regions in Figure 7.9a.

(b)

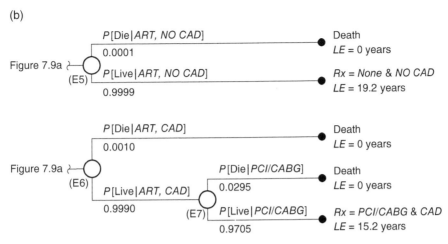

Figure 7.9 (*Continued*)

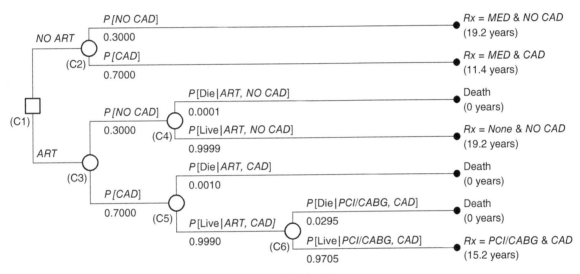

Figure 7.10 Copy of Figure 6.11 showing the alternate decision tree for Problem 2.

Assuming Ms. Maple survives the exercise stress test, chance node **E9** represents the uncertainty about the test result. Recall there are three possibilities: (1) indeterminate result, (2) negative result, and (3) positive result. The following abbreviations are used to conserve space in Figures 7.9a and 7.9b:

$EST^{\pm}$: denotes indeterminate exercise stress test result
EST^{-}: denotes negative exercise stress test result
EST^{+}: denotes positive exercise stress test result

The corresponding branch probabilities are computed using the conditional probabilities provided in the definition for Problem 3. For example,

$$P\left[EST^{\pm}\right] = \left(P\left[EST^{\pm} \mid NO\ CAD\right] \times P\left[NO\ CAD\right]\right) + \left(P\left[EST^{\pm} \mid CAD\right] \times P\left[CAD\right]\right)$$
$$= \left(0.3317 \times 0.3000\right) + \left(0.2639 \times 0.7000\right) = 0.2842$$

Similarly,

$$P\left[EST^{-}\right] = \left(0.6154 \times 0.3000\right) + \left(0.2787 \times 0.7000\right) = 0.3797$$

$$P\left[EST^{+}\right] = \left(0.0529 \times 0.3000\right) + \left(0.4575 \times 0.7000\right) = 0.3361$$

The portion of the tree following chance node **E9** represents the three different arteriography decisions that would be faced after the exercise stress test result is known. These three decisions (decision nodes **E10**, **E13**, and **E16**) each have the same two alternatives **ART** and **NO ART**. What differs between these three decisions is the probability of coronary artery disease given the corresponding exercise stress test result.

For example, decision node **E10** represents the arteriography decision if the exercise stress test result is indeterminate. That test result determines the probabilities for the branches originating from the subsequent disease chance nodes (**E11** and **E12**). We use Bayes' formula from Chapter 4 to compute those branch probabilities:

$$P\left[NO\,CAD\,|\,EST^{\pm}\right] = \frac{P\left[NO\,CAD\right] \times P\left[EST^{\pm}\,|\,NO\,CAD\right]}{P\left[NO\,CAD\right] \times P\left[EST^{\pm}\,|\,NO\,CAD\right] + P\left[CAD\right] \times P\left[EST^{\pm}\,|\,CAD\right]}$$

$$= \frac{0.3000 \times 0.3317}{0.3000 \times 0.3317 + 0.7000 \times 0.2720} = 0.3501$$

which means

$$P\left[CAD\,|\,EST^{\pm}\right] = 1 - P\left[NO\,CAD\,|\,EST^{\pm}\right] = 1 - 0.3501 = 0.6499$$

Similar calculations determine the branch probabilities for the disease chance nodes (**E14**, **E15**, **E17**, and **E18**) following the other two test results.

The remainder of the decision tree for Problem 3 represents the uncertainty about surviving arteriography and the resulting treatment. For example, if Ms. Maple does not undergo coronary arteriography, she will remain on her current drug-based therapy, denoted by $Rx = MED$ in the decision tree. Her actual disease state is denoted by CAD and $NOCAD$ in the decision tree. The corresponding life expectancies in the definition for Problem 3 determine what Ms. Maple's life expectancy will be without arteriography.

On the other hand, if Ms. Maple does undergo arteriography, she faces the small risk to her survival from the procedure. Chance nodes **E5** and **E6** in Figure 7.9b represent this uncertainty. Chance node **E5** represents Ms. Maple's risk of death from the procedure if she does not have coronary artery disease (0.0001). Chance node **E6** represents Ms. Maple's risk of death if she does have coronary artery disease (0.0010).

Arteriography could discover that Ms. Maple does not have coronary artery disease. This would mean she is not a candidate for more aggressive treatment. Moreover, her medical therapy would be discontinued. As discussed in the previous chapter, this would mean she faces the life expectancy that is roughly of a 65-year-old woman in the general population.

If arteriography discovers significant narrowing in her coronary arteries Ms. Maple will undergo either a percutaneous coronary intervention (PCI) or coronary artery bypass graph surgery (CABG), depending on additional assessments of her heart. Chance node **E7** represents the uncertainty about surviving the subsequent treatment. Problem 3 assumes the probability of a perioperative death is 0.0295 for Ms. Maple.

The decision tree for Problem 3 has more nodes and branches than the decision tree for Problem 2. However, more importantly, the life expectancies for the decision options in this more complicated tree can no longer be determined by simply multiplying the branch probabilities on each of the paths. Calculating the outcome probabilities must account for how the exercise stress test affects the subsequent arteriography decision. This requires the folding-back operation.

7.2.5 Folding-back operation applied to two-stage coronary artery disease decision problem

The folding-back operation starts with part 2 of this decision tree, which is reproduced in Figure 7.11. The two fragments of the decision tree shown in Figure 7.11 represent the uncertainty about the consequences of arteriography for Ms. Maple. If Ms. Maple does not have coronary artery disease, the only uncertainty with arteriography is the small probability that she will die during the procedure. Otherwise, arteriography would reveal the patency of Ms. Maple's coronary arteries. This result would indicate that further treatment is unnecessary. Problem 3 assumes Ms. Maple's life expectancy without treatment and with disease would be 19.2 years. Therefore, the life expectancy for node **E5** in Figure 7.11 is determined by the expression.[2]

$$LE = \left(0.0001 \times 0\,\text{years}\right) + \left(0.9999 \times 19.2\,\text{years}\right) = 19.1981\,\text{years}$$

---

[2] The unrealistic number of significant figures are required to show how undergoing arteriography reduces her life expectancy.

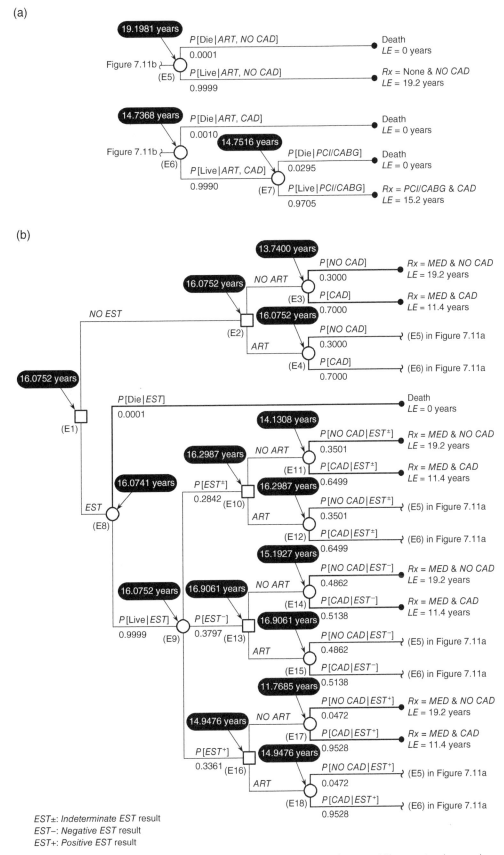

(a)

(b)

EST±: *Indeterminate EST* result
EST−: *Negative EST* result
EST+: *Positive EST* result

Figure 7.11 (a) Folding-back operation applied to part 2 of the decision tree for Problem 3. Computed life expectancies are shown in the black cartouches attached to the nodes. (b) Folding-back operation applied to part 1 of the decision tree for Problem 3. Computed life expectancies are shown in the black cartouches attached to the nodes.

Chance node **E6** represents the slightly more complicated consequences of arteriography if Ms. Maple does have coronary artery disease. She faces a higher risk of dying because of the procedure. Survival will lead to more aggressive treatment, which also implies a risk of death (0.0295). If Ms. Maple survives the procedure, Problem 3 assumes her life expectancy would be 15.2 years. Therefore, the life expectancy for chance node **E6** is

$$LE = (0.9990 \times 0.9705 \times 15.2 \, \text{years}) = 14.7368 \, \text{years}$$

These life expectancies are shown in the black cartouches that have been added to Figure 7.11. Figure 7.11b shows the similar folding-back operations applied to the rest of the decision tree for Problem 3.

7.2.6 Conclusion of the folding-back operation

If life expectancies expressed with four significant figures can be believed, the preferred alternative for decision node **E1** is to forgo the exercise stress test. That is because the life expectancy for *NO EST* is 16.0752 years whereas the life expectancy for *EST* is 16.0741 years. Of course, the difference between the two life expectancies is less than 10 hours for Ms. Maple. A difference this small is far less than the precision of the approximations assumed for this problem.

Therefore, the analysis is showing that exercising stress testing would have virtually no effect on Ms. Maple's outcome. This is surprising. Problem 3 represents the exercise stress test as costless procedure, with no risk of morbidity to Ms. Maple and almost no risk of death. One would expect that the information provided by such a test should provide at least some benefit to Ms. Maple.

Later chapters provide a more detailed analysis of how testing affects outcomes; however, note the following in Figure 7.11b. Focusing on the arteriography decision represented by decision node **E2**, having arteriography is the preferred option for Ms. Maple if she does not have an exercise stress test. Decision nodes **E10**, **E13**, and **E16** show the same decision based on the exercise test result. For these decision nodes, arteriography is preferred, regardless of the test result. In other words, the exercise stress test does not affect Ms. Maple's decision. This means the test's only effect on her life expectancy is the minimal risk of fatal complications if she has coronary artery disease. That minimal risk amounts to the 10-hour reduction in her life expectancy.

7.2.7 Comment on number of significant figures used in calculations

Perhaps, this would be a good place to discuss the number of significant figures that will be shown for parameter values and calculations. Confidence in most parameter values seldom justifies more than one or two numbers to the right of the decimal point. The probability of 0.0001 for exercise stress test fatalities, is an exception since this number is derived from a national survey involving approximately half a million tests (Stuart and Ellestad, 1980). However, most other probabilities are derived from prevalence observed in populations that include at most a few thousand patients. This means that any conclusions reached by decision tree analysis should be based on final results that have been rounded to, at best, the nearest hundredths, or even the nearest tenths. For example, a final probability should be expressed in parts per hundred and a final life expectancy should be expressed in tenths of a year.

On the other hand, prematurely rounding the parameter values used to calculate those final results will conceal differences that could lead to valid conclusions about a decision problem. Representing the risk during exercise stress testing is an example. In order to be consistent with the lower precision for the other probabilities, this risk might be rounded to zero. However, doing so would eliminate an important consideration for patients who actually have coronary artery disease since these are the patients who might die during the procedure.

Therefore, the following convention will be adopted in this book. Normally probabilities used as parameter values, or as the results of intermediate calculations, will be expressed in parts per ten thousand. In other words, these probabilities will be shown with four digits to the right of the decimal point. Similarly, lengths of life or a life expectancy normally will be expressed as hundredths of a year. Exceptions will be made when necessary to show the differences between two calculated life expectancies. On the other hand, a final outcome probability always will be expressed with two digits to the right of the decimal point. Similarly, a final life expectancy will be expressed with one digit to the right of the decimal point or a tenth of a year.

7.3 Sensitivity analysis

Returning to the conclusion of the folding-back operation, recall that some of the values for the life expectancies and probabilities used in the decision tree for Problem 3 have limited empirical support. We called those the *low confidence parameter values*. For example, death during arteriography for a patient with a healthy heart is extremely rare.

Undoubtedly, it can happen. However, none was reported in the study used to estimate the risk of death during arteriography (Peterson *et al.*, 2010). All patients with fatal complications in that study had coronary artery disease. Therefore, our decision tree analysis assumed the risk of death during arteriography for a disease-free patient is 10% of what was reported for patients with diseased hearts. Of course, that is just a guess. Similarly, Ms. Maple's life expectancy, if she does not have coronary artery disease and she does not receive treatment, probably falls somewhere between 19.2 and 24.2 years. The analysis assumed the lower bound for this range.

Questionable assumptions about the values for parameters are inevitable in the analysis of any real medical decision. Indeed, coronary artery disease was chosen for the examples in these chapters because this disease has been so widely studied. The resulting reports comprise a large body of empirical evidence for determining the required parameter values for analyzing the management of this common disease. In contrast, most medical decisions involve uncertainties that are less well characterized. Even when a relevant study does exist, its application to a specific patient's decision often requires some adjustment. Estimating Ms. Maple's life expectancy when she is disease free is an example.

A process called *sensitivity analysis* can determine the importance of a low confidence parameter value. Precise knowledge about the values for these parameters may not be necessary to make a credible comparison of the alternatives in a decision problem. The systematic examination of how possible values for the parameter in question affect the final analysis can determine when this is the case. In other words, we can determine the sensitivity of the analysis to the values for the problematic parameter. Our exploration of this important component to decision tree analysis will begin with Problem 2 which was analyzed in the previous chapter.

> **Definition: sensitivity analysis**
>
> The systematic exploration of how uncertainty about an estimated value affects the analysis of a decision.

7.3.1   One-way sensitivity analysis for simple decision problems

We will start our exploration of sensitivity analysis with Problem 2. Recall that Problem 2 concerned the decision to perform coronary artery disease on a patient who probably had coronary artery disease. The invasive diagnostic procedure was being considered because of the possibility that the patient should have a more aggressive treatment. Problem 2 is chosen as the starting point for the discussion of sensitivity analysis because this problem has only one decision node. We will see that sensitivity analysis is easiest for problems with only one decision node. For this reason, we called Problem 2 a *simple* decision problem.

Figure 7.12 demonstrates sensitivity analysis for Ms. Maple's disease-free life expectancy, which is one of the questionable parameter values in Problem 2. Recall that actuarial data for 65-year-old women would place her life expectancy at 24.2 years. The CASS study data implied a 19.2-year life expectancy if Ms. Maple is disease free.

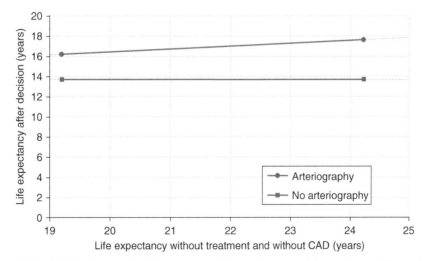

Figure 7.12 Sensitivity analysis for Problem 2 comparing life expectancy with arteriography to life expectancy without arteriography, for possible values of Ms. Maple's life expectancy when she receives no treatment and does not have coronary artery disease.

Figure 7.12 shows how Ms. Maple's overall life expectancy with and without arteriography changes with the value for her disease-free life expectancy. The horizontal axis shows the range of possible values for the disease-free life expectancy. The vertical axis shows the corresponding life expectancies with and without arteriography. The leftmost points on the two curves correspond to the value assumed in the analysis for Ms. Maple's disease-free life expectancy.

Notice that the curve representing the decision to undergo arteriography always falls above the curve for the decision to not undergo arteriography. Therefore, the recommendation that Ms. Maple should have arteriography is not affected by the value for this problematic parameter. That is, we have shown that the conclusion of the decision tree analysis is not sensitive to the range of reasonable values for Ms. Maple's disease-free life expectancy.

The trick to drawing sensitivity analysis curves for a simple decision tree is recognizing that these curves always are straight lines when the parameter under examination is a branch probability or an outcome value. The curves are straight lines because the life expectancy calculation is what mathematicians call a linear function of the values used in the decision tree. This means the increase in the contribution of the parameter to the life expectancy calculation is proportional to the value of the parameter. Doubling the parameter value doubles the contribution.

For example, recall the expression, from the previous chapter, used to compute Ms. Maple's life expectancy if she has arteriography:

$$LE[ART] = (0.3000 \times 0.0001 \times 0 \text{ years}) + (0.3000 \times 0.9999 \times 19.17 \text{ years}) + (0.7000 \times 0.0010 \times 0 \text{ years})$$
$$+ (0.7000 \times 0.9990 \times 0.0295 \times 0 \text{ years}) + (0.7000 \times 0.9990 \times 0.9705 \times 15.21 \text{ years})$$
$$= 16.06 \text{ years}$$

The value for Ms. Maple's disease-free life expectancy (19.2 years) is shown with a boldface font in this expression. With a little arithmetic, this expression becomes

$$LE[ART] = 0 + (0.3000 \times 19.17 \text{ years}) + 0 + 0 + 10.31 \text{ years}$$
$$= 16.06 \text{ years}$$

which simplifies to

$$LE[ART] = 0.3000 \times \mathbf{19.17 \text{ years}} + 10.31 \text{ years}$$

Therefore, the contribution of Ms. Maple's disease-free life expectancy to her overall life expectancy with arteriography is

$$0.3000 \times \mathbf{19.17 \text{ years}} = 5.31 \text{ years}$$

If Ms. Maple's disease-free life expectancy is doubled to 38.34 years, the contribution to her overall life expectancy with arteriography also doubles:

$$0.3000 \times \mathbf{28.34 \text{ years}} = 10.62 \text{ years}$$

In other words, the contribution of this parameter to Ms. Maple's life expectancy is proportional to the value of the parameter. In turn, this proportionality makes the corresponding curve a straight line. This means that only two points are needed to determine one of the curves in Figure 7.12, such as 19.2 and 24.2 years.

Note that the two curves in Figure 7.12 are not parallel. This means that for some values of the disease-free life expectancy, the corresponding values for LE[ART] and LE[NO ART] will cross, which in turn means that the preferred option will switch from ordering the arteriography to forgoing the arteriography. The crossover occurs when the value for LE[ART] equals the value for LE[NO ART]. A little algebra can be used to determine this crossover – or threshold – value for the parameter.

In general, let X denote the parameter of interest in the sensitivity analysis. For example, in Figure 7.12, X is Ms. Maple's disease-free life expectancy. Let $X1$ and $X2$ be two possible values for X, such as $X1$ equals 19.2 years and $X2$ equals 24.2 years. Finally, let X^* denote the threshold value the parameter. Also, let $T1$ and $T2$ denote two possible treatment options. The corresponding life expectancies for these two treatments can be denoted $LE[T1, X]$ and $LE[T2, X]$ for a given value of X. The threshold value for the parameter X is determined by setting $LE[T1, X]$ equal to $LE[T1, X]$ and solving for X. The result is the following messy expression

$$X^* = \frac{(X1 \times (LE[T1, X2] - LE[T2, X2])) - (X2 \times (LE[T1, X1] - LE[T2, X1]))}{(LE[T1, X2] - LE[T2, X2]) - (LE[T1, X1] - LE[T2, X1])}$$

This expression can be simplified by setting

$$\Delta(X) = LE[T1 \mid X] - LE[T2 \mid X]$$

For example, $\Delta(X)$ is the vertical distance between the two curves in Figure 7.12 for a given value of the parameter X. The expression for the threshold value can then be written as

$$X^* = \frac{(X1 \times \Delta(X2)) - (X2 \times \Delta(X1))}{\Delta(X2) - \Delta(X1)}$$

When the parameter X is a probability, it is natural to pick the values $X1 = 0.0$ and $X2 = 1.0$. In this case, the threshold expression reduces to

$$X^* = \frac{\Delta(X1)}{\Delta(X1) - \Delta(X2)}$$

A version of this last expression for X^* will reappear in Chapter 13 in the discussion of threshold probabilities and test selection.

Returning to the sensitivity analysis for Ms. Maple's disease and treatment-free life expectancy, from Figure 7.12

$$\Delta(19.2\,\text{years}) = 16.1\,\text{years} - 13.7\,\text{years} = 2.3\,\text{years}$$

$$\Delta(24.2\,\text{years}) = 17.6\,\text{years} - 13.7\,\text{years} = 3.9\,\text{years}$$

Inserting these values into the expression for the X^*

$$X^* = \frac{(X1 \times \Delta(X2)) - (X2 \times \Delta(X1))}{\Delta(X2) - \Delta(X1)} = \frac{(19.2\,\text{years} \times 3.9\,\text{years}) - (24.2\,\text{years} \times 2.3\,\text{years})}{3.9\,\text{years} - 2.3\,\text{years}}$$

$$= 11.4\,\text{years}$$

In other words, in order for the decision tree recommendation to switch from ordering arteriography to forgoing arteriography, Ms. Maple's disease-free life expectancy would have to be less than what her life expectancy would be if she had coronary artery disease and it was treated by placement of a stent or bypass surgery (15.2 years), which clearly is not the case. Therefore, for Problem 2, the recommendations of the decision tree analysis would not be changed by plausible values for Ms. Maples' disease and treatment-free life expectancy.

7.3.2   Two-way sensitivity analysis for simple decision problems

The sensitivity analysis summarized in Figure 7.12 demonstrates the effects of varying the value for a single parameter. However, some decision tree parameters might be linked so that changes in one parameter affect the value of the other parameter. In this case, two-way analysis, in which two parameters are varied, is required.

Figure 7.13 shows another one-way sensitivity analysis, this time for the risk of death during arteriography if Ms. Maple does have coronary artery disease. Problem 2 assumes that the risk of death during arteriography depends on Ms. Maple's disease state. If she has coronary artery disease, the probability of death during the procedure is estimated to be 0.0010. There are no large studies of fatal complications for disease-free patients undergoing arteriography. Therefore, Problem 2 assumes that the risk of death during the procedure is 0.0001 if Ms. Maple does not have coronary artery disease.

Notice in Figure 7.13 that the threshold for switching between preferring arteriography or no arteriography is a probability of 0.2271. In other words, switching to no arteriography would require a risk of death for diseased patients that is over 200 times what is reported in the literature. In this analysis, the risk of death during arteriography if Ms. Maple does not have coronary artery disease has been held constant at 0.0001.

It follows that the decision to prefer arteriography would not be affected by reasonable values in the two model parameters tested in Figures 7.12 and 7.13. But what if both of these parameters changed? Could it be possible that no arteriography would become the preferred alternative for a combination of different values for the risk of death from arteriography with and without coronary artery disease?

Figure 7.14 shows a two-way sensitivity analysis that explores the answer to this question. The light-colored surface in this figure shows how life expectancy with arteriography varies for combinations of values for the risk of death with and without coronary artery disease. The dark-colored surface shows how life expectancy without arteriography varies for combinations of values for the risk of death with and without coronary artery disease.

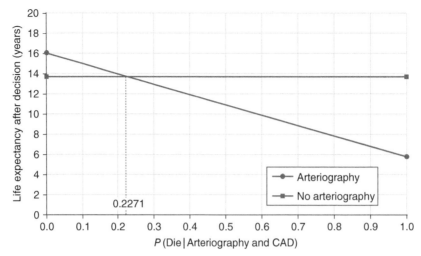

Figure 7.13 Sensitivity analysis for Problem 2 comparing life expectancy with arteriography to life expectancy without arteriography for possible values for the risk of arteriography death if Ms. Maple has coronary artery disease.

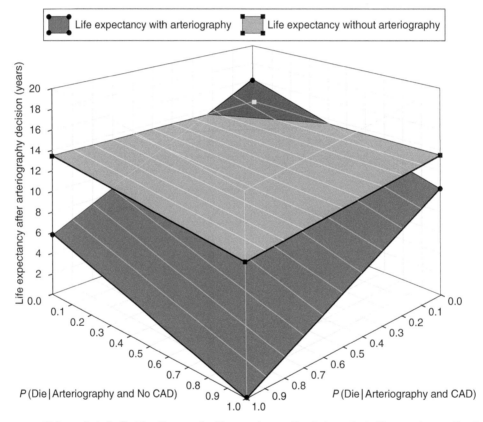

Figure 7.14 Two-way sensitivity analysis for Problem 2 comparing life expectancy with arteriography to life expectancy without arteriography for possible probabilities of death because of arteriography, with and without coronary artery disease.

Notice in Figure 7.14 that the curves for the life expectancies have changed from lines to surfaces. However, the same linearity trick used to draw the figure for the one-way analysis also applies to two-way analysis. The two surfaces were drawn by setting a value for the risk of death from arteriography with coronary artery disease and then conducting a one-way sensitivity analysis for the other parameter – the risk of death from arteriography without coronary artery disease. The resulting intersection between the two surfaces indicates that arteriography is always the preferred alternative given the small risks of death for the procedure located in the back corner of the figure.

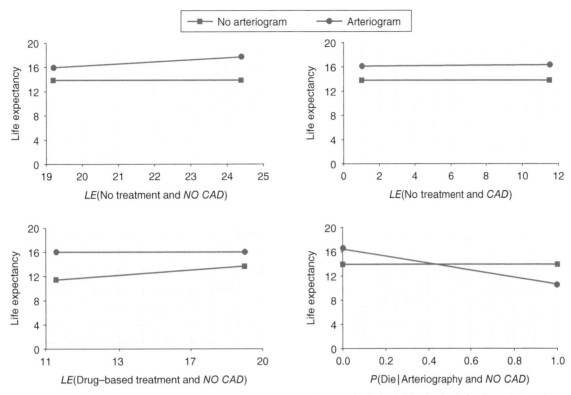

Figure 7.15 One-way sensitivity analysis for parameters in the definition for Problem 2 with limited objective basis for determining value.

Returning to the definition for Problem 2, recall the four problematic parameter values were shown with a boldface font. Figure 7.15 shows the one-way sensitivity analysis for each of these parameters. The analysis of the risk of arteriography death has already been discussed. There would be no change in recommendation for reasonable values for any of the other three parameters. Therefore, reasonable values for the four problematic parameters would not change the conclusion that arteriography is the preferred option for Ms. Maple.

7.3.3 Sensitivity analysis for problems with two decisions

Sensitivity analysis for problems involving more than one decision is more complicated because life expectancy no longer varies linearly with respect to the model parameters. The goal of sensitivity analysis is still the same – determine if changes in the value used for a problematic parameter will affect the recommendation. However, because the relationship between life expectancy and parameters is no longer linear, the life expectancy curves must be evaluated at multiple points, rather than just two points.

Figure 7.16 illustrates this behavior for Problem 3. The curve in Figure 7.15 shows how life expectancy without an exercise stress test varies with changes in the probability of death from arteriography if the patient has coronary artery disease. Notice the point where the probability of arteriography death equals 0.2271. This value coincides with the threshold value in Figure 7.13. Recall that the curves in Figure 7.13 showed a preference for undergoing arteriography if the chance of death from the procedure is low. With a low arteriography risk, the survival benefits of the changing treatment outweigh the risks of the procedure. Those benefits decrease as the risk of arteriography death increases. At some point, the risk of dying from the procedure exceeds the possible benefits of the treatment change. This switch between the two arteriography options results in the change in slope for the curve in Figure 7.16.

Therefore, when analyzing a complex decision tree with more than one decision node, the life expectancy for a decision option may depend on the threshold values where subsequent decisions in the problem switch between their alternatives. This was easy to determine for the option of forgoing the exercise stress test. Finding the threshold can be more complicated for other options. Sensitivity analysis applied to problems with multiple decisions can be difficult.

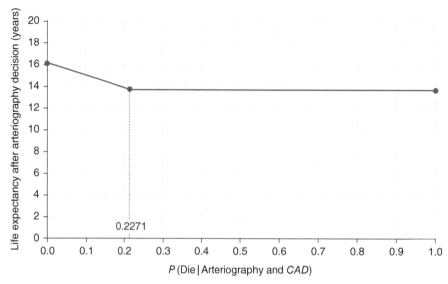

Figure 7.16 Life expectancy with exercise stress test in Problem 3, for possible values of the risk of arteriography death if Ms. Maple has coronary artery disease.

7.3.4 Sensitivity analysis and clinical policies

This chapter has used an individual patient's problem to illustrate decision tree analysis. In principle, the same analysis could be applied to any challenging clinical decision. However, drawing individual decision trees for each patient's decision and estimating the necessary branch probabilities is not practical in most clinical settings. Currently, the important application of these methods is the development of clinical policies or practice guidelines that are applied to populations rather than individuals. Presumably, those policies or guidelines are designed to optimize the care of the individuals in the population in much the same way as Ms. Maple's decision was optimized in this chapter.

Later chapters in this book will discuss the development of clinical policies; however, the principles are similar to the analysis that has been applied to the hypothetical Ms. Maple. Sensitivity analysis plays a crucial role in the extension of this analysis to policy development. A physician caring for an individual patient only needs to determine the parameter values that represent what that physician and that patient believe. Ideally, those opinions will reflect the available data, but decisions are still made in the absence of data. Given enough time, and attention to the cognitive biases discussed in Chapter 3, subjective probability assessment can be used to fill in the gaps in the available data.

This is less true for policy development. Expert opinion still plays a role in policy development; however, the trend is toward evidence-based policies that derive their credibility from the use of data-based probabilities. Sensitivity analysis can extend the reach of evidence-based policy development by showing when missing data does not affect the validity of the recommended policies.

Summary

This chapter has focused on the use of decision trees to analyze medical decisions.

- When the goal is maximization of the patient's life expectancy, the folding-back operation can be used to determine the optimal decision. The folding-back operation reduces the original decision tree to an equivalent trivial decision tree using a step-by-step process that replaces each node using one of the following two processes:
  Chance node: Replaced by an outcome with life expectancy equal to the life expectancy computed for the possible outcomes that can follow the node.
  Decision node: Replaced by an outcome with life expectancy equal to the maximum life expectancy for the possible alternatives that can follow the node.
- When ordering the chance nodes in a decision tree, the relative position of one chance node relative to another chance node is arbitrary. However, the position of chance node A relative to a decision node B must be such that if node A is placed before node B, then, in the actual decision problem, the uncertainty represented by node A must be fully resolved before the decision represented by node B would be made.

- Sensitivity analysis is the systematic exploration of how uncertainty about the value of a branch probability or life expectancy affects the conclusion reached by analyzing the decision tree.
- In the case of decision problems with a single decision node, the life expectancy computed for a decision varies linearly with the value for any single model parameter. This means that one-way sensitivity analysis for simple decision problems requires evaluation of the decision tree for only two values of the model parameter in question. Linearity does not necessarily apply to the problem that involves multiple decisions.

Epilogue

Some readers might be troubled by the policy implications of the examples used in this chapter. These examples clearly show a strong preference for the use of coronary arteriography in the evaluation of Ms. Maple. The corresponding policy would recommend an expensive diagnostic procedure, involving significant morbidity and discomfort, for any 65-year-old woman with the symptoms of stable angina and a 70% chance of having coronary artery disease. Indeed, one-way sensitivity analysis, applied to the probability of coronary artery disease, finds a threshold probability of 0.04. In other words, the policy would recommend arteriography for virtually any 65-year-old woman with the symptoms of stable angina. Most would consider this to be an overly aggressive policy for management of a very common disease.

The shortcomings of the analysis leading to this troubling conclusion partly are the dependence on life expectancy as an outcome measure. Length of life is important to most patients. However, even ignoring the complicated issue of cost, patients also want healthcare that optimizes the quality of their lives. Most patients also would like to avoid risk. A low-risk good outcome often is preferred to a higher-risk better outcome. The simple idea of measuring outcomes by the corresponding life expectancy misses these considerations.

The next three chapters will show how to extend decision tree analysis to incorporate a more complete view of how outcomes are valued by those who will have to live with the results of the decisions that are made.

Bibliography

Bartel, A.G., Behar, V.S., Peter, R.H. *et al.* (1974) Graded exercise stress tests in angiographically documented coronary artery disease. *Circulation*, **49**, 348–56.

Peterson, E.D., Dai, D., DeLong, E.R. *et al.* (2010) Contemporary mortality risk prediction for percutaneous coronary intervention: results from 588,398 procedures in the national cardiovascular data registry. *Journal of the American College of Cardiology*, **55**, 1923–32.

Stuart, R. and Ellestad, M.H. (1980) National survey of exercise stress testing facilities. *Chest*, **77**, 94–7.

CHAPTER 8

Outcome utility – representing risk attitudes

8.1 Introduction

This chapter describes risk attitudes and their role in medical decision making. Our risk attitudes determine how our preferences are affected by uncertainty. For example, suppose that a choice must be made between the following two options:

Option A: Receive one million dollars
Option B: Receive two million dollars if the toss of a fair coin lands heads up

Behavioral psychologists who study decision making find that people usually prefer Option A over Option B. That is not surprising. Winning two million dollars would be nice but most of us would prefer to settle for the one million dollars because that choice avoids the possibility the tossed coin will land tails up, leaving us with nothing.

Preference for Option A over Option B demonstrates a type of risk attitude that is called *risk aversion*. Option A is preferred to Option B because the latter has a risky outcome. More concisely, Option A is preferred to Option B even though both have the same expected value of winning one million dollars. With Option A receiving that expected value is certain. With Option B the same expected value comes with the risk of receiving nothing. Most of us choose Option A because we want to avoid the risk of Option B.

> **Definition: risk attitudes with monetary outcomes**
>
> Risk attitudes are how preferences for alternatives are affected by the uncertainty in those alternatives. In the case of monetary outcomes, an individual is *risk averse* if they prefer receiving the expected value of a gamble over the gamble itself.

To understand the role of risk attitudes in medicine, consider the treatment decision faced by someone like Ms. Maple in Chapters 6 and 7. Ms. Maple probably has coronary artery disease. Some types of coronary artery disease are best treated by surgery because longer life is more likely than would be expected with less invasive treatments, like drug-based management. However, treatments involving surgery also include a risk of perioperative death for Ms. Maple. Choosing surgery would mean accepting that risk in exchange for a greater likelihood of still being alive in 10 years.

Medical Decision Making, Third Edition. Harold C. Sox, Michael C. Higgins, Douglas K. Owens, and Gillian Sanders Schmidler.
© 2024 John Wiley & Sons Ltd. Published 2024 by John Wiley & Sons Ltd.

Ms. Maple certainly would like to be alive in 10 years. This means she agrees that the increased long-term survival with successful surgical treatment is an advantage. However, avoiding an immediate perioperative death might also be very important to Ms. Maple. The pending completion of a major project she has led at work, the expected birth of a grandchild, and even the arrival of Spring after a hard Winter – these are all possible reasons why Ms. Maple might want to minimize the risk of her death in the near term. Clearly, a decision about Ms. Maple's care should respect her desire to avoid a near-term risk to her life. The challenge is how to balance her concerns about that near-term risk with her desire to live a longer life.

This chapter describes how to assign values to outcomes so that risk attitudes are reflected in the analysis of a decision. In the previous two chapters, recall how outcome values were combined with outcome probabilities to calculate an expected value for each alternative in a decision problem. The decision analysis described in those earlier chapters identified the best alternative based on which alternative had the greatest expected value. Those examples used the patient's length of life for the outcome values in the calculations. This meant the analysis found the alternative that maximized the patient's life expectancy.

One problem with life expectancy analysis is its indifference toward how Ms. Maple might feel about the risks in the options she faces. As an extreme example, suppose Ms. Maple was choosing between living 9 years for certain or risking a 50% chance of dying today in exchange for a guaranteed 20 years of life if she survives the risk. The life expectancy for the first option is 9 years whereas the life expectancy for the second option is 0.5 times 20, or 10 years. Therefore, life expectancy analysis would recommend the second option even though it would mean a significant chance that Ms. Maple would not live to see the sun rise tomorrow.

The discussion in this chapter describes a published study of how actual patients felt about the balance of near-term risks versus long-term benefits in a real treatment decision. The study demonstrated that, depending on individual attitudes toward risk, some patients preferred the treatment that minimized near-term risk whereas other patients were willing to accept near-term risk in exchange for better long-term survival. The comparison in this study borrowed a concept from economics called *utility*. The calculations in the study used utility, rather than length of life, to represent the outcome values for comparing the treatment options faced by these patients.

The word "utility" may sound familiar to readers who took economics in college. Economists use a concept they call "utility" to explain how supply and demand drive market behavior. That utility concept differs from the utility concept described in this chapter. In formal terms, this chapter is about what is called *von-Neumann-Morgenstern utility*, named after the mathematician and economist who first proposed its use in the analysis of decisions involving uncertainty.

The focus of this chapter is on the conceptual foundations for using utility to analyze decisions. The next chapter describes the mathematics that could turn the concept of utility into a clinically useful tool. A third chapter concludes the discussion of utility by showing how the analysis can be adjusted to reflect the patient's concerns about the quality of their life.

8.2   What are risk attitudes?

Returning to the choice between Option A and Option B in the introduction, consider how we might quantify risk aversion in the world of monetary gambles. Figure 8.1 represents that choice as a decision tree. One approach to quantifying risk aversion would be to change the option based on the coin toss (Option B) to include a bonus of X dollars that would be paid regardless of how the coin landed. Suppose that an individual was risk averse, meaning they preferred the option without the coin toss (Option A) when X equals zero. Undoubtedly, this same individual would switch to preferring Option B if the bonus X was one million dollars, since then either outcome of the coin toss would be at least

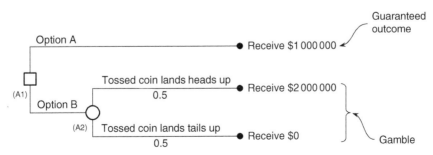

Figure 8.1 Decision tree illustrating risk aversion with a monetary gamble.

as good as Option A. As the value for X is reduced from one million, at some point, the individual would switch back to referring Option A with its guaranteed outcome of one million dollars.

The value for X, where that switch takes place, quantifies this individual's risk aversion. For some individuals, the value for X where Option B becomes the preferred option is close to one million. We might call these individuals highly risk averse. Others would choose Option B for values of X closer to zero. These individuals have lower risk aversion.

This approach to quantifying risk attitudes can reveal how individuals differ when it comes to the importance they place on the risks they might face in a decision problem. The next section describes a study that demonstrated how quantifying risk attitudes applies to medical decisions.

8.2.1 Risk-tolerant preferences

However, before moving on to a medical example, some mention first should be made of what are called *risk-tolerant* preferences. These are the risk attitudes demonstrated by someone who chooses Option B over Option A. In other words, a risk-tolerant individual, when faced with a choice between the two options in Figure 8.1, would choose the gamble over the guaranteed outcome.

Risk tolerance is the often-misunderstood twin of risk aversion. The confusion partly derives from the different reasons for choosing risky alternatives. Some risk-tolerant behavior is motivated by an attraction to the risk itself. In the extreme, this behavior can lead to habitual gambling – a behavior that has damaged countless lives. For this reason, risk tolerance sometimes is known by the more judgmental labels of "risk seeking" or "risk preferring."

However, a risk-tolerant individual might also be someone who simply places more importance on the good outcomes possible with a risky alternative. Consider the choice between Option A and Option B from the perspective of a small business owner facing bankruptcy because of a $1.5 million debt. Choosing Option A would only add to what the business owner will lose in the bankruptcy settlement. On the other hand, Option B could keep the business alive. This individual would not be foolish to choose the risky possibility of Option B over the certainty of Option A. That risk-tolerant individual is not seeking the risk they are choosing. They simply are in a situation where the possible good outcome of Option B is more important than the possible bad outcome.

Unfortunately, patients sometimes find themselves in similar situations. Consider the case of an otherwise healthy young person who unexpectedly finds themselves diagnosed with a highly aggressive cancer that will not respond to established treatments. Suddenly, the promise of the future is lost for this unfortunate patient. Would it not be reasonable for this patient to accept a highly risky experimental treatment, even if the low probability of a cure meant an overall life expectancy that is less than the few months they would otherwise live?

> **Definition: risk-tolerant preferences with monetary outcomes**
>
> An individual is *risk tolerant* if they prefer the gamble over receiving the expected value of the gamble.

Medical decisions usually are not as dramatic as what is faced by that young person with an aggressive cancer. However, risk is a common element in many patient care decisions. How we feel about risk – our risk attitudes – is how we can differ as individuals. The fundamental premise of the methods described in these chapters is that whenever possible, the analysis of decisions should reflect those differences.

8.3 Demonstration of risk attitudes in a medical context

In 1978, Barbara McNeil, Ralph Weichselbaum, and Stephen Pauker published a study in the New England Journal of Medicine demonstrating the effects of risk attitudes on treatment decisions (McNeil *et al.*, 1978). Their paper titled, "The Fallacy of the Five-Year Survival in Lung Cancer," explored how patients felt about the risks involved in lung cancer treatments.

At the time of the study, two options were available for the treatment of Stage I or Stage II lung cancer. One treatment was a surgical procedure with a substantial perioperative mortality rate. At that time, lung cancer perioperative mortality rates in older patients varied from 5 to 20%. Combined with the risk of perioperative death, the overall 5-year survival rate for surgical treatment was reported to range from 24 to 33%. The other treatment at the time of McNeil's study was radiotherapy. This option avoided the risk of perioperative death but also had a lower 5-year survival rate of only 21%.

Therefore, the advantage of the surgical treatment was a better 5-year survival rate and a longer life expectancy. However, that advantage came with a higher risk of near-term death. The focus of the McNeil study was to determine how patient preferences for length of life affected the choice between these two treatments.

8.3.1   Depicting choice of lung cancer treatment as a decision tree

The tree shown in Figure 8.2 depicts the decision faced by patients with lung cancer at the time of the study. Both treatment options resulted in an uncertain length of life. That uncertainty is represented by branch probabilities for the different number of years the patient might live. Note that the outcomes in the decision tree are represented by years of life. Therefore, the decision tree assumes the patient will live exactly 1, 2, or 3 years, and so forth, following treatment. Because of the risk of perioperative death, the branches emanating from the surgery chance node (**B3**) include a branch leading to the outcome of immediate death. With this outcome, the patient would live 0 years.

Figure 8.2 only shows a portion of the possible outcomes for the decision tree. Assuming an age of 60 years, the patient might live another 45 years. Therefore, a full rendering of the decision tree would show at least 45 outcomes for each of the two treatment alternatives.

8.3.2   Branch probabilities for the lung cancer treatment decision

The complex tree for this decision might be difficult to show on a single page, but it is easy to analyze. Figure 8.3 shows the survival curves for a 60-year-old man undergoing either of the two treatments. The survival curve shown for surgery assumes a 10% risk of perioperative death. The life expectancies for these two survival curves are 6.7 years for surgery and 6.3 years for radiotherapy.

The two survival curves in Figure 8.3 can determine the corresponding branch probabilities for the decision tree. How this is done will be described in a later chapter; however, that process is straightforward. The resulting branch probabilities become the outcome probabilities for the possible lengths of life. Combining those outcome probabilities with outcome values to produce an expected value for each treatment option requires only simple arithmetic. The challenge is how to select outcome values that reflect the patient's risk attitudes.

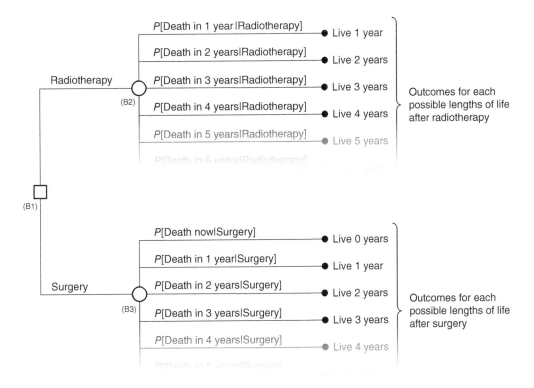

Figure 8.2 Decision tree for choice between radiotherapy and surgery for treatment of Stage I or Stage II lung cancer.

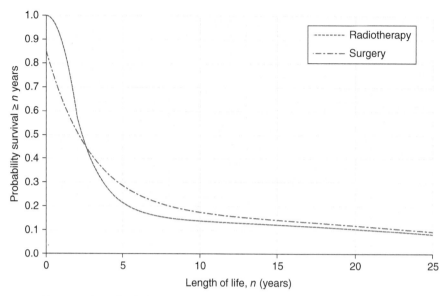

Figure 8.3 Survival curves used in comparison of radiotherapy and surgical treatment for a 60-year-old male lung cancer patient, assuming a perioperative mortality rate of 10%.

8.3.3 von Neumann-Morgenstern utility and the outcome values

A key step in the study undertaken by McNeil and her colleagues was assigning outcome values that quantify a patient's risk attitudes. They used a discovery of John von Neumann and Oskar Morgenstern to complete this step. Von Neumann's and Morgenstern's discovery was based on the recognition that the strength of someone's preference for an outcome is not always proportional to the numerical value of that outcome.

For example, consider two outcomes in which the patient lives either 2 or 4 years. Living 4 years is better than living only 2 years. However, is living 4 years twice as good as living only 2 years? In other words, in an expected value calculation, are we correct to assume that an outcome that means the patient will live 4 years should contribute twice as much as an outcome that means the patient will live only 2 years?

That assumption of proportionality is central to a life expectancy calculation. But as we saw in the earlier discussion of risk aversion, the proportionality assumption is not always true. Winning two million dollars is better than settling for one million dollars. However, that is no longer the case once we discount the possible two-million-dollar win by the 50% chance of winning nothing. That 50% chance reduces our preferences for the possible two million dollars to less than our preferences for the guaranteed one million dollars.

Instead of the proportionality assumption, von Neumann and Morgenstern proposed a concept they called utility to measure the strength of preferences for an outcome. That preference measure becomes the value for an outcome in a decision analysis. Their utility assigns numerical values to outcomes so that the calculated expected value – what we will call the *expected utility* – is greatest for the most preferred alternative. In other words, an expected utility calculation incorporates the individual's risk attitudes.

More precisely, von Neumann and Morgenstern showed that under a reasonable set of assumptions, we can always find outcome utilities that quantify risk attitudes so that the expected utility will be greatest for the most preferred alternative (von Neumann and Morgenstern, 1947). The claim that we can always find what we need to solve a decision problem may seem unbelievable. However, with this remarkable result, von Neumann and Morgenstern established the foundation for how decisions involving uncertainty can be analyzed.

Von Neumann's and Morgenstern's proof is abstract and will not be covered in this book. However, buried in their proof is a practical method for determining the outcome utilities for a decision problem.

Definition: von Neumann-Morgenstern utility

Von Neumann-Morgenstern utility is a numerical value assigned to an outcome such that the expected utility, when computed for each alternative in the decision problem, is always greatest for the preferred alternative.

8.3.4 Using standard gamble assessment questions to determine outcome utilities

Von Neumann's and Morgenstern's method for determining the utility for outcome x starts with two additional outcomes we will denote by x_A and x_B. The only requirement for selecting these two additional outcomes is that outcome x_A must be preferred to outcome x and outcome x must be preferred to outcome x_B. Given this requirement, the process that determines the utility for outcome x is based on the following comparison of outcome x and a gamble between outcomes x_A and x_B:

Just to be clear, the gamble shown on the right will result in outcome x_A with probability p and outcome x_B with probability $1-p$.

Suppose a choice must be made between the gamble and outcome x. The gamble would be preferred over outcome x if probability p is close to 1 since that would mean outcome x_A is almost certain and outcome x_A is preferred to outcome x. On the other hand, outcome x would be preferred over the gamble if probability p is close to 0 since that would mean outcome x_B is almost certain and outcome x is preferred to outcome x_B.

At some intermediate value for probability p, the gamble and outcome x will be equivalent. That is, neither option is preferred more than the other. We call this value for p the *indifference probability* for outcome x.

The importance of the indifference probability is that we can use it to determine the utility for outcome x relative to the utilities for outcomes x_A and x_B. Denote the indifference probability by $p^\star$ and the utility for outcome x by $U(x)$. Saying that outcome x and the gamble are equivalent means that the utility for outcome x must equal the expected utility for the gamble. Since outcome x and the gamble are equivalent when probability p equals $p^\star$, it follows that

$$U(x) = p^\star U(x_A) + (1-p^\star)U(x_B)$$

Notice that the indifference probability captures how outcome x compares to outcomes x_A and x_B in the presence of the uncertainty represented by the gamble. For example, suppose that outcome x is live 5 more years, outcome x_A is live 10 more years, and outcome x_B is die immediately. Living 10 more years is preferred to living only 5 more years. However, the risk of dying offsets our preference for that longer possible lifetime. If the probability of immediate death is small, most people would prefer a gamble that would double the length of life. If the probability of immediate death is large, that preference is diminished. How much it is diminished depends on how the individual feels about risk. Put in other words, the indifference probability captures the individual's risk attitudes.

This approach to quantifying risk attitudes applies equally to any number of outcomes. Suppose we are analyzing a decision problem with n possible outcomes. Let $x_1, \ldots, x_n$ denote these outcomes. In particular, let x_{Best} denote most preferred outcome and let x_{Worst} denote the least preferred outcome. Then we can determine the utility for any outcome x_i by using the following comparison

The following expressions determine the utility for outcome x_i if $p_i^\star$ denotes the indifference probability in this comparison:

$$U(x_i) = p_i^\star U(x_{\text{Best}}) + (1-p_i^\star)U(x_{\text{Worst}})$$

We can assign any values we want to the outcome utilities for the best and worse outcomes as long as the utility for the former is more than the utility for the latter. However, the arithmetic is much simpler if we assign $U(x_{Best})$ the value of 1 and $U(x_{Worse})$ the value of 0. Then

$$U(x_i) = p_i^\star U(x_{Best}) + (1 - p_i^\star) U(x_{Worst}) = p_i^\star \times 1 + (1 - p_i^\star) \times 0 = p_i^\star$$

In other words, if we use these two convenient values as the utilities for the best and worst outcomes, the utility for the other outcomes becomes the corresponding indifference probabilities. This approach to determining outcome utilities is called *standard gamble assessment*.

Whichever values we use as the utilities for the best and worse outcomes, von Neumann's and Morgenstern's key insight is that the outcome utilities derived from the indifference probabilities encode enough about the individual's risk attitudes so that those outcome utilities have a critical property for decision making: the alternative with the greatest expected utility is the alternative that should be preferred.

For example, suppose that outcomes are expressed as the remaining years of life for the patient and we are analyzing a choice between Treatment A and Treatment B. Recall the notation for conditional probabilities used in the previous chapters and let $P[x_1 | A], \ldots, P[x_n | A]$ denote the outcome probabilities for Treatment A. That is

$$P[\text{Length of life} = x_i \text{ with Treatment A}] = P[x_i | A]$$

A similar notation represents the outcome probabilities for Treatment B. We then can use the following expressions to determine the expected utility for the two treatments:

$$\text{Expected Utility for Treatment A} = P[x_1 | A] \times U(x_1) + \ldots + P[x_n | A] \times U(x_n)$$
$$\text{Expected Utility for Treatment B} = P[x_1 | B] \times U(x_1) + \ldots + P[x_n | B] \times U(x_n)$$

where $U(x_i)$ is the utility for living x_i years. Once again, the important property of an expected utility is that the treatment with the greatest expected utility will be the treatment preferred by a patient whose risk attitudes are represented by the outcome utilities used in the calculation. Therefore, the expected utilities calculated by these two expressions identify the treatment preferred by this patient.

So far we have discussed a probability-based approach to standard gamble assessment. This approach is probability-based in the sense that it depends on determining the indifference probability for an outcome. In other words, probability p is the unknown in the standard gamble:

The process that captures the individual's risk attitudes does so by determining a probability that would mean the two options are equivalent.

The same comparison can be reversed with the probability p set equal to a known value, like 0.5, and the value for outcome x left as an unknown. For example, suppose again that outcome x_A is live 10 more years, and outcome x_B is die immediately. The outcome-based approach to standard gamble assessment asks what guaranteed length of life x would be equivalent to the gamble with a known probability p. Let $x^\star$ denote the answer to this question. Using the same convention that assigns $U(x_A)$ the value of 1 and $U(x_B)$ the value of 0, it follows that

$$U(x^\star) = pU(x_A) + (1 - p)U(x_B) = p \times 1 + (1 - p) \times 0 = p$$

In other words, the mathematics is the same for outcome-based standard gamble assessment as they are for probability-based standard gamble assessment. The only difference is that we have determined what outcome has a given utility rather than what utility applies to a given outcome. Some individuals are more comfortable deciding on the outcome that is equivalent to a gamble rather than a gamble that is equivalent to an outcome. For this reason, McNeil and her colleagues used outcome-based standard-gamble assessment in their study of patient preferences for lung cancer treatments.

Definition: standard gamble assessment

With standard gamble assessment the utility for outcome x relative to the utilities for outcomes x_A and x_B is determined by the values for outcome x and probability p such that the following two alternatives are equivalent

When the two alternatives are equivalent

$$U(x) = pU(x_A) + (1-p)U(x_B)$$

Standard gamble assessment when the outcome x is known is called *probability based*. With probability-based assessment, the value for the probability p where the guaranteed outcome and the gamble are equivalent is called the *indifference probability*. Standard gamble assessment when the probability p is known is called *outcome based*.

Before returning to the study by McNeil and her colleagues, a comment should be made about using arbitrary values as the utilities for outcomes x_{Best} and x_{Worst}. This may seem peculiar; however, much like a physical measurement such as temperature, utility is expressed according to a relative scale. In scientific measurements, temperature typically is expressed so that the temperature of freezing water is $0°C$ and the temperature of boiling water is $100°C$. The choice of the two reference values 0 and $100°C$ is arbitrary, but essential, for a temperature measurement to have a meaning.

Similarly, utility is always expressed relative to any two arbitrary reference values. The only requirement is that the ranking of the reference values used must match how the corresponding outcomes are ranked by preference. In other words, the utility for x_{Best} must be greater than the utility for x_{Worst}. For much of this chapter, the reference values of 1 and 0 are used to scale utility because these values simplify the arithmetic.

8.3.5 Determining the outcome utilities for the lung cancer decision problem

Returning to the study by McNeil and her colleagues, their goal was to demonstrate how risk attitudes affect a patient's preference for the two lung cancer treatments. Traditionally, cancer treatments are compared based on 5-year survival rates. The treatment with the highest 5-year survival is assumed to be the best option for a patient. However, a 5-year survival rate applies to a population, which means that all patients who match the characteristics of that population would be assigned the same treatment.

Instead, McNeil and her colleagues recognized that different patients have different risk attitudes. Outcome utilities determined using standard gamble assessment represent those different risk attitudes. Therefore, the differences in the expected utilities calculated for a patient will demonstrate how that patient's treatment preferences differ from those of other patients. In particular, those differences demonstrate the hypothesis that using 5-year survival rates to select the same treatment for all patients ignores how patients view risk.

In order to demonstrate this hypothesis the researchers recruited fourteen patients with Stage I or Stage II lung cancer. The average age for these patients was 67 years, with a range of 48 to 80 years. The patients were recruited for the study after they had selected their lung cancer treatment.

The range of lifetimes faced by these fourteen patients is represented by the survival curves shown in Figure 8.3. Those survival curves imply the outcome probabilities for the decision tree shown in Figure 8.2. Using the outcome utilities determined for a patient, the decision tree can be analyzed to determine which treatment that patient prefers.

McNeil and her colleagues used outcome-based standard gamble assessment to determine a patient's utilities for different lengths of life. They started by setting the utility for immediate death to be 0 and the utility for living 25 more years to be 1. Next, they determined which lengths of life had utilities of 0.25, 0.50, and 0.75. This required each patient to answer three questions.

The answer to the first question determined the length of life that had a utility of 0.50. The following is a wording for this question:

Suppose that you are faced with a risky treatment that has a 50% chance of causing your immediate death. You will live another 25 years if you survive the treatment. Your alternative is a second treatment that has no risk of immediate death but provides a shorter length of life. For what guaranteed length of life (X_1) following the second treatment would you be exactly indifferent between the two treatments?

Figure 8.4 shows a decision tree representing the first question. The term X_1 in the decision tree denotes the answer provided by the patient. In other words, in Figure 8.4, X_1 is the length of life for the guaranteed outcome that is equivalent to the gamble between either living 25 years or dying immediately.

By definition, the value for X_1 is the length of life such that the two alternatives at decision node **C1** in Figure 8.4 are equivalent. This means the expected value for the two alternatives must be equal. However, recall that *value* in our analysis is measured by the utility for an outcome, rather than the numerical length of life.

Recall that the following reference values were used to scale utility in this problem:

$$U(0 \text{ years}) = 0.0 \text{ and } U(25 \text{ years}) = 1.0$$

This means

$$U(X_1 \text{ years}) = 0.50 \times U(25 \text{ years}) + 0.50 \times U(0 \text{ years}) = 0.5 \times 1.0 + 0.5 \times 0.0 = 0.5$$

The average response for the 14 participants in the study was 5.0 years with a standard deviation of 3.7 years. Therefore, on the average,

$$U(5 \text{ years}) = 0.5$$

But risk attitudes describe an individual rather than a population. This was demonstrated by the standard deviation for the responses provided by the fourteen participants. Not all of the participants provided the same answer to this question. Later, we will see why the range of answers was important to McNeil and her colleagues. However, for the moment, we will assume the point of view of a hypothetical patient who stated their value for X_1 was 5 years. We will refer to this individual as Patient A.

Recall that this study characterized the risk attitudes for the fourteen patients by determining for each patient which outcomes had the utilities of 0.25, 0.50, and 0.75. The answer to the first question determined that for Patient A, living 5 years had a utility of 0.50.

The following is a wording of the second question. The answer to this question determines the outcome that has a utility of 0.25 for Patient A:

Suppose that you are faced with a treatment that has a 50% chance of causing your immediate death. You will live another 5 years if you survive the treatment. Your alternative is a second treatment that has no risk of immediate death but provides a shorter length of life. For what guaranteed length of life (X_2) following the second treatment would you be exactly indifferent between the two treatments?

Figure 8.5 depicts this second question as a decision tree. Note that the 5-year outcome included as a possible outcome for the gamble (decision node **D2**) is Patient A's answer to the first question (X_1). The answer to the first question

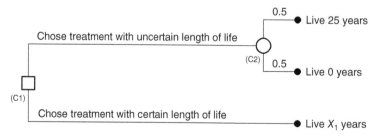

Figure 8.4 Decision tree representation of the first question asked each participant.

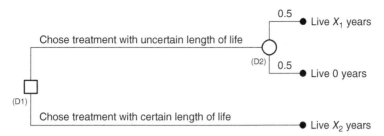

Figure 8.5 Decision tree representation of the second question asked each participant. X_2 is the participant's answer to this question and X_1 is the same participant's answer to the first question shown in Figure 8.4.

determined that a lifetime of 5 years has a utility of 0.50 for Patient A. The patient's answer to the second question is X_2, which in Figure 8.5 is the length of life for the guaranteed outcome.

Suppose Patient A's answer to the second question (X_2) is 2 years. Repeating the same reasoning used to interpret the first question,

$$U(2\,\text{years}) = 0.5 \times U(0\,\text{years}) + 0.5 \times U(X_1\,\text{years})$$
$$= 0.5 \times U(0\,\text{years}) + 0.5 \times U(5\,\text{years})$$
$$= 0.5 \times 0.0 + 0.5 \times 0.5$$
$$U(2\,\text{years}) = 0.25$$

Therefore, Patient A's answer to the second question implies this patient believes that 2 years has a utility of 0.25.

Finally, the answer to the third question determines the outcome that has a utility of 0.75 for Patient A. This question would be worded:

Suppose that you are faced with an uncertain treatment that has a 50% chance of leaving you with a life that lasts 25 years. Otherwise, this treatment will result in you living another 5 years. Your alternative is a second treatment that has no uncertainty. For what guaranteed length of life (X_3) following the second treatment would you be exactly indifferent between the two treatments?

Figure 8.6 depicts this third question as a decision tree. As with sthe second question, the 5-year outcome, included as a possible outcome for the gamble (decision node **E2**), is Patient A's answer to the first question. Let X_3 denote the patient's answer to this third question.

Suppose that Patient A's answer to the third question (X_3) is 10 years. Following the same reasoning used to interpret the other questions,

$$U(10\,\text{years}) = 0.5 \times U(5\,\text{years}) + 0.5 \times U(25\,\text{years}) = 0.5 \times 0.5 + 0.5 \times 1.0 = 0.75$$

In summary, the answers to the three questions have determined the utilities for three outcomes:

$$U(2\,\text{years}) = 0.25$$

$$U(5\,\text{years}) = 0.50$$

$$U(10\,\text{years}) = 0.75$$

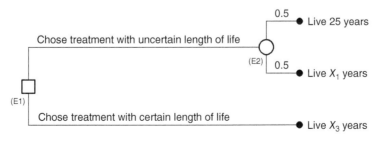

Figure 8.6 Decision tree representation of the third question asked each participant. X_3 is the participant's answer to this question and X_1 is the same participant's answer to the first question shown in Figure 8.4.

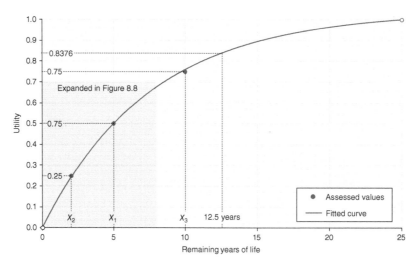

Figure 8.7 Utility for length of life for Patient A based on their answers to the three questions represented by the decision trees shown in Figures 8.3, 8.4, and 8.5. For this hypothetical participant, the answers to the three questions were $X_1 = 5$ years, $X_2 = 2$ years, and $X_3 = 10$ years.

We also assumed the following reference outcome utilities

$$U(0\,\text{years}) = 0.00$$

$$U(25\,\text{years}) = 1.00$$

These five outcome utilities have been plotted in Figure 8.7, along with a curve fitted to these utilities. How that curve was fitted will be described in the next chapter. The resulting curve determines the utilities needed to complete the comparison of the two treatment alternatives for Patient A.

Before showing how to make use of the outcome utilities shown in Figure 8.7, we will first consider an interesting implication of what we have learned about Patient A's risk attitudes.

Recall the earlier discussion about proportionality and how an outcome's numerical value often does not fully reflect the contribution of that outcome to the patient's preferences for an alternative. For example, the monetary example used in the introduction noted that winning two million dollars is not twice as good as winning half that amount.

The curve in Figure 8.7 demonstrates this same absence of proportionality for length-of-life outcomes. Notice that 12.5 years is the midpoint for a 25-year lifetime. As shown in Figure 8.7, the utility for this midpoint is 0.8376. In comparison, the utility for the full 25 years, by assumption is 1.0, which is only 0.1624 more than 0.8376. Therefore, the first 12.5 years add far more than the second 12.5 years to the utility for a 25-year lifetime. In short, the strength of preference for an outcome, like a lifetime, is not proportional to the numerical value of that lifetime. That lack of proportionality is what simple life expectancy calculations overlook and expected utility calculations capture.

8.3.6 Computing Patient A's expected utility for each of the treatments

The outcome utilities we have determined for Patient A can now be used to find the treatment alternative most preferred by this individual. Suppose that Patient A is a 60-year-old man. These outcome utilities combine with the corresponding outcome probabilities to calculate the expected utilities for the treatment alternatives. The alternative with the greater expected utility will be the treatment preferred given Patient A's risk attitudes.

Table 8.1 shows the details of the expected utility calculations for Patient A. The leftmost column, labeled x_i, contains the possible numbers of years that might remain in Patient A's life. Notice that the calculations have been carried out to 45 years, which includes the longest possible remaining years for most 60-year-old men. The corresponding utility for each of these lifetimes is shown in the column labeled $U(x_i)$.[1]

---

[1] Notice in Table 8.1 that the outcome utilities for 0, 5, and 25 years line up exactly with the corresponding utilities determined from Patient A's answer to the first question. On the other hand, the outcome utility shown for 2 years (0.2399) is slightly less than the utility of 0.25 determined from Patient A's answer to the second question. Similarly, the outcome utility for 10 years (0.7502) is slightly more than the utility of 0.75 determined from Patient A's answer to the third question. These deviations are because the outcome utilities shown in Table 8.1 are from the fitted curve, which does not exactly match the outcome utility values determined from the questions asked of Patient A. The justification for using this fitted curve is discussed in the next chapter.

The next pair of columns in Table 8.1 contains the terms in the expected utility calculation for surgery. The column labelled $P(x_i|Rx)$ in this pair contains the outcome probabilities for surgery. These probabilities were determined from the survival curve for surgery shown in Figure 8.3. The column labelled $P(x_i|Rx) \times U(x_i)$ contains the product of the outcome probability and the outcome utility for each of the possible lifetimes. As shown in the last row of the second surgery column, the total of those products is 0.3900. This total is Patient A's expected utility for undergoing surgery.

The two rightmost columns in Table 8.1 contain the same expected utility calculations for radiotherapy. Patient A's expected utility for radiotherapy determined by the calculations in these columns is 0.4115. Since 0.4115 is greater than 0.3900, we can conclude Patient A would prefer radiotherapy over surgery for treatment of their lung cancer.

Table 8.1 Expected utility calculations for lung cancer treatment decision using outcome utilities for Patient A.

Lifetime		Rx = Surgery		Rx = Radiotherapy	
x_i	$U(x_i)$	$P(x_i|Rx)$	$P(x_i|Rx) \times U(x_i)$	$P(x_i|Rx)$	$P(x_i|Rx) \times U(x_i)$
0	0.0000	0.1000	0.0000	0.0000	0.0000
1	0.1278	0.2387	0.0305	0.1073	0.0137
2	0.2399	0.1605	0.0385	0.3198	0.0767
3	0.3382	0.1081	0.0366	0.1929	0.0652
4	0.4244	0.0730	0.0310	0.1065	0.0452
5	0.5000	0.0496	0.0248	0.0591	0.0296
6	0.5663	0.0339	0.0192	0.0332	0.0188
7	0.6245	0.0235	0.0147	0.0190	0.0119
8	0.6754	0.0165	0.0112	0.0113	0.0076
9	0.7202	0.0119	0.0086	0.0071	0.0051
10	0.7594	0.0089	0.0068	0.0049	0.0037
11	0.7938	0.0070	0.0055	0.0038	0.0030
12	0.8240	0.0058	0.0047	0.0032	0.0027
13	0.8504	0.0050	0.0043	0.0030	0.0026
14	0.8736	0.0046	0.0040	0.0030	0.0026
15	0.8940	0.0044	0.0039	0.0031	0.0027
16	0.9118	0.0043	0.0039	0.0032	0.0029
17	0.9275	0.0044	0.0040	0.0034	0.0031
18	0.9412	0.0045	0.0042	0.0035	0.0033
19	0.9532	0.0046	0.0044	0.0037	0.0036
20	0.9638	0.0048	0.0047	0.0039	0.0038
21	0.9730	0.0050	0.0049	0.0041	0.0040
22	0.9812	0.0053	0.0052	0.0043	0.0043
23	0.9883	0.0049	0.0049	0.0041	0.0040
24	0.9945	0.0057	0.0056	0.0047	0.0047
25	1.0000	0.0058	0.0058	0.0049	0.0049
26	1.0048	0.0060	0.0060	0.0050	0.0050
27	1.0090	0.0062	0.0062	0.0051	0.0052
28	1.0127	0.0063	0.0064	0.0052	0.0053
29	1.0159	0.0063	0.0064	0.0053	0.0054
30	1.0188	0.0064	0.0065	0.0053	0.0054
31	1.0213	0.0063	0.0065	0.0053	0.0054
32	1.0235	0.0063	0.0064	0.0052	0.0053
33	1.0254	0.0061	0.0063	0.0051	0.0052
34	1.0271	0.0059	0.0061	0.0049	0.0051
35	1.0285	0.0057	0.0058	0.0047	0.0049
36	1.0298	0.0054	0.0055	0.0045	0.0046
37	1.0310	0.0050	0.0052	0.0042	0.0043
38	1.0320	0.0046	0.0047	0.0038	0.0040
39	1.0328	0.0042	0.0043	0.0035	0.0036
40	1.0336	0.0037	0.0038	0.0031	0.0032
41	1.0343	0.0032	0.0033	0.0027	0.0028
42	1.0349	0.0027	0.0028	0.0023	0.0024
43	1.0354	0.0023	0.0024	0.0019	0.0020
44	1.0358	0.0018	0.0019	0.0015	0.0016
45	1.0362	0.0015	0.0015	0.0012	0.0013
			EU (Surgery) = 0.3900		EU (Radiotherapy) = 0.4115

In other words, both the life expectancy and the 5-year survival rate may be greater for surgery. However, radiotherapy is the preferred treatment given Patient A's attitudes toward the risk that surgery could lead to near-term death.

8.3.7 Risk attitudes matter

Recall that McNeil's and her colleague's goal was to test the hypothesis that risk attitudes affect the treatment a patient prefers. Their test of this hypothesis used the risk attitudes assessed for fourteen different patients. Outcome-based standard gamble assessment determined the risk attitudes of the patients. This meant that different outcome utilities were determined for each of the 14 patients participating in the study.

Once the outcome utilities were determined, the preferred treatment was determined for each patient using 16 different clinical scenarios. These scenarios were designed to represent what might be encountered by patients with lung cancer at the time of the study. The analysis was repeated for each of the fourteen participants, assuming each of those 16 scenarios.

The scenarios were defined according to three variables:

Age of the patient: Set as either 60 years of age or 70 years of age. The value for this variable affected the survival curve for the patient assuming they did not succumb to the lung cancer or the treatment.

Surgical mortality rate: Set as either 5, 10, 15, or 20%.

Surgical results: Set as either *typical* or *excellent*. With *typical* surgical results, the survival curve was adjusted to achieve a 5-year survival rate of 24% after surviving surgery. With excellent surgical results, the survival curve was adjusted to achieve a 5-year survival rate of 33% after surviving surgery.

Table 8.2 shows how preference for radiotherapy varied for each of the sixteen scenarios. For each scenario, the percentage of patients preferring radiotherapy is shown based on either the 5-year survival rate or expected utility. For example, the two percentages shown in the upper left-hand corner of the table are for a 60-year-old patient facing a 5% perioperative mortality rate and excellent surgical results. If comparison of the treatment alternatives is based on the 5-year survival rate, none of the fourteen patients would have chosen radiotherapy. On the other hand, if the comparison of the treatments is based on expected utility analysis, 7% of the participants had risk attitudes which meant a preference for radiotherapy over surgery.

For 60-year-olds facing excellent surgical results, the percentage of participants with risk attitudes implying a preference for radiotherapy climbs from 7 to 64% as the perioperative mortality rates climb from 5 to 20%. This same trend is evident in the other combinations of age and surgical results.

On the other hand, when using 5-year survival as the basis for comparing treatments, radiotherapy only becomes the preferred alternative when the perioperative mortality rate reaches 15% and the surgical results become what McNeil and her colleagues called "typical." In other words, accounting for risk attitudes implies significantly different preferences for the treatment of an important disease.

This landmark study showed that a patient's risk attitudes can matter when making treatment decisions. More specifically, as the title of the paper suggests, the traditional approach of selecting treatment based on 5-year survival rates

Table 8.2 Percentage of patients preferring radiotherapy over surgery for the treatment of Stage I or Stage II lung cancer, based on the comparison of 5-year survival and expected utility. Comparison of the two treatments is considered for 16 different scenarios based on age, perioperative mortality rate, and surgical result.

| Age | Outcome measure | Excellent surgical results | | | | Typical surgical results | | | |
| | | Perioperative mortality rate | | | | Perioperative mortality rate | | | |
		5%	10%	15%	20%	5%	10%	15%	20%
60 years	5-year survival	0%	0%	0%	0%	0%	0%	100%	100%
	Expected utility	7%	21%	43%	64%	64%	71%	100%	100%
70 years	5-year survival	0%	0%	0%	0%	0%	0%	100%	100%
	Expected utility	14%	43%	50%	71%	71%	100%	100%	100%

Adapted from McNeil *et al.* (1978).

ignores what often is important to the patients living with the outcome of those decisions. Demonstrating that insight alone is a remarkable contribution.

> ### Result: risk attitudes can matter when selecting treatment
>
> Treatment alternatives with a risk of death in the near term are overvalued in comparison with less risk of death in the near term if the analysis does not account for risk aversion.

McNeil and her colleagues also demonstrated an important methodologic advance in medical decision analysis. This method combines the probability concepts described in earlier chapters, with something new called an outcome utility. The remainder of this chapter, and the two chapters that follow, will show how the concept of utility can be turned into a clinically relevant tool for analyzing decisions.

8.4   General observations about outcome utilities

The utility concept discovered by von Neumann and Morgenstern quantifies risk attitudes. We just saw the usefulness of that quantification when analyzing decisions involving risk and risk is common with choices between treatments. However, that usefulness only matters if credible values for the outcome utilities can be determined.

By their very nature, outcome utilities are subjective. This means the outcome utilities for one individual may not be the same as the outcome utilities for another individual. That is because the risk attitudes quantified by utilities often differ between individuals.

This subjectivity becomes a problem when the goal of a decision analysis is the formulation of a clinical policy. Clinical policies are applied to a population rather than an individual. When using outcome utilities to formulate a clinical policy, whose risk attitudes should be quantified?

Also, what does the expected utility for an alternative mean in tangible terms? The life expectancy for an alternative is a length of life. That length of life is highly tangible for most of us. On the other hand, an expected utility is only a number. We can use those numbers to compare the alternatives in a decision. Therefore, utility does have a relative meaning because two utilities can be compared. However, the lack of tangibility complicates how to decide if the difference between two utilities is meaningful.

These are the challenges that must be addressed if the concept of utilities is to be more than an intellectual curiosity. That is (1) we need a credible method for determining an individual's utilities, (2) we must decide how to think about the subjective nature of utilities in the context of a clinical policy, and (3) we need a tangible perspective so that we can judge the clinical significance of an expected utility difference.

Addressing these three challenges is the focus for the remainder of this chapter and the two chapters that follow. The discussion begins with the tangibility issue.

8.4.1   Certainty equivalent – providing a tangible meaning for expected utility analysis

Recall the analysis of the lung cancer decision for hypothetical Patient A. The analysis summarized in Table 8.1 found that for this individual, the expected utility is 0.3900 for surgery and 0.4115 for radiotherapy. What do these expected utilities mean? Since 0.4115 is greater than 0.3900, the analysis concluded that radiotherapy is the treatment preferred by Patient A. However, does this difference indicate a strong preference for radiotherapy over surgery?

Figure 8.8 shows an expanded portion of the utility curve in Figure 8.7. We can determine from Figure 8.8 that 0.4115, the expected utility for radiotherapy, is also the utility for a lifetime of 3.84 years. This means that for Patient A, facing the uncertainty of radiotherapy would be equivalent to facing a guaranteed lifetime of 3.84 years since both would have the same utility. For this reason, we call 3.84 years Patient A's *certainty equivalent* for radiotherapy.

Referring again to Figure 8.8, we can see that 0.3900, the expected utility for surgery, is the utility for a lifetime of 3.64 years. This means Patient A's certainty equivalent for surgery is 3.58 years.

These certainty equivalent calculations provide what for many is a more tangible comparison of the two treatment alternatives. In effect, the certainty equivalent for an alternative is a risk-adjusted outcome measure. With radiotherapy, that risk-adjusted measure is 3.84 years. Switching to surgery would reduce that measure by the difference between 3.84 and 3.64 years, Patient A's certainty equivalent for surgery. That works out to roughly a 3-month difference for someone with Patient A's risk attitudes.

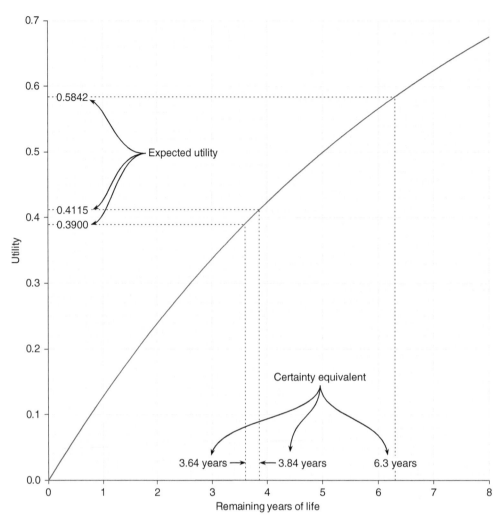

Figure 8.8 Expanded portion of utility curve Figure 8.7 showing example of how a certainty equivalent can be determined for an expected utility.

In summary, certainty equivalent provides a tangible perspective for thinking about alternatives with uncertain outcomes. When the outcomes correspond to lifetimes, a certainty equivalent is a length of life. However, unlike a life expectancy, a certainty equivalent also reflects the risk attitudes of the individual.

Definition: certainty equivalent

The *certainty equivalent* for an uncertain alternative is the guaranteed outcome that has the same utility as the expected utility of the uncertain alternative.

8.4.2 Risk attitudes revisited

We now will show how the concept of a certainty equivalent can be used to characterize someone's risk attitudes. We also will consider how risk attitudes are reflected in the shape of a utility curve.

The initial discussion of risk attitudes, earlier in this chapter, defined risk aversion for monetary gambles. Someone who is risk averse prefers to have the expected winnings for a gamble over the gamble itself. That definition can be extended to outcomes expressed as lifetimes. A risk-averse patient prefers a guaranteed life of a given length over a risky treatment with the same life expectancy.

For example, Patient A, the 60-year-old man in the earlier discussion, would have a life expectancy of 6.3 years with radiotherapy. If Patient A is risk averse, they would rather be guaranteed a lifetime of 6.3 years, then face the

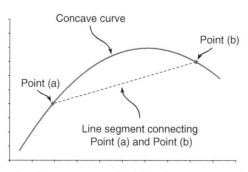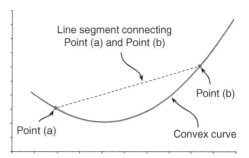

Figure 8.9 Examples of a concave curve (on left) and a convex curve (on right).

uncertainty of radiotherapy, even though the procedure leads to the same life expectancy. This means for this patient the life expectancy for surgery must be less than the certainty equivalent for surgery.

Therefore, certainty equivalent provides another way to define risk aversion. By definition, a risky treatment is equivalent to a guaranteed length of life that equals the risky treatment's certainty equivalent. That was the point of the discussion in the previous subsection. This means that with risk aversion, the certainty equivalent must be less than the life expectancy for a treatment. Otherwise, the treatment would be preferred to its life expectancy, which contradicts the definition of risk aversion.

For example, in the analysis of Patient A's preferences, we saw that their certainty equivalent for radiotherapy is 3.84 years. This certainty equivalent is less than their life expectancy of 6.3 years with this treatment. Therefore, Patient A is risk averse, at least in the context of the lung cancer treatment decision.

Note that what we have said so far about risk aversion applies only to specific choices involving a specific range of possible outcomes. However, a broader statement about someone's risk aversion can be made based on the shape of the curve for their outcome utilities.

Consider the shape of Patient A's curve for their outcome utilities shown in Figures 8.7 and 8.8. This curve is what mathematicians call a *concave* curve. In simple terms, a concave curve has the property that a straight line drawn between any two points on the curve always falls below the curve. The panel on the left in Figure 8.9 shows an example of a concave curve.

The reason for mentioning this seemingly abstract geometric concept is that someone is risk averse for all gambles if and only if their utility curve is concave. The proof of this useful result requires a long and not very interesting discussion that will not be presented here. However, this result provides a visual method for recognizing when someone is risk averse. For example, because Patient A's utility curve is concave from 0 to 25 years, we know that Patient A will have risk-averse preferences for any risky treatment that could result in outcomes over this range of lifetimes.

Definition: risk-averse preferences

When faced with decisions involving risky alternatives, an individual demonstrates *risk-averse* preferences for length of life outcome if
1. They prefer a guaranteed lifetime that equals the life expectancy for a risky alternative rather than actually facing the uncertainty of that alternative.
2. Their certainty equivalent for a risky alternative is less than what their life expectancy would be with that alternative.
3. The shape of their utility curve over the range of outcomes is concave.

A parallel discussion applies to risk tolerance. Recall that with monetary gambles, someone is risk tolerant if they would rather take their chances with a gamble than accept the guaranteed expected winnings for that gamble. In a medical context, risk tolerance means facing the uncertainty of a risky treatment is preferred to a guaranteed lifetime that equals the life expectancy for that treatment. It follows that someone also is risk tolerant if their certainty equivalent for a risky treatment is greater than what their life expectancy would be with that treatment. Therefore, switching from risk aversion to risk tolerance reverses the ordering of life expectancy and certainty equivalent.

The shape of the utility curve for someone who is risk tolerant has a similar reversal from what was seen with risk aversion. To visualize this reversal, consider the preferences of a second hypothetical patient with lung cancer, who is risk tolerant. We will call this individual Patient B. Recall the first of the three questions used by McNeil and her colleagues to quantify risk attitudes. That question asked their participants to consider a risky treatment that had an even chance of resulting either in a life lasting 25 years or immediate death. The question asked the participants to state their certainty equivalent for this risky treatment.

As we have just seen, when a participant was risk averse, like Patient A, their answer to the first question was a length of life less than the life expectancy of 12.5 years offered by the risky treatment. In fact, we supposed that Patient A stated their certainty equivalent for the risky treatment was 5 years, which is considerably less than 12.5 years. However, for someone like Patient B, who is risk tolerant, the answer to the first question would be a length of life greater than 12.5 years. Therefore, suppose Patient B replied that they would be indifferent between a guaranteed 20 years of life or the risky treatment. Note that 20 years is greater than 12.5 years, as it should be for someone who is risk tolerant.

Referring back to the decision tree representation of the first question, shown in Figure 8.4, Patient B's answer means that their value for X_1 is 20 years. Suppose that Patient B's response to the other two questions means that X_2 is 15 years and X_3 is 23 years. Based on these answers, Figure 8.10 shows what the curve would look like for Patient B's outcome utilities.

The shape of the utility curve in Figure 8.10 is no longer concave. Instead, this curve is what mathematicians call a *convex curve*. In general, a convex curve has the property that a straight line drawn between any two points on the curve always falls above the curve. Note how this definition is the inverse of how a concave curve was defined earlier. The right-hand panel in Figure 8.9 shows example of a convex curve in addition to a concave curve.

The significance of a convex utility curve is that this shape means Patient B is risk tolerant for all decisions resulting in possible lengths of life between 0 and 25 years. That is because a convex utility curve always implies risk tolerance.

Definition: risk-tolerant preferences

When faced with decisions involving risky alternatives, a patient demonstrates *risk-tolerant* preferences for length of life outcome if
1. They prefer to face the uncertainty of a risky alternative over a guaranteed lifetime that equals the life expectancy for the risky alternative.
2. Their certainty equivalent for a risky alternative is more than what their life expectancy would be with that alternative.
3. The shape of their utility curve over the range of outcomes is convex.

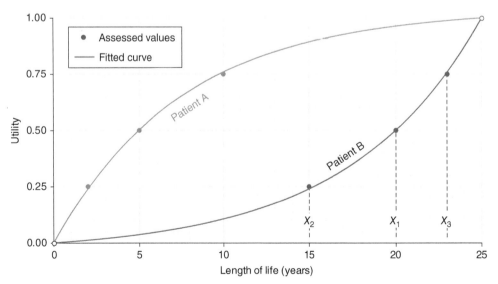

Figure 8.10 Outcome utilities for Patient B, who is risk tolerant, based on their answers to the three questions represented by the decision trees shown in Figures 8.3, 8.4, and 8.5. For this hypothetical participant, the answers to the three questions are $X_1 = 20$ years, $X_2 = 15$ years, and $X_3 = 23$ years.

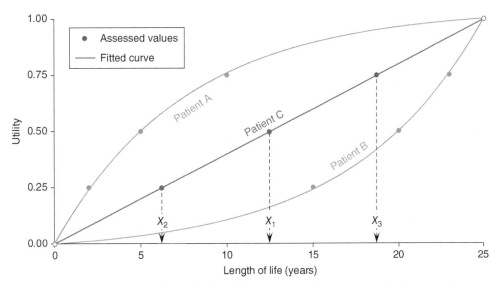

Figure 8.11 Example of outcome utilities for Patient C, who is risk indifferent, based on their answers to the three questions represented by the decision trees shown in Figures 8.3, 8.4, and 8.5. For this hypothetical participant, the answers to the three questions are $X_1 = 6.25$ years, $X_2 = 12.5$ years, and $X_3 = 18.75$ years.

Finally, before leaving this discussion of risk attitudes, some mention should be made of what is called *risk indifferent* or *risk-neutral* preferences. When faced with a monetary gamble, someone who is risk indifferent considers the gamble to be equivalent to the expected winnings. In a medical context, someone who is risk indifferent compares risky alternatives based only on life expectancy. In other words, the certainty equivalent for a risky treatment equals the life expectancy for the treatment.

For example, suppose that Patient C is a risk indifferent patient with lung cancer. This individual's answer to the first utility assessment question would be 12.5 years because that is the life expectancy for the treatment that would result in either a life lasting 25 years or immediate death. This would mean Patient C's value for X_1 was 12.5 years. The second assessment question would ask Patient C what guaranteed length of life is equivalent to a gamble that has a 50% of causing immediate death and a 50% chance of resulting in a life lasting 12.5 years – Patient C's answer to the first question. Because Patient C is risk indifferent their answer would be 6.25 years since that is the life expectancy for the gamble in this question. Similarly, Patient C's answer to the third question would be 18.75 years. Figure 8.11 shows the resulting curve for Patient C's outcome utilities.

Note that the utility curve for this risk-indifferent individual is a straight line. That shape for a utility curve is the hallmark of risk indifference. When someone is risk indifferent their utility curve is a straight line. Conversely, when we use a straight line to represent someone's utility curve, we are assuming that they are risk indifferent.

Definition: risk indifferent preferences

When faced with decisions involving risky alternatives an individual demonstrates *risk-indifferent* preferences for length of life outcome if
1. They are indifferent between facing the uncertainty of a risky alternative and having a guaranteed lifetime that equals the life expectancy for the risky alternative.
2. Their certainty equivalent for a risky alternative equals what their life expectancy would be with that alternative.
3. The shape of their utility curve over the range of outcomes is a straight line.

8.5 Determining outcome utilities – underlying concepts

This last section begins the discussion of how to determine outcome utilities. The discussion of this important topic will only begin in this section. A more complete description of how to determine outcome utilities appears in the next chapter. The goal here is to describe the basic concepts underlying how risk attitudes are quantified.

Keep in mind that risk attitudes are a characteristic of an individual. This means that determining someone's outcome utility requires the assessment of how uncertainty affects their preferences for an outcome. The discussion that follows considers two different forms of the utility assessment process.

8.5.1 Lifetime-tradeoff assessment

As was noted earlier, McNeil and her colleagues used an outcome-based version of standard gamble assessment. Their assessment method was outcome-based in the sense that the participant provided outcomes, such as live 5 years, when responding to the assessment question. We will call this method *lifetime-tradeoff assessment*. To understand the reason for this label, recall the first question the study participants were asked. That question asked participants to consider a gamble that had an even chance of resulting either in a life lasting 25 years or immediate death. The response was a guaranteed outcome that the participant felts was equivalent to this gamble. The decision tree representation for this question has been repeated in Figure 8.12.

Consider the question depicted in Figure 8.12 from the perspective of someone like Patient A. With the risky procedure, Patient A faces the life expectancy of 12.5 years. This risk-averse individual would be willing to reduce their lifetime to a guaranteed 5 years to avoid the uncertainty of the gamble with the possible 25-year lifetime. That is, Patient A would tradeoff some of their lifetime to avoid risk. On the other hand, someone like Patient B, who is risk tolerant, would only be willing to reduce their lifetime to a guaranteed 20 years to avoid the same uncertainty. This means that Patient B would trade off less of their lifetime to avoid risk. In other words, the greater the importance placed on uncertainty the greater the acceptable lifetime tradeoff.

The question posed in Figure 8.12 also can be thought of as asking the participants to state their certainty equivalent for the risky treatment used in the assessment question. The certainty equivalent for a risky treatment is the guaranteed outcome that is equivalent to facing the uncertainty of that risky treatment. As we saw in the previous section, someone's risk attitudes are characterized by the difference between their certainty equivalent for a risky option and their life expectancy with that same option.

There are tricks for how best to ask assessment questions. So far, this discussion has implied that individuals answer lifetime-tradeoff assessment questions by directly stating their equivalent guaranteed lifetimes. For example, recall Patient A who had an equivalent guaranteed lifetime of 5 years for the first assessment question. That question asked the patient to consider a risky treatment that had an even chance of resulting either in a life lasting 25 years or immediate death. The implication has been that someone like Patient A would simply provide a value for the guaranteed outcome in response to this question.

The questions used by lifetime-tradeoff assessment can be difficult to answer with a specific value for the certainty equivalent. Often using a series yes-no questions provides a more effective approach. For example, an answer to that first question can be reached by starting with the following:

Suppose that you are faced with a risky treatment that has a 50% chance of causing your immediate death. You will live another 25 years if you survive the treatment. Your alternative is a second treatment that has no risk of immediate death but only guarantees a shorter lifetime of 1 year. Would you prefer this second treatment over the risky first treatment?

Presumably, the patient would answer "no" to this question, meaning that X_1 is greater than 1 year for the individual. The next question in the series would change the outcome of the treatment with a guaranteed outcome to a longer lifetime, such as 20 years. Expect for someone who is very risk tolerant, the answer to this second question most likely would now be "yes." This second answer provides an upper bound of 20 years for the value of X_1. By alternating between successively shorter and longer lifetimes for the second treatment, the bounds for X_1 can be narrowed. At the same time, the difficulty in answering the question becomes more difficult as the possible range for X_1 decreases. Ideally, the required level of precision for the outcome utility is reached before the individual becomes too unsure of their answers.

The sensitivity analysis described in Chapter 7 can be used to determine the required precision. The outcome utilities determined by assessment become part of the calculations performed during a decision analysis. Recall that sensitivity analysis shows how uncertainty about the values in those calculations affects the confidence we have in the conclusions that are reached. In turn, this implies the required level of precision for the outcome utilities.

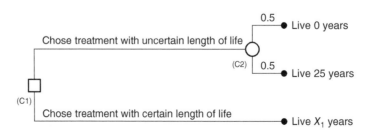

Figure 8.12 Decision tree representation of the first question asked each participant in the lung cancer treatment study. The value for X_1 is the participant's answer. This figure is a copy of Figure 8.4.

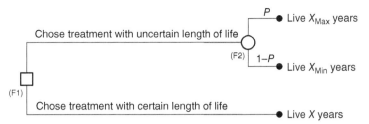

Figure 8.13 Decision tree representation of the general form for the assessment question. The values for the outcomes are chosen so that X_{Max} is greater than X and X is greater than X_{Min}. The value for P represents a level of uncertainty.

Using a series of questions to assess an outcome utility has another advantage over directly asking the individual to state their certainty equivalent in an assessment question. People who think of themselves as mathematically informed often will simply calculate the life expectancy for the risky alternative and mistakenly believe this calculation has determined the "correct" answer for the assessment question. Of course, some people are risk indifferent so their answer to the assessment question should be equal to calculated life expectancy. However, risk indifference is rare. Most likely these folks are just attempting to give what they believe is the correct answer to a question they do not fully understand.

The advantage of using the series of questions is that it requires the individual to think about risk in a variety of scenarios. Hopefully, this will help the individual understand more deeply what risk actually means to them.

So far, the discussion of lifetime-tradeoff assessment has shown how this approach was used to assess outcome utilities for a specific decision problem. Figure 8.13 shows the decision tree representing a general form for the questions used in lifetime-tradeoff assessment. Note that this is just the outcome-based standard gamble assessment question described earlier. The following three values in Figure 8.13 can adjust the assessment question to a represent different clinical contexts:

X_{Max} Maximum length of life in the risky treatment
X_{Min} Minimum length of life in the risky treatment
P Probability of the length of life will equal X_{Max} with the risky treatment

Someone in their eighties probably will not relate to an assessment question with a possible 50-year lifetime. This would suggest a smaller value for X_{Max}. Similarly, someone facing a decision with a very small probability of death may not be comfortable contemplating questions with large values for P. Patients should be asked to consider their risk attitudes in a context that is consistent with their clinical circumstances. Adjusting the parameter values can establish a clinical context that is meaningful for the individual.

The value for X in Figure 8.13 is provided by the individual and equals their certainty equivalent for the risky treatment. Given a value for X the following expression determines the utility for X relative to the utilities for X_{Max} and X_{Min}:

$$U(X) = P \times U(X_{max}) + (1-P) \times U(X_{min})$$

Definition: lifetime-tradeoff assessment

Lifetime-tradeoff assessment determines an individual's outcome utility by asking what guaranteed length of life X would be equivalent to a risky option that would result in one of two different lengths of life X_{Max} and X_{Min} with probability P and $1-P$, respectively. The decision tree presentation for this question is:

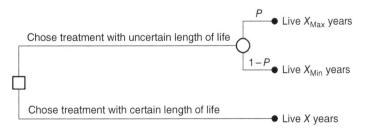

The following expression can be used to determine the utility for living X years relative to the utility for living X_{Max} years and X_{Min} years:

$$U(X) = P \times U(X_{Max}) + (1-P) \times U(X_{Min})$$

8.5.2 Survival-tradeoff assessment

McNeil and her colleagues chose to use lifetime-tradeoff assessment because their questions asked subjects to state something tangible – a length of life. Next, we will consider an alternate assessment approach that uses probabilities to express risk attitudes. We will call this second approach *survival-tradeoff assessment*. Note that survival-tradeoff assessment is just a renaming of the probability-based standard gamble assessment, which was discussed earlier. In the next two chapters, we will find that this naming convention highlights the relationship between the different forms of utility assessment that will be described.

Recall the first question used by McNeil and her colleagues. This was the question that asked the patient to consider a risky treatment that had an even chance of resulting either in a life lasting 25 years or immediate death. Figure 8.14 shows the decision tree representation for a version of this question expressed for use in a survival-tradeoff assessment. The structure of the decision tree for this question is much like the structure of the tree for the corresponding lifetime-tradeoff assessment question, shown in Figure 8.12. However, there are two differences. First, the guaranteed length of life has been changed from a variable (X) to a fixed value (5 years). Second, the probability for the outcome of living 25 years has been changed from a fixed value (0.5) to a variable (P). The answer to this question is a value for the probability P.

The following is a possible wording for the question:

Suppose that you are faced with a risky treatment that has a chance of causing your immediate death. You will live another 25 years if you survive this first treatment. Your alternative is a second treatment that has no risk of immediate death but provides a shorter length of life of only 5 years. For what probability of survival with the first treatment (P) would you be exactly indifferent between the two treatments?

The participant's answer to this question is a value for the survival probability P. That value for P is called the participant's *indifference probability* for the choice posed in the question. The following discussion shows how the indifference probability quantifies the participant's risk attitudes.

Consider how Patient A would answer this question. Recall that Patient A is risk averse. From the lifetime-tradeoff question, we know Patient A believed that being guaranteed 5 years was equivalent to the risky treatment when P is equal to 0.5. This means that Patient A's certainty equivalent is 5 years for the risky treatment when the survival probability is 0.5. However, the life expectancy for the risky treatment is 12.5 years when the survival probability of is 0.5. Someone who is risk averse has a certainty equivalent for a risky treatment that is less than what their life expectancy would be the treatment. Therefore, an indifference probability of 0.5 for Patient A is consistent with Patient A's risk aversion.

In general, we can determine the range of values for the indifference probability with risk aversion. Once again, using the test for risk aversion described in the previous section, when someone is risk averse their certainty equivalent for the risky treatment is less than their life expectancy with the treatment. The assessment question states that the certainty equivalent for the risky treatment is 5 years when the survival probability equals the individual's indifference probability. Moreover, for any value of the survival probability P the life expectancy for the risk treatment is calculated by the expression:

Life expectancy $= P \times 25$ years

For the risk-averse person, since life expectancy is greater than the certainty equivalent for a gamble. Therefore, it follows that

Certainty equivalent $= 5$ years $<$ Life expectancy $= P \times 25$ years

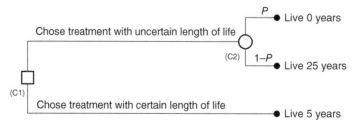

Figure 8.14 Decision tree representation of a version of the first question used in the lung cancer treatment study, expressed as a survival tradeoff assessment question. The value for *P* is the participant's answer.

which can be rearranged to show that

$$P > \frac{5\,\text{years}}{25\,\text{years}} = 0.2$$

In other words, anyone who is risk averse will have an indifference probability that is greater than 0.2 for this assessment question.

Now consider how someone who is risk tolerant would answer the same question. Recall that by definition, with risk tolerance, the certainty equivalent for a risky treatment is greater than the life expectancy. Once again, the certainty equivalent for the risky treatment in the question is 5 years when the value for P equals the individual's indifference probability. Using the same logic as for the risk-averse example, it follows that

$$P < \frac{5\,\text{years}}{25\,\text{years}} = 0.2$$

when someone is risk tolerant.

Finally, the same logic shows that the indifference probability for someone who is risk indifferent would be exactly 0.2.

This shows that there are values for the indifference probability that indicate risk aversion. There are values for the indifference probability that indicate risk tolerance. And there is a value for the indifference probability that indicates risk indifference. In short, the indifference probability captures the participant's risk attitudes.

Definition: survival-tradeoff assessment

Survival-tradeoff assessment determines an individual's outcome utility by asking what survival probability P would mean that a risky option is equivalent to a guaranteed length of life X, when the risky option will result in one of two different lengths of life X_{Max} and X_{Min} with probability P and $1-P$, respectively. The decision tree representing this question is:

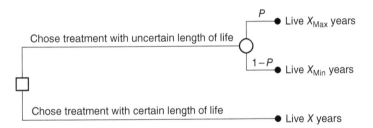

The value for P when the equivalence is true is called the *indifference probability*. Given a value for P, the following expression can be used to determine the utility for living X years relative to the utility for living X_{Max} years and X_{Min} years:

$$U(X) = P \times U(X_{\text{Max}}) + (1-P) \times U(X_{\text{Min}})$$

The decision tree for the generalization of the survival-tradeoff assessment question looks the same as the tree for the generalization of the lifetime-tradeoff assessment question shown in Figure 8.13. The only difference is that the survival probability P is now a variable and the length of life for the guaranteed outcome X is a constant, such as 5 years. Given a value for P, the same expression determines the outcome utility for the guaranteed outcome X:

$$U(X) = P \times U(X_{\text{Max}}) + (1-P) \times U(X_{\text{Min}})$$

Also, the same comments about the advantages of a series of yes-no assessment questions apply to survival-tradeoff assessment. Many people find it difficult to answer a direct question about their indifference probability in an assessment question. A series of questions starts the process with questions that typically are easier to answer.

Finally, as mentioned earlier, McNeil and her colleagues chose lifetime-tradeoff assessment because it required the participants to provide a highly tangible answer – a length of life. They also had more confidence in their subjects' understanding of assessment questions involving uncertain outcomes when the survival probability was a probability that had a more familiar value, such as 0.5. However, survival-tradeoff assessment also has been used successfully, at least in one research project involving large numbers of individuals (Attema *et al.*, 2013).

Summary

This chapter described the conceptual foundations for incorporating risk attitudes into the analysis of a decision

- Risk attitudes are how preferences for alternatives are affected by the uncertainty in those alternatives. In the case of monetary outcomes, an individual is *risk averse* if they prefer receiving the expected value of a gamble over the gamble itself.
- An individual is *risk tolerant* if they prefer the gamble over receiving the expected value of the gamble.
- von Neumann Morgenstern utility is a numerical value assigned to an outcome such that the expected utility, when computed for each alternative in the decision problem, is always greatest for the preferred alternative.
- With *standard gamble assessment*, the utility for outcome x relative to the utilities for outcomes x_A and x_B is determined by the values for outcome x and probability p such that the following two alternatives are equivalent.

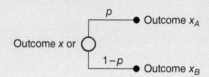

When the two alternatives are equivalent

$$U(x) = pU(x_A) + (1-p)U(x_B)$$

Standard gamble assessment when the outcome x is known is called *probability based*. With probability-based assessment, the value for the probability p where the guaranteed outcome and the gamble are equivalent is called the *indifference probability*. Standard gamble assessment when the probability p is known is called *outcome based*.
- Treatment alternatives with a risk of death in the near term are overvalued in comparison with less risk of death in the near term if the analysis does not account for risk aversion.
- The *certainty equivalent* for an uncertain alternative is the guaranteed outcome that has the same utility as the expected utility for the uncertain alternative.
- When faced with decisions involving risky alternatives, an individual demonstrates *risk-averse* preferences for length of life outcome if
  1. They prefer a guaranteed lifetime that equals the life expectancy for a risky alternative rather than actually facing the uncertainty of that alternative.
  2. Their certainty equivalent for a risky alternative is less than what their life expectancy would be with that alternative.
  3. The shape of their utility curve over the range of outcomes is concave.
- When faced with decisions involving risky alternatives, a patient demonstrates *risk-tolerant* preferences for length of life outcome if
  1. They prefer to face the uncertainty of a risky alternative over a guaranteed lifetime that equals the life expectancy for the risky alternative.
  2. Their certainty equivalent for a risky alternative is more than what their life expectancy would be with that alternative.
  3. The shape of their utility curve over the range of outcomes is convex.

- When faced with decisions involving risky alternatives, an individual demonstrates *risk-indifferent* preferences for length-of-life outcome if
  1. They are indifferent between facing the uncertainty of a risky alternative and having a guaranteed lifetime that equals the life expectancy for the risky alternative.
  2. Their certainty equivalent for a risky alternative equals what their life expectancy would be with that alternative.
  3. The shape of their utility curve over the range of outcomes is a straight line.
- *Lifetime-tradeoff assessment* determines an individual's outcome utility by asking what guaranteed length of life X would be equivalent to a risky option that would result in one of two different lengths of life X_{Max} and X_{Min} with probability P and $1-P$, respectively. The decision tree representing this question is:

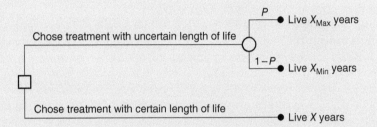

The following expression can be used to determine the utility for living X years relative to the utility for living X_{Max} years and X_{Min} years:

$$U(X) = P \times U(X_{Max}) + (1-P) \times U(X_{Min})$$

- *Survival-tradeoff assessment* determines an individual's outcome utility by asking what survival probability P would mean that a risky option is equivalent to a guaranteed length of life X, when the risky option will result in one of two different lengths of life X_{Max} and X_{Min} with probability P and $1-P$, respectively. The decision tree presentation for this question is:

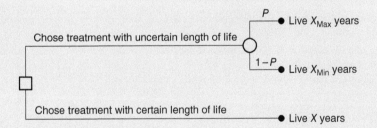

The value for P when the equivalence is true is called the *indifference probability*. Given a value for P the following expression can be used to determine the utility for living X years relative to the utility for living X_{Max} years and X_{Min} years:

$$U(X) = P \times U(X_{Max}) + (1-P) \times U(X_{Min})$$

Epilogue

The focus of this chapter has been the question: how do we fully capture the preferences of the patient who will live with the consequences of a risky treatment? Decision analysis quantifies preferences as numerical values that are assigned to each of the possible outcomes of a decision. The analysis finds the treatment that maximizes life expectancy when those outcome values are assigned based solely on length of the patient's life.

However, life expectancy provides an imperfect comparison of risky treatments. One shortcoming is the omission of quality of life as a consideration when comparing treatment options. How to adjust an analysis to reflect how patients feel about the quality of their lives will be covered in a later chapter. Another shortcoming of life expectancy, as an outcome measure, is its failure to account for risk attitudes. The chapter focused on addressing this second shortcoming by showing how risk attitudes can be reflected in the analysis of a decision.

Risk attitudes are an intangible but inevitable part of how we think about uncertainty. Achieving a given length of life because that was the only possibility is not the same as facing that same lifetime as the life expectancy for a risky treatment that also could result in much shorter lifetimes. Some individuals will prefer the risky treatment when it also includes the possibility of a significantly longer lifetime. Those individuals have what we called "low risk aversion," or even "risk tolerance." Even fewer individuals ignore the risk differences and prefer a treatment based solely on the life expectancy. We called these preferences "risk indifference." However, most of us prefer to avoid risk. When faced with multiple alternatives we usually chose the one that minimizes the risk of bad outcomes. We called this behavior "risk aversion."

The work by McNeil and her colleagues showed that risk attitudes mattered to patients when faced with a choice between treatments for lung cancer. The method they used demonstrated how to quantify risk attitudes based on the theoretical work of two brilliant thinkers John von Neumann and Oskar Morgenstern. We called the method used by McNeil and her colleagues "expected utility analysis."

The expected utility analysis demonstrated by McNeil and her colleagues could generalize to many of the decisions encountered in care of patients. However, a key step in this form of analysis is determination of something we called "outcome utilities." The practical challenges in determining outcome utilities are a key barrier to making expected utility analysis a useful clinical tool. The next chapter will show how those challenges can be reduced.

Bibliography

Attema, A., Brouwer, W., and l'Haridon, O. (2013) Prospect theory in the health domain: a quantitative assessment. *Journal of Health Economics*, **32**, 1057–65.

Hawkins, N.V. (1975) Panel discussion of glottic tumors. VIII. The treatment of glottic carcinoma: an analysis of 800 cases. *Laryngoscope*, **85**, 1485–93.

McNeil, B.J., Weichselbaum, R., and Pauker, S.G. (1978) Fallacy of the five-year survival in lung cancer. *New England Journal of Medicine*, **299**, 1397–1401.

McNeil, B.J., Weichselbaum, R., and Pauker, S.G. (1981) Speech and survival. Tradeoffs between quality and quantity of life in laryngeal cancer. *New England Journal of Medicine*, **304**, 982–7.

Stokes, M.E., Thompson, D., Montoya, E.L. *et al.* (2008) Ten-year survival and cost following breast cancer recurrence: estimates from SEER-Medicare data. *Value in Health*, **11**, 213–20.

von Neumann, J. and Morgenstern, O. (1947) *Theory of Games and Economic Behavior*, 2nd ed., Princeton University Press, Princeton, NJ.

CHAPTER 9

Outcome utilities – clinical applications

9.1 Introduction

This chapter shows how expected utility analysis could be used in clinical settings. We noted in the previous chapter that adding uncertainty to an alternative can change how we compare that alternative to other alternatives. That change reflects what we call our risk attitudes. An analysis that ignores our risk attitudes will leave out a consideration that most of us feel is important.

More precisely, the previous chapter showed how to quantify risk attitudes in medical decision problems. The key idea is that something called utility can measure preferences for the possible outcomes of a decision. Those measures, called outcome utilities, reflect how the individual feels about risk. Combining outcome utilities with outcome probabilities calculates the expected utility for the alternatives in a decision. John von Neumann and his colleague Oskar Morgenstern showed that the most-preferred alternative will be the one with the greatest expected utility. This means the comparison of alternatives based on expected utilities accounts for risk attitudes.

The previous chapter discussed a study conducted in 1987 that used expected utility analysis to demonstrate how a patient's preference in a choice between lung cancer treatments can depend on that patient's risk attitudes. While the available treatments for lung cancer have changed significantly since 1987, the underlying notion that risk attitudes matter has not. The paper describing this result was titled *The Fallacy of Five-Year Survival* (McNeil *et al.*, 1978).

Therefore, outcome utilities represent something important for many patient care decisions. Despite this importance, major challenges confront the clinical use of expected utility analysis. Perhaps foremost among those challenges are the time constraints in most clinical settings. Assembling the necessary numbers and performing the calculations is time consuming.

A partial solution may be found in the vast amounts of available clinical data resulting from electronic medical record adoption. That data will aid the discovery of credible values for the necessary probabilities. Electronic medical record systems also provide computational resources that could automate the necessary calculations. Therefore, a data-driven application, fully integrated into an electronic medical record system, could use automation to address the time barrier constraint faced by the clinical use of expected utility analysis.

Nevertheless, once the time challenge has been addressed, the clinical use of expected utility analysis still must address an important cognitive barrier. Risk attitudes may be an inevitable part of how we view risky outcomes. However, most people do not understand how risk attitudes can be quantified. The utility assessment concepts described in the previous chapter provide a theoretical framework for addressing that lack of understanding.

Medical Decision Making, Third Edition. Harold C. Sox, Michael C. Higgins, Douglas K. Owens, and Gillian Sanders Schmidler.
© 2024 John Wiley & Sons Ltd. Published 2024 by John Wiley & Sons Ltd.

Answering an assessment question forces the individuals to express their intangible concerns about risk as a concrete number.

But that concrete number is only meaningful if the patient fully understands the assessment question. Moreover, the multitude of outcomes possible after a treatment requires a corresponding number of assessment questions. The number of required questions further complicates the clinical use of expected utility analysis.

This chapter focuses on how to simplify the utility assessment process. The approach described uses a mathematical expression called a *parametric utility model*. This expression determines outcome utilities by using patterns in how most people think about risk. The result is a simple way to determine someone's outcome utilities based on their answer to a single assessment question. Moreover, that question often can be expressed in scenarios that will be more familiar to many patients.

Therefore, the parametric utility model described in this chapter improves the chances that meaningful outcome utilities can be determined in clinical settings. This approach also addresses the challenge in how to use expected utility analysis in the design of clinical policies. A clinical policy sets patient care for a population rather than an individual. As noted in Chapter 8, utility is the property of an individual rather than a population. This raises the question – whose outcome utilities should be represented in the design of a clinical policy? The use of a parametric utility model addresses this problem by simplifying how a clinical policy can be adjusted to the risk preferences of a population member. This adjustment is much like how clinical policies often are adjusted to reflect the patient's clinical attributes that are relevant to their care.

The first section in this chapter describes parametric utility models and their use in the analysis of decisions for individual patients. The second section extends the discussion to clinical policy design. Finally, the third section turns to a slightly different topic and discusses the implications of risk attitudes in how treatment options should be communicated to patients.

9.2   A parametric model for outcome utilities

One goal of this book is individualization of medical decisions. The subjectivity of utility is key to achieving this goal. The assessment process used to determine someone's utility means the analysis will represent how that individual feels about risk. But then, as has just been discussed, the complexity of the assessment process also interferes with the clinical use of utility-based decision analysis.

It should be mentioned that one solution would be to simply ignore risk aversion. Risk-averse and risk-tolerant utility curves are as varied as the individuals who make up our world. On the other hand, there is only one risk *indifferent* utility curve – the straight line. This singularity is appealing to the analyst – if all risk-indifferent people have the same utility curve, why not simplify the problem of quantifying preferences by assuming everyone is risk indifferent? This assumption reduces the conceptual complexity of an analysis, but it ignores the individuality in how different people see the same problem. As *The Fallacy of Five-Year Survival* demonstrated, differences in how individuals view uncertainty can be important to finding the preferred alternative in a choice between treatments.

Utility assessment is not easy. However, it might be easier if it were possible to predict the shape of a person's utility curve with sufficient accuracy using a minimal number of assessment questions. This section demonstrates such an approach based on parametric models. These mathematical expressions minimize the number of assessment questions and still retain the conceptual power of von Neumann-Morgenstern utility as a representation of risk attitudes.

9.2.1   What is a parametric model?

In general, a parametric model is a mathematical expression that can be adjusted to fit a real-world phenomenon by changing a few values that are part of the expression. Those values are the model parameters. Parametric models play a central role in statistical inference by reducing the number of observations needed to fully characterize a population property.

The normal or Gaussian distribution provides an important example of how parametric models simplify data analysis. Consider a property of a real-world phenomenon, such as the size of a measurement error. If that property has a Gaussian distribution, then the possible values for the property can be fully described just by knowing the two Gaussian distribution parameters of mean and variance. Determining values for those two parameters completely describes the full range of possible values for the property, even when extended to the entire population.

> **Definition: parametric utility model**
>
> A parametric utility model determines the values for outcome utilities by using a mathematical expression that includes terms, called parameters, that can be adjusted to match someone's risk attitudes.

9.2.2   The exponential utility model

The parametric model we will use to represent outcome utilities is called the *exponential utility model*. One of its functional forms is:

$$U(x) = 1 - e^{-\gamma x}$$

where x is the length of life, and γ is the model parameter.[1] The exponential utility model has not been widely discussed in the medical decision-making literature. However, this parametric model is frequently used when utility analysis is applied to other fields. A traditional reference is Howard Raffia's **Decision Analysis Introductory Lectures on Choices under Uncertainty** (Raffia, 1968).

Figure 9.1 shows the curve of an exponential utility model. The value for the parameter γ in this example is 0.13/year. Later sections in this chapter discuss several approaches for determining a value for the parameter. We will see that a parameter value of 0.13/year represents the risk attitudes of the typical participant in the study of patient preferences by McNeil and her colleagues.

In fact, the curve shown in Figure 9.1 may look familiar. Recall Patient A, the hypothetical patient used in the discussion of risk attitudes in the previous chapter. We supposed that Patient A provided answers to each of the three assessment questions used by McNeil and her colleagues in their study of risk attitudes. Patient A's supposed answers matched the average responses among the participants in the study. In the previous chapter, we saw that Patient A's answers implied the three outcome utilities that were plotted in Figure 8.6. The exponential utility model curve in Figure 9.1 is the curve fitted to those outcome utilities in Figure 8.6.

More precisely, the curve in Figure 9.1 is the exponential utility model fitted to Patient A's answer to the first of the three assessment questions. This was the question that asked the patient what guaranteed length of life is equivalent

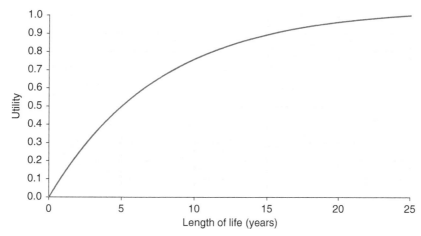

Figure 9.1 Example of an exponential utility model for length of life with a parameter value of 0.13/year. The utility values have been scaled so that the utility for 0 years of life is 0 and the utility for 25 years of life is 1.

---

[1] The term e in the exponential utility model is a constant called Euler's number. The value for e is 2.7183. Readers probably encountered this useful constant back in the first math class they took that discussed logarithms. For complicated reasons e also appears in mathematical representations for medical phenomenon that depend on the accumulation of events, such as drug elimination in pharmacology, radioactive decay in nuclear medicine, or hazard rates in epidemiology. We will see this constant again when we talk about survival models in a later chapter.

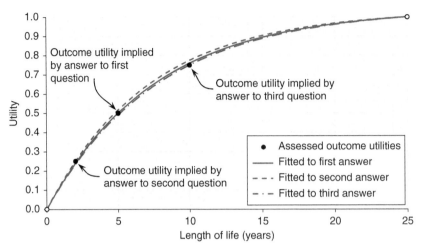

Figure 9.2 Three exponential utility models fitted to hypothetical Patient A's answers to the three utility assessment questions used in the lung cancer treatment decision study.

to a risky treatment that had an even chance of resulting either in a lifetime of 25 years or immediate death. We assumed Patient A's answer to this question was 5 years implying Patient A's utility for living 5 years is 0.50. The exponential utility model shown in Figure 9.1 is matched to this assessed outcome utility. Figure 9.2 shows the three outcome utilities implied by Patient A's answers to the three assessment questions. Figure 9.2 shows the three exponential utility models fitted to the corresponding utilities.

Later in this chapter, we will describe how to adjust the parameter γ so that an exponential utility model matches a single assessed outcome utility. However, for now, notice the close agreement between the three utility curves. This agreement is not a coincidence. Patient A matches the average of the responses for the 14 participants in the lung cancer study. Those responses illustrate a pattern often found in how we feel about risk. That pattern is the assumption underlying the use of the exponential utility model and will be discussed after some observations about how the outcome utilities shown in Figures 9.1 and 9.2 have been scaled.

9.2.3 Scaling exponential utility models

Recall the discussion in the previous chapter of how outcome utilities are scaled according to the utilities for two reference outcomes. Typically, we select immediate death as the worst possible outcome and set the corresponding utility equal to 0. In principle, the maximum length of life would be the obvious choice for the other reference outcome. However, the maximum possible length of life is a fuzzy concept for most patients. Instead, we often pick an arbitrary value for the second reference outcome that suits our purposes.

For example, Figures 9.1 and 9.2 show outcome utilities for lengths of life between 0 and 25 years. Therefore, 25 years was used at the second reference outcome and given the utility of 1. This meant the values for the utility curve shown in Figures 9.1 and 9.2 will range from 0 to 1. Life can last longer than 25 years. The outcome utilities will be greater than 1 for these longer lifetimes. However, that does not matter as long as we are consistent in how we define all outcome utilities relative to the same two reference values.

Mathematically, this means the utility curves in Figures 9.1 and 9.2 show the values for the following version of the exponential utility model:

$$U(x) = \frac{1 - e^{-\gamma x}}{1 - e^{-\gamma \, 25 \, years}}$$

Recall that for any nonzero value x, raising x to the zeroth power equals 1. That is

$$x^0 = 1$$

Therefore, this second version of the exponential utility model equals 0 when x equals 0. Note the expression also equals 1 when x equals 25 years.

This second version of the exponential utility model is the same as the first version except that we have divided by a value that is a positive constant with respect to the outcome measure x. Dividing or multiplying all outcome values by the same positive constant does not change the meaning of an analysis based on the resulting outcome utilities any more than switching from a Fahrenheit scale to a Celsius scale changes the meaning of a temperature.

This discussion of utility scaling may seem like an unnecessary diversion; however, scaling can lead to confusion when we use still another version of the exponential utility model:

$$U(x) = \frac{1 - e^{-\gamma x}}{\gamma}$$

This novel version of the exponential utility model may look different; however, it is just the same expression we started with, only divided by the parameter γ. And γ is just another constant so far as changes in x are concerned. This means that an analysis using this third form of the exponential utility model will have the same results as an analysis based on the original form. Later in this chapter, we will find that using this third form of the exponential utility model greatly simplifies how we calculate expected utilities.

Definition: exponential utility model

The exponential utility uses the following formula to express an individual's utility for an outcome measured by the variable x.

$$U(x) = 1 - e^{-\gamma x}$$

For example, x might be the length of the individual's life. The term γ quantifies the individual's risk attitudes and is expressed in units that are one over the units of x.

The exponential utility model also can be scaled so that $U(A) = 0$ and $U(B) = 1$ by the following form:

$$U(x) = \frac{e^{-\gamma A} - e^{-\gamma x}}{e^{-\gamma A} - e^{-\gamma B}}$$

The following is a third form of the exponential utility function:

$$U(x) = \frac{1 - e^{-\gamma x}}{\gamma}$$

9.2.4 Assumption underlying the exponential utility model

The exponential utility model provides an exact match for the outcome utilities of someone whose preferences follow a simple pattern called the *delta property*. Perhaps this pattern is most easily understood in the context of a monetary gamble.

Suppose the following equivalence is true:

Win $400 equivalent to ○ ─┬─ p ──● Win $800
                          └─ $1-p$ ──● Win $0

The pattern justifying the exponential utility model holds if the same equivalence is true even if the same fixed amount is added to each of the three possible outcomes in the question. That is, this equivalence means for any Δ, it also is true that:

Win $400 + \Delta$ equivalent to ○ ─┬─ p ──● Win $800 + \Delta$
                                     └─ $1-p$ ──● Win $0 + \Delta$

This pattern is called the *delta property*.

When the delta property is true for someone's preferences, the utilities for that individual can be presented by an exponential utility model. The opposite also is true. Not only does the delta property imply an exponential utility model, but it also is true that an exponential utility model requires the delta property.

Proof of the relationship between the delta property and the exponential utility model is beyond the scope of this book. The interested reader can find a proof in the reference by Howard Raffia mentioned early (Raffia, 1968). However, this result establishes a simple representation for someone's utility. When the delta property is true, an individual's utility for all possible outcomes is determined by establishing the value for the parameter γ. For reasons that will be explained shortly, the parameter γ will be called the *risk parameter*.

Definition: delta property and constant risk attitudes

An individual's preferences have the delta property if for any outcomes X_A, X_B, and X_C and probability p, the following equivalence:

implies the same equivalence if Δ is added to each of the outcomes. That is, for any Δ, it also is true that:

Someone whose risk attitudes have the delta property is also said to have *constant risk attitudes*.

When an individual's risk attitudes match the delta property, their outcome utilities can be determined by an exponential utility model.

Assuming the delta property also can be thought of as assuming risk attitudes are constant. In effect, the Δ in the definition of the delta property establishes a context in which the gamble between the guaranteed outcomes X_A is compared to the gamble between outcomes X_B and X_C is considered. As we saw in the previous chapter, when the guaranteed outcome and gamble are equivalent, the value for the probability p characterizes an individual's risk attitudes.

This equivalence can be depicted by the following diagram:

The greater the individual's risk aversion, the greater the value for p in this diagram. The delta property assumes that p does not change when the value for Δ changes. In other words, the delta property assumes that risk attitudes are constant across changes in context.

As one might expect, assuming the delta property, or constant risk attitudes, is not always accurate. Consider a monetary gamble with prizes ranging from $0 to $1000 from the perspective of someone who owns only a few dollars. That individual's attitudes toward the gamble might change significantly if they suddenly inherited a million dollars. This dramatic change in wealth probably would reduce their concerns about an adverse outcome for the gamble, which would mean a change in that individual's risk attitudes. In other words, in the extreme, the constant risk attitudes assumption of the exponential utility model may not always be true.

Nonetheless, the delta property is part of a descriptive model of preferences called *Prospect Theory*. We will discuss this model of decision making later in this chapter when we consider how best to communicate risk to patients. Daniel Kahneman and Amos Tversky developed Prospect Theory by observing how individuals make choices between gambles. One of the observations they made when formulating their model is that individuals typically do ignore context when choosing between gambles and guaranteed alternatives. In other words, Prospect Theory assumes risk attitudes are constant across contexts.

9.2.5 Determining the exponential utility model parameter – first approach

We will now consider how to determine the exponential utility model parameter from the answer to an assessment question. Recall the lifetime-survival assessment question described in the previous chapter. This question uses the outcome-based form of standard gamble assessment to determine the guaranteed outcome that has a given utility. For example, suppose that lifetime-survival assessment determined the following equivalence for Patient A:

This would mean that Patient A believes living 5 years has an outcome utility of 0.5 if immediate death has a utility of 0 and living 25 years has a utility of 1. What does this tell us about Patient A's value for exponential utility model parameter γ?

From the definition of outcome utilities, we know this equivalence can be expressed as follows:

$$U(5\,\text{years}) = 0.5 \times U(25\,\text{years}) + 0.5 \times U(0\,\text{years})$$

The term on the left side of the equal sign is the utility for the guaranteed outcome in the assessment question. The term on the right side of the equal sign is the expected utility for the gamble.

Since we are using the exponential utility model to express Patient A's outcome utilities, for any length of life x, we have

$$U(x\,\text{years}) = 1 - e^{-\gamma x}$$

where γx in this expression is: just the product of the parameter γ and the length of life x. In particular,

$$U(5\,\text{years}) = 1 - e^{-\gamma 5}$$

Therefore, we can express the equivalence learned from the lifetime-survival assessment question as

$$\left(1 - e^{-\gamma 5}\right) = 0.5 \times \left(1 - e^{-\gamma 25}\right) + 0.5 \times \left(1 - e^{-\gamma 0}\right)$$

But

$$e^{-\gamma 0} = e^0 = 1$$

This means we can simplify the expression for lifetime-survival assessment question as follows

$$\left(1 - e^{-\gamma 5}\right) = 0.5 \times \left(1 - e^{-\gamma 25}\right) + 0.5 \times (1 - 1) = 0.5 \times \left(1 - e^{-\gamma 25}\right)$$

or rearranging terms

$$\frac{1 - e^{-\gamma 5}}{1 - e^{-\gamma 25}} = 0.5$$

This is as far as we can go with simple algebraic manipulations. The correct value for γ must satisfy this last expression; however, it is not possible to turn this expression into an equation with γ on one side of the equal sign and everything else on the other side.

However, there are several other approaches for determining the value for γ that satisfies this equation. Perhaps the simplest is a trial-and-error process that evaluates the ratio on the left for different values of γ until the ratio equals 0.5. Done correctly, this brute force approach will find that the ratio is close to the target of 0.5 when γ equals 0.13/year. In other words, based on Patient A's answer to the lifetime-survival assessment question that started this example, the value for γ is approximately 0.13/year. Appendix A.9.1 presents a nomogram that also determines the exponential utility model parameter from the answer to the assessment question.

Result: determining the exponential utility model parameter

Suppose that someone's risk attitudes mean the following equivalence is true:

The value of the exponential utility model parameter γ satisfies the following expression:

$$\frac{1-e^{-\gamma X_A}}{1-e^{-\gamma X_B}} = p$$

The value for γ satisfying this expression can be solved by trial-and-error methods that evaluate the ratio on the left for different values of the parameter γ until the ratio equals the probability on the right.

To summarize what has been established so far,
1. Risk attitudes can be important when deciding between treatment alternatives.
2. Von Neuman–Morgenstern utility incorporates risk attitudes into the analysis of treatment decisions.
3. A mathematical expression called the exponential utility model can determine the von Neumann–Morgenstern utilities for a problem.
4. The answer to a single assessment question fully specifies the exponential utility model that matches an individual's risk attitudes.

However, there still remains a problem with the utility assessment process. The required assessment questions ask the individual to consider choices in hypothetical scenarios. In order for meaningful responses, those scenarios must be meaningful to the individual. The problem is that, so far, the utility assessment questions used in this discussion are based on scenarios that are far removed from the normal human experience.

For example, consider the following wording of the assessment question that has been used to illustrate how the exponential utility model parameter is determined:

> Suppose you have a disease that will cause your death in 5 years. Also suppose that if this disease were cured you could expect to live another 25 years. If there is a risky treatment that will either cure the disease or cause your immediate death, how small would the risk of death have to be for you to choose the treatment?

Note that this question includes outcomes like *death in 5 years* and *live another 25 years*, meaning that the individual will *live exactly 5 years* or *live exactly 25 years*. Few people have any familiarity with outcomes like *live exactly 5 years* or *live exactly 25 years*. Does an outcome that guarantees 5 years of life mean the individual no longer has to worry about stepping off the curb in front of a car and dying tomorrow? This wording of the assessment question depends on an unrealistic scenario. There are few real-world situations in which someone knows exactly how long they will live. This means we are asking the patient to make difficult choices between very unfamiliar options.

Fortunately, the exponential utility model supports an alternative form for assessment questions that minimizes the use of unrealistic scenarios. Moreover, we will see that these alternative assessment questions avoid the complexity of how the exponential utility model parameter is determined.

9.2.6 Determining the exponential utility model parameter – alternate assessment approach
The following is a natural rewording of the assessment question discussed earlier:

> Suppose that you have a disease that will cause your death, <u>on average</u>, in 5 years. Also suppose that if this disease were cured you could expect to live, <u>on average</u>, another 25 years. If there is a risky treatment that will either cure your disease or cause your immediate death, how small would probability of death have to be for you to choose this treatment?

The underlined portions in this second wording of the assessment question emphasize that each of the unrealistic guaranteed lifetimes has been replaced by an average lifetime. In other words, the assessment question now has been asked in a way that is more like the world in which patients actually live. A treatment can change the average length of life; however, a treatment does not remove the uncertainty about whether that change takes place. The patient can still step off that curb in front of a car.

Treating these two wordings of the assessment question as equivalent is tempting. However, the two wordings actually describe very different situations. The first wording will be called *guaranteed outcome assessment* because it compares outcomes that will be experienced with certainty. The second wording of the question will be called *uncertain outcome assessment* because it involves outcomes that are themselves driven by chance occurrences. The expected value for those gambles may equal the corresponding value for the guaranteed outcome in the first version of the question. However, the fundamental principle underlying utility analysis is that a gamble is not the same as its expected value. Recall that earlier example with a choice between 50% of winning $2 000 000 or a guaranteed outcome $1 000 000. That difference between the options in that choice is the main motivation for considering expected utility analysis in the first place.

> **Definition: guaranteed outcome assessment**
>
> Guaranteed outcome assessment uses questions that ask the individual to compare outcomes that are guaranteed lengths of life.

This presents a dilemma. The guaranteed outcome assessment question aligns with how von Neumann–Morgenstern utility assigns values to specific lengths of life. The uncertain outcome assessment question avoids unrealistic scenarios but does not immediately lead to a utility for a given outcome. This is where a property of the exponential utility model becomes useful.

> **Definition: uncertain outcome assessment**
>
> Uncertain outcome assessment uses questions that ask the individual to compare outcomes that are uncertain, typically expressed as a life expectancy or a survival model.

As a first step in resolving the dilemma, consider Figure 9.3. This figure shows a decision tree representation for the first version of the assessment question – what we call guaranteed outcome assessment. The only uncertainty is the patient's survival if Option B is chosen. That uncertainty is represented by the chance node **A2**. Assuming the patient survives the hypothetical treatment represented by **A2**, the outcome is a guaranteed lifetime of 25 years. Otherwise, if Option A is chosen, the patient faces a guaranteed lifetime of 5 years. Those guaranteed lifetimes are why the assessment process represented in Figure 9.3 is called *guaranteed* outcome assessment.

Now consider the decision tree shown in Figure 9.4. This decision tree depicts what we are calling an *uncertain* outcome assessment question. Option B still includes the uncertainty about survival, as represented by chance node **B3**. However, even if the hypothetical treatment is survived, the individual still faces uncertainty about how long they will live afterward. This additional uncertainty is represented by chance node **B4**. If the patient survives the treatment, they can die during the following first year, second year, third year, and so forth. The probability of dying during each of those following years is such that the patient's life expectancy, after surviving the hypothetical treatment, is 25 years.

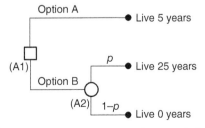

Figure 9.3 Decision tree representing guaranteed outcome assessment expressed as a survival-tradeoff assessment question. The individual provides the value for the probability *p* such that Option A and Option B are equivalent.

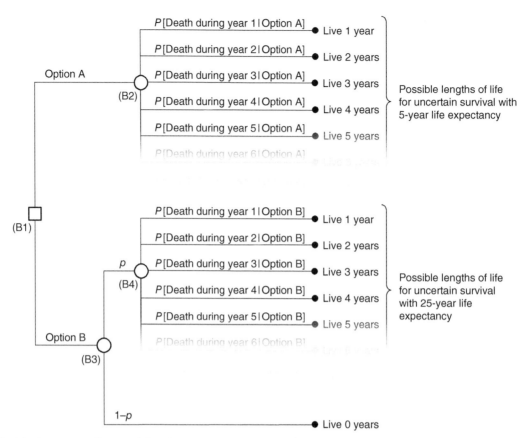

Figure 9.4 Decision tree representing uncertain outcome assessment expressed as a survival-tradeoff assessment question. The individual provides the value for the probability *p* such that Option A and Option B are equivalent.

The patient faces a similar uncertainty about the length of their life with Option A. This uncertainty is represented by chance node **B2**. The difference is that the probabilities for the different possible lifetimes are such that the life expectancy is 5 years.

At first glance, the decision tree shown in Figure 9.4 may look intimidating because of all the branches. However, this decision tree is very similar to the tree used in the previous chapter to represent the lung cancer treatment decision (see Figure 8.2). The necessary branch probabilities in that earlier decision tree came from the observed survival models for surgical treatment and radiotherapy (see Figure 8.3). Based on those branch probabilities, the expected utilities were easily computed for the lung cancer treatment alternatives.

Therefore, computing the expected utilities for the two options shown in Figure 9.4 is not difficult. However, our real interest in this decision tree is how to determine the value for the exponential utility model parameter γ when those two expected utilities are equal. That turns out to be easier than it may appear; however, we first need to understand some properties of survival models.

Survival models are mathematical representations of the uncertainty about the length of a patient's life. Different examples of survival models are discussed extensively in Chapter 11. The discussion of utility assessment in this chapter focuses on one particularly useful example called the *exponential survival model*.

In general, a survival model shows the probability the patient will survive until given times in the future. In turn, those survival probabilities depend on the risk of death the patient faces during each time interval prior to one of those given times. The probability of death during a time interval is called the *hazard rate*. For example, a hazard rate might measure the probability the patient dies during a 1-year time interval – what is called the *annual mortality rate*.

The exponential survival model assumes the hazard rate remains constant for the remainder of the patient's life. In general, this assumption obviously is false – the hazard rate typically increases as the patient ages. However, in later chapters, we will see that assuming a constant hazard rate provides a useful approximation for the survival probabilities faced by many patients.

The following is the functional form for the exponential survival model

$$P\left[\text{Alive at time } t\right] = 1 - e^{-\lambda t}$$

where t is time measured relative to now and λ is that constant hazard rate. The hazard rate is expressed in the time units of t. For example, suppose that t is 20 years. Then λ is the probability of dying during a year and $1 - e^{-\lambda 20}$ equals the probability that the patient will still be alive in 20 years.

For our purposes, the exponential survival model has two important properties. First, with the exponential survival model, the patient's life expectancy is 1 over the hazard rate. For example, if a patient faces an annual mortality rate of 0.1/year, then the patient's life expectancy is 1 over 0.1/year or 10 years.

The second important property of the exponential survival model is how easy it is to compute expected utility when risk attitudes are represented by the exponential *utility* model. Suppose that the uncertainty for the length of a patient's life can be represented by the exponential survival model with a hazard rate of λ. In particular, we will use the third form of the exponential utility model described earlier. That is, the utility for x years of life is

$$U(x) = \frac{1 - e^{-\gamma x}}{\gamma}$$

Then

$$\text{Expected utility} = \frac{1}{\lambda + \gamma}$$

In other words, that messy expected utility calculation reduces to a simple arithmetic expression. Proving this useful result requires the use of integrals from calculus. Therefore, that proof will not be presented here. However, this means we can avoid determining all of those branch probabilities and performing that long summation. Instead, we can determine the expected utility by dividing the sum of two numbers by 1.

Armed with this simple expression, let us return to our goal of determining the value for the exponential utility model parameter γ. Recall the uncertain outcome assessment question shown in Figure 9.4. Our goal is the value for γ implied when Option A and Option B are equivalent in Figure 9.4. We will approach this goal with the assumption that the uncertainty about the length of life in the assessment question can be represented by exponential survival models.

More specifically, the uncertainty with the choice of Option A will be represented by an exponential survival model with a life expectancy of 5 years. Using that first useful property of exponential survival models, the life expectancy for an exponential survival model is 1 over the model parameter λ. Therefore, the exponential survival model with Option A has a value of 1 over 5 years, or 0.2/year, for the parameter λ. This means

$$\text{Expected utility for Option A} = \frac{1}{0.2/\text{year} + \gamma}$$

Similarly, the uncertainty with the choice of Option B in Figure 9.4, assuming the patient survives the hypothetical treatment represented by chance node **B3**, will be represented by an exponential survival model with a life expectancy of 25 years. That life expectancy implies value for λ of 1 over 25 years, or 0.04/year.

The stated probability for surviving the hypothetical treatment represented by chance node **B3** in Figure 9.4 is 0.5. This means

$$\text{Expected utility for Option B} = 0.5 \times \frac{1}{0.04/\text{year} + \gamma} + 0.5 \times U(0 \text{ years})$$

$$\text{Expected utility for Option A} = \frac{0.5}{0.04/\text{year} + \gamma}$$

Recall that our goal is to determine the value for the utility model parameter γ such that Option A and Option B are equivalent. These two options are equivalent if their expected utilities are equal. This means we want to determine the value for γ such that

$$\frac{1}{0.2/\text{year} + \gamma} = \frac{0.5}{0.04/\text{year} + \gamma}$$

A little algebra can be used to solve this expression for γ. The result is

$$\gamma = \frac{0.5 \times 0.2 / \text{year} - 0.04 / \text{year}}{1 - 0.5} = \frac{0.1 / \text{year} - 0.04 / \text{year}}{0.5} = \frac{0.06 / \text{year}}{0.5} = 0.12 / \text{year}$$

In other words, the equivalence of the two options in the uncertain outcome assessment question implies the value of 0.12/year for the exponential utility model parameter.

Recall that earlier we used guaranteed outcome assessment to determine a value of 0.13/year for the exponential utility model parameter. The difference between this value for γ and the value determined by uncertain outcome assessment is not surprising because the two forms of assessment are asking different questions. One is asking about the patient's preferences for options that ultimately result in guaranteed lifetimes. The other is asking about the patient's preferences for options that ultimately result in outcomes that are survival models. Survival models can be thought of as gambles in the sense that the actual length of life is not known with certainty. As we have said before, gambles are not the same as their expected values any more than a 50% chance of winning $2 000 000 is the same as a guaranteed $1 000 000.

Finally, Figure 9.5 shows a general form for the uncertain outcome assessment question. The patient's life expectancy (X_B) with a favorable outcome for the gamble is set to a value that is meaningful to the patient. A typical value might be the patient's life expectancy if they were free of disease. The rest of the assessment question in Figure 9.5 can be expressed as a lifetime-tradeoff assessment question by setting the probability p equal to a constant and asking the patient for the value of the life expectancy X_A such that the two options are equivalent. Or the question can be expressed as a survival-tradeoff assessment question by setting the life expectancy X_A equal to a constant and asking the patient for the value of the probability p such that the options are equivalent. In either case, the corresponding expression for determining the value of the exponential utility parameter is

$$\gamma = \frac{p / X_A - 1 / X_B}{1 - p}$$

Result: exponential utility model parameter

Suppose the following equivalence is determined by an assessment question in which outcomes are expressed as the life expectancies for exponential survival models, as shown in the following diagram:

Life expectancy = X_A equivalent to ○ — p — ● Life expectancy = X_B

 — $1-p$ — ● Live 0 years

The patient's risk parameter then is given by

$$\gamma = \frac{p / X_A - 1 / X_B}{1 - p}$$

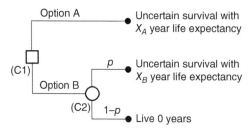

Figure 9.5 Decision tree representing a general form of the uncertain outcome assessment question. The value for X_{Max} is specified. If the value for X also is specified, the individual provides the value for the probability p such that Option A and Option B are equivalent. If the value for p is specified, the individual provides the value for X such that Option A and Option B are equivalent.

9.2.7 Exponential utility model parameter and risk attitudes

Shortly, we will see how to incorporate risk attitudes into the design of clinical policies. However, before turning to that important topic, we first will examine what the exponential utility model parameter tells us about someone's risk attitudes.

Figure 9.6 shows the curves for exponential utility models with different parameter values. Notice that each of these utility models has been scaled so the utility for 20 years of life is 1.0.

Recall the discussion in the previous chapter of how risk attitudes affect the shape of someone's utility curve. With risk aversion, the curve has a concave shape, meaning that a straight line connecting any two points on the curve always falls below the curve. Conversely, when someone is risk tolerant, their utility curve is convex meaning that a straight line connecting any two points on the curve always falls above the curve. Individuals who are risk indifferent have a utility curve that is a straight line.

Notice that each type of risk attitude is represented in Figure 9.6. The four curves with positive values for γ are concave so they show risk averse preferences. The four curves with negative values for γ are convex so they show risk-tolerant preferences. One curve – the straight line – showing risk-indifferent preference.

Also notice how the magnitude of γ changes the shapes of the utility curves in Figure 9.6. Starting with the curve for $\gamma = 0.4/\text{year}$, the shape of the curves approaches the straight line as γ decreases in value. Put another way, the greater the value of γ for an individual, the more risk averse that individual is. A similar trend applies to negative values for γ and risk tolerance.

Therefore, we will call γ the *risk parameter* because it characterizes – and in a sense quantifies – an individual's risk preferences. Positive values for γ indicate risk-averse preferences. The greater the value of γ, the stronger the individual's risk aversion. Negative values for γ indicate risk tolerance. The greater the magnitude of a negative γ, the stronger the individual's risk tolerance.

Definition: risk parameter

The parameter γ for the exponential utility model is called the *risk parameter*. When γ is positive, the individual is risk averse. When γ is negative, the individual is risk tolerant. When γ is zero, the individual is risk indifferent.

Of course, the risk parameter γ is an imperfect measure of risk attitudes because its validity depends on the validity of the exponential utility model as a representation of someone's risk attitudes. In turn, the validity of the exponential

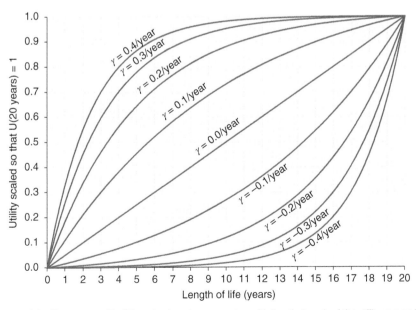

Figure 9.6 Curves for exponential utility curves with different values for parameter γ. Notice that each of the utility curves has been scaled so that the utility for 20 years of life is 1.0.

utility model depends on the assumption that risk attitudes do not change with context for an individual. Suppose that a patient was indifferent between a guaranteed survival of 5 years or a gamble that would result in a lifetime of 10 years with probability 0.9 or death with probability 0.1. This choice can be represented by the following comparison:

Would the same patient be indifferent if that choice would come after living ten more years? In other words, what if the choice was between a guaranteed life of 15 years or a gamble that would result in a lifetime of 20 years with probability 0.9 or a lifetime of 10 years with probability 0.1. This different context can be represented by the comparison:

The exponential utility model assumes that this change in context – the adding of 10 years to all of the outcomes – does not change the relationship between the guaranteed outcome and the gamble in this comparison.

As long as assuming constant risk attitudes does match an individual's preferences, the risk parameter summarizes how that individual feels about the risks they face. Using γ to characterize risk attitudes is similar to using body-mass index (BMI) to characterize someone's weight status. Both are imperfect summaries of something that is far too complicated to be fully represented by a single number. However, both γ and BMI provide a useful tool for managing that complexity.

9.3 Incorporating risk attitudes into clinical policies

This section is about the design of clinical policies that incorporate risk attitudes. A clinical policy prescribes care for the members of a target population. The challenge to be addressed is how to take a concept like risk attitudes, which are the characteristics of an individual, and apply it to a population, which is the focus of clinical policy.

The community developing clinical policies has long recognized the need to individualize patient care. Not all patients should receive the same care for the same problem. Partly this is because what constitutes the "same problem" can differ between patients. Those differences can involve factors such as age, sex, and comorbidities. Patients also differ in terms of preferences, as demonstrated by the study conducted by McNeil and her colleagues. Their paper *Fallacy of the Five-Year Survival in Lung Cancer* showed that different patients had different preferences for treatment of the same disease.

Another research group that included one of the coauthors of this book explored patient preferences for outcomes involved with the management of angina (Nease *et al.*, 1995). This study assessed the utilities of 220 patients for outcomes with different symptom levels. The symptom levels were defined by the type of pain and level of disability caused by angina. The study found statistically significant differences in the numerical values of the patients' outcome utilities. The implication of this result is that a clinical policy for the management of angina could rank treatment alternatives differently for patients because of these outcome utility differences.

This study of patient preferences for levels of angina focused on the quality of life rather than the duration of life. The next chapter discusses methods for representing quality of life preferences. The focus of this chapter is on risk attitudes for the duration of life. As such, this section will consider how clinical policies could be adjusted to account for a patient's risk attitudes. We will call these *risk-adjusted clinical policies*.

9.3.1 Risk-adjusted clinical policies – underlying concept
So far in this chapter, we have seen how to represent risk attitudes by a single number we call the risk parameter. The previous section demonstrated methods that determined an individual's risk parameter based on the answer to a single assessment question. Answering that assessment question requires imagining a decision about a hypothetical scenario. Depending on how we word the question, the hypothetical scenario can resemble the types of decisions many patients actually face, only in a greatly simplified context.

For example, suppose the patient is a 46-year-old man. The previous chapter described a type of assessment question that asked individuals to express their risk attitudes by stating the length of life reduction they would accept in order to avoid uncertainty about how long they will live. We called these lifetime-tradeoff assessment questions. The patient's answer to the following lifetime-tradeoff assessment question would determine the life expectancy for an outcome with a utility of 0.5 if the utility for a life expectancy of 35 years is 1 and the utility for immediate death is 0:

Imagine there is a risky treatment for a disease you have. The chances this treatment will cause your immediate death is 50%. However, if you survive the treatment, on average you will live another 35 years. Your alternative is to take your chances with the disease, which will mean a shorter average life. How short would your average life with the disease have to be before you would choose the risky treatment?

The average lifetime of 35 years was chosen as the best outcome for the gamble because, according to US actuarial tables, 34 years is the remaining life expectancy for a 46-year-old male. In theory, we should have chosen 34 years but rounding to 35 years provides a simpler question.

Using this same logic, if the patient was a 33-year-old woman, we would have chosen 50 years as the life expectancy for the surviving the gamble because 49 years is the life expectancy for a 33-year-old woman. In other words, the wording of this question has been adjusted to ask the patient what type of risk they would accept in order to restore their life to roughly what it would be without the disease.

Using the methods described in the previous section, the 46-year-old man's risk parameter can be determined from their answer to this question. This approach to utility assessment can be adapted to fit the circumstances of any patient by adjusting the life expectancy for the gamble in the question.

Returning to clinical policies, the design of clinical policies typically is about identifying patient groups for whom a specific action is optimal. The lung cancer treatment study by McNeil and her colleagues, discussed in the previous chapter, showed that risk attitudes can affect when surgery is the optimal treatment. As we have just seen, the risk parameter in the exponential utility model represents risk attitudes. Answering the proper assessment question determines the value of the risk parameter.

In this section, we will see that knowing the exact value of the risk parameter is not always necessary. Only knowing if the risk parameter falls within a certain range usually is sufficient. This means the assessment process often can be reduced to a simpler yes-no question of the following form:

Imagine there is a risky treatment for a disease you have. The chances the treatment will cause your immediate death is 50%. However, if you survive the treatment, on average you will live another 35 years. Your alternative is to take your chances with the disease, which will mean, on average, you will live another X years. Would choose the risky treatment?

The value for X in the question would be selected to test if the value for the risk parameter indicates a given action is optimal for the patient given their risk attitudes.

This section describes an approach to designing clinical policies that starts with determining when the patient's risk attitudes affect which treatment alternative is optimal. When risk attitudes matter, the corresponding range of risk parameter values will be identified. In turn, that range of risk parameter values will correspond to specific assessment questions. When properly worded, those assessment questions can be expressed as yes-no questions. The recommendations of the clinical policy can be personalized by adjusting the assessment question to the patient's specific age, sex, and any other factor affecting their baseline survival. The result is a clinical policy that is adjusted to a patient's risk attitudes by answers to a single yes-no question.

Definition: risk-adjusted clinical policies

A risk-adjusted clinical policy includes the patient's risk attitudes in the treatment alternative recommended for the care of the patient.

9.3.2   Clinical context for illustrating risk-adjusted clinical policy design

This personalized approach to clinical policy design will be illustrated by analyzing the same treatment decision used by McNeil and her colleagues in their study of risk attitudes. Recall from the discussion in the previous chapter, the decision they analyzed concerned the choice of treatment for Stage I or Stage II lung cancer. At the time of the study, the available treatments for lung cancer were limited to surgery or radiotherapy. Our design goal will be a policy that

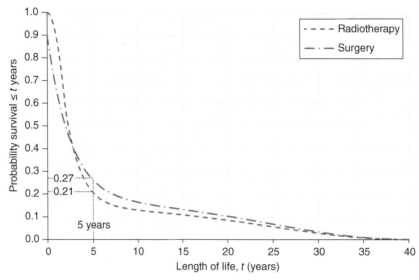

Figure 9.7 Surgery and radiotherapy survival curves for 60-year-old man used to illustrate parametric clinical policies.

recommends either surgery or radiotherapy for a patient with Stage I or Stage II lung cancer. Of course, lung cancer treatment has advanced far beyond the limited options available in the 1970s. However, the concepts that will be demonstrated still apply today.

The average age for the patients in the lung cancer study was 60 years. Figure 9.7 shows the surgery and radiotherapy survival curves for a 60-year-old man with Stage I or Stage II lung cancer. Notice that the 5-year survival with surgery (0.27) is substantially greater than the 5-year survival with radiotherapy (0.21). Therefore, based on the 5-year survival rates, surgery would be the recommended treatment.

However, McNeil and her colleagues showed that some of the patients in their study had risk attitudes that implied radiotherapy would be their preferred treatment. This interaction between preferred treatment and risk attitudes provides the foundation of the clinical policy that will be designed.

9.3.3 Determining the risk parameter threshold

Focusing for a moment on the case of a 60-year-old man, suppose that we use the following question to assess this patient's risk attitudes:

Suppose there is a risky treatment for a disease you have. The chances the treatment will cause your immediate death is 50%. However, if you survive treatment you will live, on average, another 20 years. Your alternative is to take your chances with the disease, which will mean a shorter average life. How short would your average life with the disease have to be before you would choose the risky treatment?

Once again, 20 years was selected as the life expectancy for the risk treatment because this approximates the life expectancy of a typical 60-year-old man. In effect, this assessment question asks the patient to express their risk attitudes in terms of the gamble they would accept in order to restore what their life would be if they did not have lung cancer.

The comparison in this question can be represented by the following diagram:

Life expectancy = X years equivalent to ◯ 0.5 ● Life expectancy = 20 years
0.5 ● Live 0 years

The gamble on the right in this comparison implies a life expectancy of 10 years. Therefore, someone who is risk averse would choose the guaranteed outcome on the right unless their life expectancy with the guaranteed outcome was less than 10 years. The greater their risk aversion, the shorter their acceptable life expectancy for the guaranteed outcome.

As we saw in the previous section, the answer to this question implies a value for the parameter γ used in an exponential utility model. We called γ the risk parameter because it characterizes the patient's risk attitudes. Recall that if X denotes the patient's answer to the assessment question, the expression we derived for determining the value for γ from X is:

$$\gamma = \frac{0.5/X - 1/20 \text{ years}}{1 - 0.5}$$

where 0.5 is the probability of surviving the gamble and 20 years is the patient's resulting life expectancy.

For example, suppose that our 60-year-old man was risk averse and responded that having a life expectancy of 4 years was equivalent to the gamble. That is X equals 4 years. The value for the patient's risk parameter then would be

$$\gamma = \frac{0.5/X - 1/20}{1 - 0.5} = \frac{0.5/4 \text{ years} - 1/20 \text{ years}}{0.5} = 0.15/\text{year}$$

On the other hand, suppose the 60-year-old man was highly risk averse and responded with a life expectancy of only 2 years. The value for the patient's risk parameter would then be

$$\gamma = \frac{0.5/2 \text{ years} - 1/20 \text{ years}}{0.5} = 0.40/\text{year}$$

Therefore, as discussed in the previous section, the value for the risk parameter γ increases as risk aversion increases. Figure 9.8 shows how the risk parameter value changes with the response to the assessment question we are using with this patient.

The risk parameter value of 0.15/year we have determined for our patient may seem like just another number derived from a complicated equation using an answer to a hypothetical question. However, this value provides us with an understanding of how this patient feels about the two treatments. Recall that the risk parameter value adjusts an exponential utility model to match this patient's risk attitudes. We can combine the resulting utility model with probabilities from the two survival models to determine the patient's expected utilities for the two treatments. The optimal treatment for the patient will be the treatment with the greater expected utility.

When we discuss the details of survival models in Chapter 11, we will see that survival curves like those shown in Figure 9.8 are not exponential survival models. This means computing the expected utilities for the two treatments

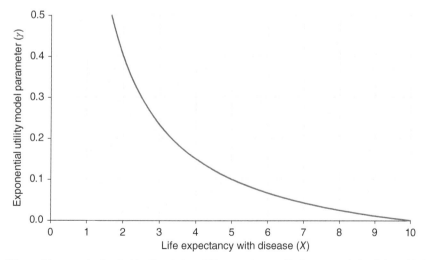

Figure 9.8 Exponential utility model parameter implied by the choice of life expectancy with disease such that living with the disease is equivalent to a risky treatment that has a 50% chance of causing immediate death and a 50% of leading to a life expectancy of 20 years.

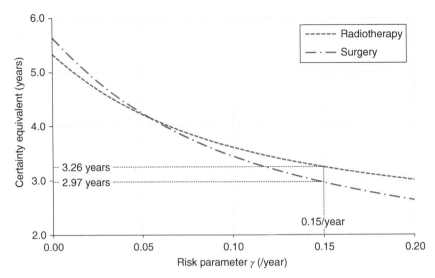

Figure 9.9 Comparison of surgery and radiotherapy as treatments for lung cancer in a 60-year-old man based on risk parameter value. Vertical axis expresses the difference between the two treatments as certainty equivalents.

requires the longer calculations demonstrated in the previous chapter (see Table 8.1). When we do those calculations, the results are

$$EU(Surgery) = 2.3989$$

$$EU(Radiotherapy) = 2.5785$$

Since EU(Radiotherapy) is greater than EU(Surgery), it follows that radiotherapy is the preferred treatment for a 60-year-old man with a risk parameter value of 0.15/year.

Figure 9.9 uses certainty equivalents to compare the two treatment alternatives based on different risk parameter values. Recall that a certainty equivalent summarizes a gamble, like a survival model, by determining the guaranteed outcome that has the same utility as the expected utility for the gamble. The certainty equivalent and the gamble are equivalent because they have the same utility given the patient's risk attitudes.

With an exponential utility model, determining a certainty equivalent is a straightforward calculation that depends on the form of the exponential utility model that has been used.

For example, suppose that u is the expected utility for one of the survival curves. The certainty equivalent for that survival curve is the value x such that the utility for x equals u. Recall that there are three forms of the exponential utility model. The expected utilities for the two treatments shown above were computed using the following form of the exponential utility model:

$$\text{Utility of } x = \frac{1 - e^{-\gamma x}}{\gamma}$$

Therefore, the certainty equivalent x for a gamble with expected utility u satisfies the following equation:

$$u = \frac{1 - e^{-\gamma x}}{\gamma}$$

Using a little high school algebra, this equation can be rearranged to show that

$$x = -\frac{\ln(1 - \gamma u)}{\gamma}$$

Similar expressions are used to compute the certainty equivalent for the other two forms of the exponential utility model.

Result: Certainty equivalent for the exponential utility model

The following expressions determine the certainty equivalent (CE) for the corresponding exponential utility model form

$$EU = 1 - e^{-\gamma x} = u \qquad\qquad CE = -\frac{\ln(1-u)}{\gamma}$$

$$EU = \frac{1 - e^{-\gamma x}}{\gamma} = u \qquad\qquad CE = -\frac{\ln(1-\gamma u)}{\gamma}$$

$$EU = \frac{e^{-\gamma A} - e^{-\gamma x}}{e^{-\gamma A} - e^{-\gamma B}} = u \qquad\qquad CE = -\frac{\ln\left(e^{-\gamma A} - \left(e^{-\gamma A} - e^{-\gamma B}\right)u\right)}{\gamma}$$

Returning to our 60-year-old patient, we can use this result to determine the certainty equivalents for each of the two treatment options. Recall that the expected utility we calculated for surgery is 2.3989 (u) and 0.1500/year is this patient's risk parameter (γ). Therefore,

$$CE \text{ for surgery} = -\frac{\ln(1-\gamma u)}{\gamma}$$

$$= -\frac{\ln(1 - 0.1500/\text{year} \times 2.3989)}{0.1500/\text{year}}$$

$$CE \text{ for surgery} = 2.97 \text{ years}$$

Similarly,

$$CE \text{ for radiotherapy} = -\frac{\ln(1 - 0.1500/\text{year} \times 2.5785)}{0.1500/\text{year}} = 3.26 \text{ years}$$

In other words, for a 60-year-old man who answered the assessment question with a 4-year life expectancy, the uncertainty they face with surgery has the same utility as facing a guaranteed 2.97 years of life. Similarly, the uncertainty of facing radiotherapy has the same utility as facing a guaranteed 3.26 years of life. This means for this patient the loss from undergoing surgery rather than radiotherapy is approximately the difference between living 3.26 or 2.97 years. That difference works out to about 3 months.

9.3.4   A simpler assessment question

We have just seen that the answer to an assessment question provides enough information about the patient's risk attitudes to identify which treatment they preferred. The process requires that the patient provides a specific value as the answer to the following question:

Suppose there is a risky treatment for a disease you have. The chances the treatment will cause your immediate death is 50%. However, if you survive treatment you will live, on average, another 20 years. Your alternative is to take your chances with the disease, which will mean a shorter average life. How short would your average life with the disease have to be before you would choose the risky treatment?

Some patients will be unable to provide an exact value when answering this question. However, that value is needed to determine the risk parameter. The value for the risk parameter is then used in the expected utility calculations which completes the comparison of the treatments. What if the patient is unable to fully answer the assessment question? What if they cannot decide what the exact life expectancy with disease must be so that living with the disease would be equivalent to the gamble posed in the assessment question?

It turns out we do not actually need the patient's exact answer to the assessment question. Looking at Figure 9.10, notice that the patient in this example would prefer radiotherapy over surgery as long as their risk parameter value is greater than 0.0533/year. This means that in order to conclude radiotherapy is the best treatment for this patient, we only need to know that their risk parameter is greater than 0.0533/year.

We might call 0.0533/year the threshold value for the risk parameter since this is where the preferred treatment switches between surgery and radiotherapy. Figure 9.11 is a copy of Figure 9.8 and shows that an answer of 6.5 years to the assessment question implies the risk parameter value of 0.0533/year. In other words, the risk parameter equals the threshold value if the patient believes that living with a life expectancy of 6.5 years is equivalent to the risky treatment in the assessment question. We will round 6.5 to 6 years to reduce the complexity of the question.

Therefore, in order to decide which treatment is best for this patient, we only need to know that their answer to the assessment question is less than 6 years. This means we can simplify the assessment question to the following yes-no question:

Suppose there is a risky treatment for a disease you have. The chances the treatment will cause your immediate death is 50%. However, if you survive treatment you will live, on average, another 20 years. Your alternative is to take your chances with the disease, which would mean the average length of life you can expect is at least 6 years. Would you choose the risky treatment?

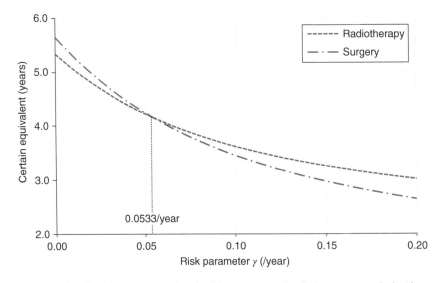

Figure 9.10 Copy of Figure 9.9 showing the risk parameter value γ implying surgery and radiotherapy are equivalent lung cancer treatments for a 60-year-old man.

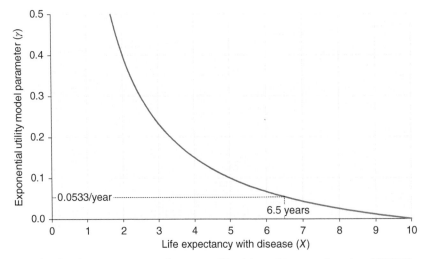

Figure 9.11 Copy of Figure 9.8 showing the assessment question answer X implying a risk parameter value of 0.0533/year, which is where surgery and radiotherapy are equivalent lung cancer treatments for a 60-year-old man.

If the patient answered "yes", surgery is their preferred treatment. If the patient answers "no" radiotherapy is the preferred treatment.

9.3.5   Generalized age- and gender-specific clinical policy

The approach we have described has determined the risk-adjusted clinical policy for a 60-year-old man. The treatment recommended by the policy uses the patient's response to a relatively simple question to determine which treatment best represents how the patient feels about risk. Extending this clinical policy to other demographic groups would involve the following changes.

The first change adjusts the survival model to reflect how the group's demographics affect the uncertainty of how long a patient in the group will live. The discussion of survival models in a later chapter shows how to make age and gender adjustments to survival curves. For example, Figure 9.12 shows the resulting surgery and radiotherapy survival curves if the demographic group consists of 30-year-old women.

The second change determines how the threshold value for the risk parameter is affected by the survival model adjustments. Figure 9.13 shows the comparison of the treatments for the example of a 30-year-old woman. Notice that

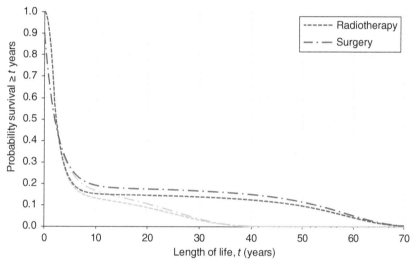

Figure 9.12 Surgery and radiotherapy survival curves for 30-year-old woman. The survival curves for a 60-year-old man, from Figure 9.7, are shown in grey.

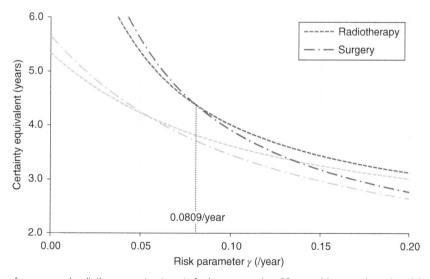

Figure 9.13 Comparison of surgery and radiotherapy as treatments for lung cancer in a 30-year-old woman based on risk parameter value. Vertical axis expresses the difference between the two treatments as certainty equivalents. Comparison of the two treatments for a 60-year-old man, from Figure 9.10, is shown in grey.

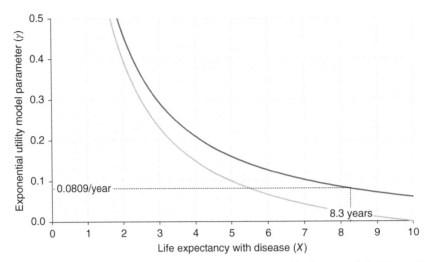

Figure 9.14 Exponential utility model parameter implied by the choice of life expectancy with disease such that living with the disease is equivalent to a risky treatment that has a 50% chance of causing immediate death and a 50% of leading to a life expectancy of 51 years. The corresponding curve used to design the clinical policy for the 60-year-old man, from Figure 9.8, is shown in grey.

the threshold value for the risk parameter has increased to 0.0809/year for this group. When the risk parameter for this patient is greater than 0.0809/year, radiotherapy is the preferred treatment. When the risk parameter is less than 0.0809/year surgery is preferred.

The other changes are to the assessment question. First, according to actuarial tables, the life expectancy for a 30-year-old woman is 51 years. Rounding this life expectancy to 50 years, the hypothetical treatment in the assessment question will now indicate a 50-year life expectancy if the patient survives the risky treatment. Figure 9.14 shows how answers to the revised assessment question affect the implied risk parameter. Notice that a response of 8.3 years to the question would imply the threshold value of 0.0809/year for the risk parameter. The second change to the assessment question incorporates this new value of 8.3 years as the life expectancy for living with the disease. Therefore, rounding 8.3 to 8.0 years, the yes-no question asked of a 30-year-old woman would be:

> *Suppose there is a risky treatment for a disease you have. The chances the treatment will cause your immediate death is 50%. However, if you survive treatment you will live, on average, another 50 years. Your alternative is to take your chances with the disease, which would mean the average length of life you can expect is at least 8 years. Would you choose the risky treatment?*

As before, answering "yes" implies risk attitudes that favor surgery, whereas answering "no" implies risk attitudes favoring radiotherapy.

Table 9.1 generalizes this approach to a range of ages for men and women. Figure 9.15 shows a decision tree representation of the assessment question that uses the values from the table. The patient's life expectancy, if they survive the hypothetical treatment in Option B (X_B), approximates the patient's disease-free life expectancy, rounded to the nearest multiple of 5 years. The life expectancy with Option A (X_A) is the corresponding life expectancy implying the threshold value for the risk parameter with Option A and Option B are equivalent.

Notice that the table contains two additional values $p = 0.25$ and $p = 0.75$. So far the discussion has focused on assessment questions where the survival probabilities were set at 0.50. Using these different survival probabilities would repeat the assessment question to verify the patient's response.

Using the notation in Figure 9.15, the assessment question can be expressed as follows.

> *Suppose there is a risky treatment for a disease you have. The chances the treatment will cause your immediate death is p. However, if you survive treatment you will live another X_B years on average. Your alternative is to take your chances with the disease, which would mean the average length of life you can expect is at least X_A years. Would you choose the risky treatment?*

9.3.6 Risk-adjusted clinical policies – what does it all mean?

In this section, we have shown how to personalize a clinical policy by the adjusting treatment recommendations according to the risk attitudes of the patient. The adjustments are tailored to the patient's demographics so that (1) the

Table 9.1 Assessment question values used to determine when surgery is preferred to radiotherapy for a patient. Option A in the question has a given life expectancy X_A. Option B is a risky treatment with a given survival probability (P) and a given life expectancy X_B with survival. Surgery is the preferred treatment if the patient prefers Option B.

	Age (years)	X_B = Life expectancy with Option B (years)	X_A = Life expectancy with Option A (years)		
			$p = 0.25$	$p = 0.50$	$p = 0.75$
Women	30	50	3	8	19
	40	40	3	8	17
	50	35	3	8	16
	60	25	3	7	14
	70	15	3	6	10
	80	10	3	5	8
	90	5	2	3	4
Men	30	45	3	8	18
	40	40	3	8	17
	50	30	3	7	15
	60	20	3	6	12
	70	15	3	6	10
	80	10	3	6	8
	90	5	2	3	4

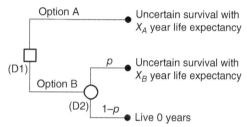

Figure 9.15 Decision tree representing general form of the assessment question for a risk-adjusted clinical policy. The value for X_B represents the patient's life expectancy without disease. The value for the survival probability is 0.25, 0.50, or 0.72 and the value for X_B is selected from Table 9.1.

survival models predicting outcomes reflect that characteristics of the patient and (2) the assessment process is framed in a clinical context that is meaningful to the patient.

9.4 Helping patients communicate their preferences

This final section shifts the focus away from determining the optimal decision for a patient and considers instead how treatment decisions should be communicated to patients. In 1979 Daniel Kahneman and Amos Tversky published a paper titled *Prospect Theory: An Analysis of Decision under Risk* (Kahneman and Tversky, 1979). This paper described a descriptive model of decision making that ultimately led to the awarding of a Nobel Prize in Economic Sciences. Prospect Theory provides a general framework for understanding how people actually make decisions. However, Prospect Theory also provides important insights into how the description of the options in a decision can distort the patient's understanding of the decision they face. Kahneman and Tversky called this the *framing problem*, which can be seen as a generalization of the cognitive biases discussed in Chapter 3. This section describes how accounting for the framing problem should be considered when discussing treatment options with patients.

Tversky and Kahneman first described the framing problem in an article published in 1981 (Tversky and Kahnman, 1981). This paper described a study in which subjects were asked to state their preferences when faced with hypothetical decision problems. The following is an example of one of the decision problems they posed:

Problem 1: Given an outbreak that will kill 600 people if untreated, choose between the following two programs:

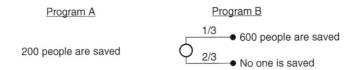

When this problem was presented to 152 subjects, 72% preferred Program A. This makes sense. All of the outcomes are expressed as gains in terms of lives saved. Moreover, both programs have the same expected value for the number saved – 200 people. However, with Program A those 200 saved lives are a certainty, whereas with Program B there is the possibility that no one will be saved. In Prospect Theory, when outcomes are gains, there is preference for a guaranteed outcome over a gamble that awards that same outcome, on average. This preference for certainty is called the *certainty effect* for gains.

Tversky and Kahneman also presented a second problem to another 155 subjects:

Problem 2: Given an outbreak that will kill 600 people if untreated, choose between the following two programs:

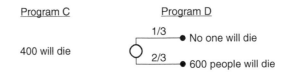

Of course, the two problems describe the same two programs. With Program C, 400 members die in the population of 600 meaning that 200 will saved. This is the same as the outcome for Program A in the first problem. Similarly, Program D is simply a rewording of Program B. However, 78% of the subjects in the second survey preferred Program D in Problem 2, which reverses the preferences stated for Problem 1.

Notice that Program C and Program D are described as losses rather than gains. Prospect Theory attributes the switch in preferences to the differences in how people view potential gains and losses. In the terminology of Prospect Theory, this change in preferences demonstrates the *framing effect.*

The clinical relevance of the framing effect is that how risks are expressed to patients can affect their choices. Mathematically, telling a patient that there is a 10% chance they will die from an operation is equivalent to telling the patient there is a 90% chance they will survive the operation. Both statements contain the same mathematical content, but they can have a very different cognitive meaning to the patient.

In 1982, a group of researchers, that included one of the coauthors of this book, published the results of a study that demonstrated the framing effect in a clinical setting (McNeil *et al.*, 1982). This study, once again, used the choice between surgery or radiotherapy for treatment of lung cancer in a 60-year-old patient. For the purposes of this study, surgical treatment was summarized by a 10% operative mortality rate with a 6.1-year life expectancy whereas radiotherapy had a 0% procedure mortality rate with a 4.7-year life expectancy. The life expectancy for surgery included the 10% mortality rate. The goal of the study was to document how the framing of the choice between the two treatments would affect preferences.

The study population included 238 patients, as well as 424 radiologists and 491 business school students. This summary focuses only on the patients, who were outpatients at the Palo Alto VA medical facility. None had lung cancer and all were male. The average age was 58 years.

Three framing factors were included in the description of how the two treatment options were described. The choice between the treatment options was described to the study participants using different framing models based on the following three factors:

Gain vs. loss: This factor expressed the treatment alternatives either in terms of gains (e.g., 90% survive the treatment) or losses (e.g., 10% die during treatment).

Life expectancy vs. cumulative survival: Treatment alternatives were characterized either by life expectancy (e.g., life expectancy with surgery is 6.1 years) or survival (e.g., 34% of patients undergoing surgery are alive after 5 years).

Treatment identified vs. treatment not identified: The actual treatment was named (e.g., treatment is surgery) or not (e.g., Treatment A is used).

Table 9.2 Percentage of patients preferring radiotherapy over surgery according to the framing model used to describe the choice between the treatment options.

Description of long-term survival	Treatment identified vs. treatment not identified	Surviving surgery expressed as gain vs. loss	Percent preferring radiotherapy
Cumulative survival	Treatment identified	10% chance of dying	40%
		90% chance of surviving	22%
	Treatment not identified	10% chance of dying	35%
		90% chance of surviving	19%
Life expectancy	Treatment identified	10% chance of dying	68%
		90% chance of surviving	31%
	Treatment not identified	10% chance of dying	50%
		90% chance of surviving	27%

Adapted from McNeil *et al.* (1982).

The third factor was used to determine how past experience (e.g., "my brother had surgery for his lung cancer and didn't do well") affected responses. The subjects were asked to state their preference for a choice between the treatments when described by combinations of the three framing factors.

For example, the following wording was used to describe the treatment decision with the three factors: (1) gain, (2) cumulative survival, and (3) treatment identified.

Of 100 people having surgery, 90 will survive the treatment, 68 will be alive by one year and 34 will have died by five years. Of 100 people having radiation therapy, all will survive the treatment, 77 will be alive by one year and 22 will be alive by five years.

On the other hand, the following wording was used to describe the treatment decision with the three factors: (1) loss, (2) life expectancy, and (3) treatment not identified.

Of 100 people having Treatment A, 10 will die during treatment, 32 will have died by one year and 66 will have died by five years. Of 100 people having Treatment B, none will die during treatment, 23 will die by one year and 78 will die by five years.

Table 9.2 shows how preference for radiotherapy changed according to the framing of the treatment decision. In all cases, the percentage of the patients preferring radiotherapy almost always doubled when the operative mortality rate for surgery was expressed as a loss rather than a gain. For example, when the long-term survival was expressed as a life expectancy and the treatments were identified, 31% of the patients preferred radiotherapy when they were told that the chances of surviving surgery were 90%. The percentage of patients preferring radiotherapy increased to 68% when the risk for surgery was described as a 10% chance of dying.

The percentages also changed if the treatments were identified in the description of the options. Patients preferred radiotherapy when they were told the decision was between radiotherapy or surgery. Expressing long-term survival as a life expectancy rather than cumulative survival probabilities also increased the attractiveness of radiotherapy to the patients. In short, the framing used to describe the options mattered to the patients when deciding which treatment they preferred. This means a patient's preferences for a treatment option can be manipulated by simply changing the wording of how the risks are expressed. When an operative risk is expressed as a probability of death rather than a probability of survival, the patient is more inclined to choose an alternative that avoids the risk of short-term mortality.

In summary, Kahneman's and Tversky's descriptive model of how individuals make decisions reveals the subtle influence using either gains or losses to describe a decision can have on how that decision is perceived. Clinicians should be aware of these cognitive biases and try to avoid unconsciously influencing the patient's choice. Explaining a choice in both frames, as either a choice between losses or a choice between gains, may help.

Summary

- A parametric utility model determines the values for outcome utilities by using a mathematical expression that includes terms, called parameters, that can be adjusted to match someone's risk attitudes.
- The exponential utility uses the following formula to express an individual's utility for an outcome measured by the variable x.

$$U(x) = 1 - e^{-\gamma x}$$

For example, x might be the length of the individual's life. The term γ quantifies the individual's risk attitudes and is expressed in units that are one over the units of x. The following is an alternate form of the exponential utility function:

$$U(x) = \frac{1 - e^{-\gamma x}}{\gamma}$$

The exponential utility model can be scaled so that $U(A) = 0$ and $U(B) = 1$ by the following form:

$$U(x) = \frac{e^{-\gamma A} - e^{-\gamma x}}{e^{-\gamma A} - e^{-\gamma B}}$$

- An individual's preferences have the delta property for numerically valued outcomes if for any outcomes X_A, X_B, and X_C and probability p, the following equivalence:

X_A equivalent to ○ — p — • X_B
 — $1-p$ — • X_C

implies the same equivalence if Δ is added to each of the outcomes. That is, for any Δ, it also is true that:

$X_A + \Delta$ equivalent to ○ — p — • $X_B + \Delta$
 — $1-p$ — • $X_C + \Delta$

Someone whose risk attitudes have the delta property is also said to have *constant risk attitudes*.

- When an individual's risk attitudes match the delta property their outcome utilities can be determined by an exponential utility model.
- Suppose that someone's risk attitudes mean the following equivalence is true:

Live X_A years equivalent to ○ — p — • Live X_B years
 — $1-p$ — • Live 0 years

The value of the exponential utility model parameter γ satisfies the following expression:

$$\frac{1 - e^{-\gamma X_A}}{1 - e^{-\gamma X_B}} = p$$

The value for γ satisfying this expression can be solved by trial-and-error methods that evaluate the ratio on the left for different values of the parameter γ until the ratio equals the probability on the right.

- Guaranteed outcome assessment uses questions that ask the individual to compare outcomes that are guaranteed lengths of life.
- Uncertain outcome assessment uses questions that ask the individual to compare outcomes that are uncertain, typically expressed as a life expectancy or a survival model.
- Suppose the following equivalence is determined by an assessment question in which outcomes are expressed as the life expectancies for exponential survival models, as shown in the following diagram:

Life expectancy = X_A equivalent to ○ — p — • Life expectancy = X_B
 — $1-p$ — • Live 0 years

The patient's risk parameter then is given by:

$$\gamma = \frac{p/X_A - 1/X_B}{1-p}$$

- The parameter γ for the exponential utility model is called the *risk parameter*. When γ is positive, the individual is risk averse. When γ is negative, the individual is risk tolerant. When γ is zero, the individual is risk indifferent.
- A risk-adjusted clinical policy includes the patient's risk attitudes in the actions recommended for the care of the patient.
- The following expressions determine the certainty equivalent (CE) for the corresponding exponential utility model form:

$$EU = 1 - e^{-\gamma x} = u \qquad\qquad CE = -\frac{\ln(1-u)}{\gamma}$$

$$EU = \frac{1-e^{-\gamma x}}{\gamma} = u \qquad\qquad CE = -\frac{\ln(1-\gamma u)}{\gamma}$$

$$EU = \frac{e^{-\gamma A} - e^{-\gamma x}}{e^{-\gamma A} - e^{-\gamma B}} = u \qquad CE = -\frac{\ln\left(e^{-\gamma A} - \left(e^{-\gamma A} - e^{-\gamma B}\right)u\right)}{\gamma}$$

- How the descriptions of options are worded can greatly change a patient's preferences for their alternatives in a decision problem. Options that are described as gains, such as the probability of surviving a procedure, are more attractive than options that are described as losses, such as the probability of dying from a procedure. Patients also tend to place more importance on outcomes that are certain when compared to options that include uncertainty. Collectively, these distortions to how possibilities are perceived, based on how they are described, are known as the framing effect.

Epilogue

The concept of utility devised by von Neumann and Morgenstern provides a method for incorporating a patient's risk preferences into the decisions affecting their lives. However, the clinical application of utility requires an assessment process that captures the patient's preferences in a mathematical expression. Utility assessment involves questions that many patients will find to be difficult to grasp. Utility assessment also can be time consuming. This chapter has described an approach to utility modeling that focuses on these two challenges.

The foundation of the approach described in this chapter is a mathematical expression called a parametric utility model. Several parametric utility models have been developed for the use of decision analysis in other domains. This chapter focused on use of the exponential utility model, which has a single parameter we called the risk parameter. An exponential utility model can be matched to the preferences of a patient by adjusting the value of the risk parameter. The input from the patient required to make this adjustment can be captured by the patient's answer to a single assessment question. Techniques for wording this question were explored that reduce the cognitive challenges in the assessment process.

This chapter demonstrated the use of parametric utility model by showing how a simple utility assessment process could be used to personalize the recommendations of a clinical policy that targets a patient population. A clinical policy can be seen as identifying patient groups for whom a particular clinical action is appropriate. When risk attitudes are used to define the boundaries for those groups, the assessment process simplifies to a relatively simple yes-no question. The structure of that question can be tailored to the patient's circumstances, further reducing the cognitive challenges of participating in the utility assessment process.

Therefore, an approach to representing patient preferences with regard to risk has been demonstrated. However, what is missing from this approach is any consideration of how decisions can affect the quality of life. How to address that consideration is the focus of the next chapter.

A.9.1 Exponential utility model parameter nomogram

This appendix presents a nomogram that simplifies determination of the exponential utility model parameter from the answer to an assessment question based on deterministic outcomes such as *live 5 years* or *live 25 years*. The following shows the structure of the assessment question:

where X_A is less than X_B. Recalling the discussion of utility assessment in Chapter 8, note that this question can be posed either as lifetime-tradeoff assessment (X_A is the unknown) or survival-tradeoff assessment (p is the unknown). That is, the patient can be asked to state their certain equivalence for a risky treatment that results in a length of life equal to X_B with a known probability of survival p. The patient's answer to the lifetime-tradeoff assessment question is X_A.

The following equality must hold when the two options represented in the assessment question are equivalent:

$$U(X_A \text{ years}) = p \times U(X_B \text{ years}) + (1-p) \times U(0 \text{ years}) = p \times U(X_B \text{ years})$$

Or, since we are using the exponential utility model

$$1 - e^{-\gamma \times X_A} = p \times \left(1 - e^{-\gamma \times X_B}\right)$$

which can be rearranged

$$\frac{1 - e^{-\gamma \times X_A}}{1 - e^{-\gamma \times X_B}} = p$$

Once again, our goal is to determine the value for γ that satisfies this expression for the values of X_A, X_B, and p in the assessment question. We can simplify our task by rescaling the lifetimes to be expressed as proportions of X_B, the lifetime if the patient survives the risky treatment in the assessment question. In effect, this eliminates one of the terms in the expression. That is let

$$\phi = \frac{X_A}{X_B}$$

The assessment question would then be expressed in terms of a new time unit that lasts X_B years.

Repeating the same steps as before leads to the expression:

$$\frac{1 - e^{-\gamma\phi}}{1 - e^{-\gamma}} = p$$

The nomogram in Figure A.9.1 shows the relationship between the exponential utility model parameter γ and the survival probability p, for given values of ϕ.

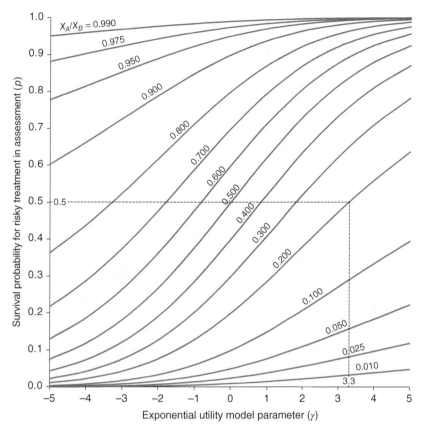

Figure A.9.1 Nomogram for determining the exponential utility model parameter γ from the answer to an assessment question that compared a guaranteed life of length X_A with a risk treatment that results in a life of length X_B with probability p. Final value for γ is determined by dividing the corresponding value on the horizontal axis by X_B.

For example, the assessment question used to illustrate the discussion in the main part of this chapter considered Patient A. This individual believed that a guaranteed lifetime of 5 years is equivalent to a risky treatment that results in a lifetime of 25 years with probability 0.5. In other words,

$X_A = 5\,\text{years}$
$X_B = 25\,\text{years}$

so

$$\phi = \frac{X_A}{X_B} = \frac{5\,\text{years}}{25\,\text{years}} = 0.2$$

This means that we are interested in the curve labelled "0.200" in the nomogram. The value for p in the assessment question is 0.5. Starting at this value on the vertical axis, we see that the corresponding value on the horizontal axis is 3.3. In other words, the exponential utility model parameter is 3.3 when lifetime is measured in 25-year time units. In order to convert time back to 1-year time units, we divide 3.3 by 25 years to show that

$$\gamma = \frac{3.3}{25\,\text{years}} = 1.3/\text{year}$$

Which is the same value for γ determined by the iterative approach described in the main part of the chapter.

Bibliography

Kahnman, D. and Tversky, A. (1979) Prospect theory: an analysis of decision under risk. *Econometrica*, **47**, 263–91.

McNeil, B.J., Weichselbaum, R., and Pauker, S.G. (1978) Fallacy of the five-year survival in lung cancer. *New England Journal of Medicine*, **299**, 1397–1401.

McNeil, B.J., Pauker, S.G., Sox, H., and Tversky, A. (1982) On the elicitation of preferences for alternative therapies. *New England Journal of Medicine*, **306**, 1259–62.

Nease, R.F., Jr, Kneeland, T., O'Connor, G.T. *et al.* (1995) Variation in patient utilities for outcomes of the management of chronic stable Angina. *JAMA*, **723**, 1185–90

Raffia, H. (1968) *Decision Analysis Introductory Lectures on Choices under Uncertainty*, Addison-Wesley, Reading, MA.

Tversky, A. and Kahnman, D. (1981) The framing of decisions and the psychology of choice. *Science*, **211**, 453–8.

CHAPTER 10

Outcome utilities – adjusting for the quality of life

10.1 Introduction

This chapter shows how to modify outcome utilities to reflect a patient's concerns about the quality of their life. The previous chapters treated the length of life as the patient's only concern. In Chapter 8, utility was introduced as a method for valuing the possible lengths of life so that a patient's risk attitudes are represented. The concepts presented in this chapter will show how to broaden the view of outcomes beyond simply on how long life will last. Life is more than just the passing of time. Life provides us with opportunities to experience what we enjoy and value as humans. The pain and disabilities caused by diseases and their treatments can reduce our access to and enjoyment of those experiences. That reduction lessens what we call the quality of life.

Anyone familiar with medicine knows that the quality of life matters to most patients. But does quality matter enough to change preferences for options that also affect how long the patient will live? Are patients willing to make tradeoffs between the length of life and its quality? A study that examined this fundamental question provides the starting point for the chapter. Not surprisingly, the study showed that patients will accept a reduction in the probability of a longer life in exchange for a better quality of life. Perhaps, more importantly, the study demonstrated a method for measuring how patients feel about the quality of the life they will live. That method is what we will call the *quality-lifetime tradeoff model.*

As the name suggests, this approach to measuring quality preferences is closely related to the lifetime-tradeoff assessment method discussed in Chapter 8. The corresponding assessment method measures how a patient feels about a symptom or disability that reduces the quality of their life by the length of life they would give up to avoid that symptom or disability. For example, a patient might believe that a life lasting 10 more years with a painful symptom would be equivalent to living only 8 more years, but without that symptom. The reduction from 10 to 8 years quantifies the importance of the painful symptom to that patient.

The previous chapter showed how mathematical expressions called parametric models can reduce the complexity of analyzing clinical decisions. In this chapter, we will see that the quality-lifetime tradeoff model can be approximated by a parametric model that extents the utility models for the length of life to reflect quality preferences. The result is a simple expression for determining outcome utilities that quantifies both risk attitudes and quality preferences. This useful expression also requires a minimal assessment process. Using this parametric model requires assumptions about the patient's preferences that will be carefully considered in this chapter.

This chapter also describes an approach to capturing quality preferences that will be called the *quality-survival trade-off model.* This second model measures how a patient feels about a symptom or disability by the risk to survival they

Medical Decision Making, Third Edition. Harold C. Sox, Michael C. Higgins, Douglas K. Owens, and Gillian Sanders Schmidler.
© 2024 John Wiley & Sons Ltd. Published 2024 by John Wiley & Sons Ltd.

would accept to avoid that symptom or disability. For example, suppose that in order to avoid a painful symptom, a patient would be willing to undergo a risky treatment that had a 5% chance of causing immediate death. If the patient survives the treatment, they will be free of that symptom for their remaining 10 years of life. In this case, the 5% risk the patient would accept quantifies the importance of the symptom to that patient.

Like the quality-lifetime tradeoff model, the quality-survival tradeoff model has a parametric form that uses a simple assessment process. However, we will see that the assumptions required for this second model are fewer in number. Both models provide an effective representation of quality preferences; however, the fewer assumptions required by the quality-survival tradeoff model suggest it is a superior approach to quality preference representation.

This chapter concludes the discussion of outcome utilities that started in Chapter 8. The discussion in these three chapters has developed a general approach to quantifying a patient's preferences for the possible outcomes of clinical decisions. The final section of this chapter concludes this discussion of outcome utilities by determining the utilities for the example used in a later chapter that describes the selection and interpretation of diagnostic tests.

10.2 Example – why the quality of life matters

Why should the analysis of medical decisions consider the importance patients place on the quality of their lives? Most patients want to avoid the unpleasant symptoms of their diseases and side effects of their treatments. However, is the desire to avoid a reduction in the quality of life important enough to risk the possibility of shortening life? McNeil, and her same two colleagues from the earlier lung cancer study, conducted a second study that explored the answer to this question.

The previous two chapters discussed the study of preferences for lung cancer treatments by McNeil and her colleagues (McNeil *et al.*, 1978). That study demonstrated the importance of risk aversion when determining the treatment a patient prefers. In their second study, McNeil and her colleagues demonstrated the importance of quality preferences in treatment decisions (McNeil *et al.*, 1981). They addressed the question: "Is the desire to avoid a reduction in the quality of life ever important enough to take a chance on shortening the length of life?"

This second study involved the treatment of laryngeal cancer localized to the vocal cords (Stage III). The 3-year survival rates for the three treatment alternatives included in the study are listed in Table 10.1.

Surgical removal of the larynx – laryngectomy – leads to better survival for patients with Stage III laryngeal cancer; however, this treatment results in the loss of normal speech. After removal of the larynx, many patients can learn an esophageal speech or adopt the use of a mechanical voice synthesizer – what we will call *artificial speech*. Depending on the level of proficiency achieved with these substitutes, verbal communication often is restored to near pre-surgery levels. However, some patients live the rest of their lives with a diminished ability to communicate. The surgery itself has little risk of fatal complications. Therefore, the survival models used by McNeil and her colleagues excluded the possibility of immediate death.

Unlike the lung cancer study, this second study interviewed healthy volunteers rather than patients with laryngeal cancer. The average age of the volunteers was 40 years. McNeil and her colleagues used a two-step process to determine their volunteers' outcome utilities. These outcome utilities quantified both the volunteers' risk attitudes as well as their quality preferences for retaining normal speech.

The first step assessed the utility for the length of life with normal speech. The same assessment questions developed for the lung cancer study were used. Recall how this was done. Each volunteer was asked the following question:

Suppose you have a disease that will cause your death in 5 years. Also suppose that if this disease were cured you could expect to live another 25 years. If there is a risky treatment that will either cure the disease or cause your immediate death, how small would the risk of death have to be for you to choose the treatment?

Table 10.1 Laryngeal cancer treatment alternative and 3-year survival rates from.

Treatment	3-year survival rate
Primary surgery	60%
Radiotherapy	30% to 40%
Radiotherapy with salvage surgery	42% to 48%

Adapted from McNeil *et al.* (1981).

The answer to this question characterized the volunteer's risk attitudes for the length of their life. Using the methods described in the previous chapter, the parameter for an exponential utility model – what we called the *risk parameter* – can be fitted to an answer to this question. Figure 10.1 shows an exponential utility model fitted to the answers provided by one of the volunteers. The risk parameter for this volunteer was 0.0815/year. We will refer to this volunteer as *Patient B*.

The second step in the assessment process determined how utility would change if normal speech were no longer possible. This was done by asking each volunteer to state the reduction in the length of their lives they would accept if it meant avoiding the loss of normal speech.

For example, a volunteer would be asked to suppose that life would continue for another 25 years but speech would be limited to the substitutes for normal speech available after laryngectomy. In order to fully understand this option, a volunteer was given a written description of the artificial or synthesized speech possible after surgery. This description of a patient's post-treatment quality state included the other effects of surgery, such as the artificial opening to the trachea necessary for breathing after laryngectomy. The volunteer also would hear recorded examples of the possible artificial or synthesized speech. After reading the description and hearing the recordings, the volunteer was asked how many years they would be willing to subtract from those 25 years with artificial speech if doing so would mean retaining normal speech. This question was repeated for several lengths of life with artificial speech.

Figure 10.2 shows the responses for the volunteer we are calling Patient B. When asked to imagine facing 25 years with artificial speech, this volunteer believed that 12.5 years with normal speech would be an equivalent outcome. The same volunteer believed that 10 years with artificial speech would be equivalent to 7 years with normal speech. Below 5 years, this volunteer would not accept any shortening of life to avoid the loss of normal speech.

By the definition of utility, believing that two outcomes are equivalent means that those two outcomes have the same utility. This means, for Patient B, the volunteer with the preferences shown in Figure 10.2, the following must be true:

$$U(5.0 \text{ years without normal speech}) = U(5.0 \text{ years with normal speech})$$
$$U(10.0 \text{ years without normal speech}) = U(7.0 \text{ years with normal speech})$$
$$U(25.0 \text{ years without normal speech}) = U(12.5 \text{ years with normal speech})$$

We already stated that Patient B's utilities for life with normal speech also match the outcome utilities shown in Figure 10.1. That is

$$U(5.0 \text{ years with normal speech}) = 0.38$$
$$U(7.0 \text{ years with normal speech}) = 0.50$$
$$U(12.5 \text{ years with normal speech}) = 0.73$$

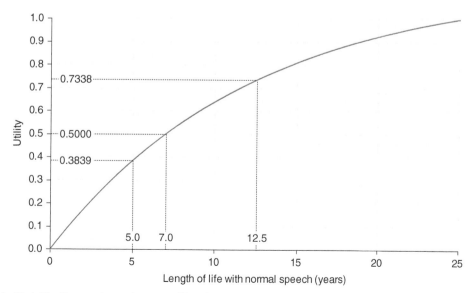

Figure 10.1 Utility for life (*u(t)*) with normal speech assessed for a laryngeal cancer study volunteer referred to as Patient B. Utility has been scaled so that the utility for 25 years of life with normal speech is 1.0.

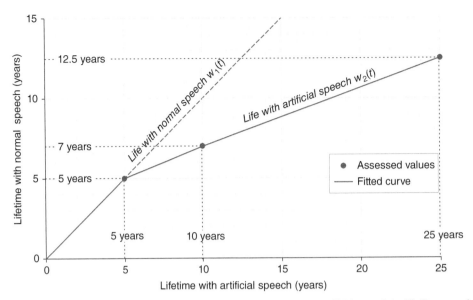

Figure 10.2 Quality-lifetime tradeoff functions for life with normal speech ($w_1(t)$) and life with artificial speech ($w_2(t)$). The curve for $w_2(t)$ is based on quality preference values assessed for volunteer referred to as Patient B.

For Patient B, it follows that:

$$U(5.0 \text{ years without normal speech}) = 0.38$$

Using the same reasoning, Patient B's utility for 10 years and 25 years of life without normal speech would be:

$$U(10.0 \text{ years without normal speech}) = 0.50$$
$$U(25.0 \text{ years without normal speech}) = 0.73$$

A smooth curve fitted to these outcome utilities is shown in Figure 10.3, together with the utility for life with normal speech first shown in Figure 10.1. The two utility curves in Figure 10.3 provide a complete set of utilities for the possible outcomes faced by Patient B when choosing between the laryngeal cancer treatment options.

McNeil and her colleagues used this two-step process to determine the outcome utilities for each of their volunteers. They then computed each volunteer's expected utility for the three treatment options. Recall that computing an expected utility requires a survival model that provides the probabilities for each of the possible lengths of life. In order to represent the range of institutional differences in the effectiveness of radiotherapy, two different survival models for radiotherapy were used. One survival model, called the *average result* for radiotherapy, was based on the lesser of the 3-year survival rates shown in Table 10.1 (30% for simple radiotherapy and 42% for radiotherapy with salvage surgery). The other survival model, called the *best result* for radiotherapy, was based on the greater of the 3-year survival rate shown in Table 10.1 (40% for simple radiotherapy and 48% for radiotherapy with salvage surgery). A single survival model for surgical treatment was used, based on the 3-year survival rate of 60% shown in Table 10.1. All three of the survival models were adjusted to reflect the normal survival model for someone who is 40 years old.

Expected utility accounts for an individual's risk attitudes when faced with an uncertain outcome. Adjusting the length of life to account for the loss of normal speech means that the expected utilities calculated by McNeil and her colleagues determined their volunteers' preferences for the resulting quality of their lives as well as the length of their lives. This means choosing the treatment with the greatest expected utility computed for a volunteer would be consistent with that volunteer's preferences.

Table 10.2 summarizes the results of the expected utility calculations for the 37 volunteers. Not surprisingly, the percentages in Table 10.2 show how preference for surgical treatment depends on the survival achieved by the alternatives based on radiotherapy. When radiotherapy would achieve what McNeill and her colleagues labelled *average*

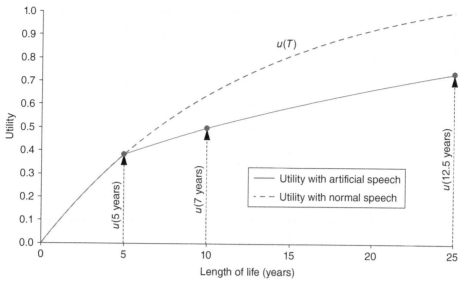

Figure 10.3 Utility for length of life with artificial speech. Utility for length of life with normal speech is shown, for comparison, as a dotted curve. The former is derived from the latter assuming the quality-lifetime tradeoff function shown in Figure 10.2. All utilities have been scaled so that the utility for 25 years of life with normal speech is 1.0.

Table 10.2 Laryngeal cancer treatment preferences determined by comparison of expected utility calculations based on utility assessments for 37 healthy volunteers.

	Treatment		
Radiotherapy result	Primary surgery	Radiotherapy	Radiotherapy with salvage surgery
Average	92%	3%	5%
Best	57%	19%	24%

results, surgery was preferred by 92% of the volunteers. When radiotherapy would achieve what was labelled *best results*, surgery was preferred by 57% of the volunteers.

This section started with the question – does quality of life matter to patients? Table 10.2 shows that the answer is "yes," at least for some of the participants in the laryngeal cancer study. Notice that none of the treatments were preferred by every participant. How these individuals weighed the importance of quality of life and the length of life affected which treatment they preferred. McNeal and her colleagues worked with healthy volunteers rather than patients actually facing the psychological trauma of a cancer diagnosis. Also, the average age of their volunteers was 40 years, which is less than the average age of patients with laryngeal cancer. Nevertheless, the assessment technique used in this study, and the subsequent analysis, show that feelings about the quality of life should influence a treatment decision even when significant reductions in survival are possible. In short, the quality of life matters.

10.3 Quality-lifetime tradeoff models

McNeil and her colleagues used what we call a *quality-lifetime tradeoff* model in their study of laryngeal cancer. The quality-lifetime tradeoff model is one of the commonly used approaches for capturing how quality-of-life preferences can affect the treatment preferred by a patient. Stated formally, a quality-lifetime tradeoff model represents the utility for an outcome that has a given length of life with a quality-reducing symptom, by determining an equivalent length of life without the symptom. The utility for the original symptomatic lifetime equals the utility for that equivalent shorter symptom-free lifetime.

Definition: quality-lifetime tradeoff model

A *quality-lifetime tradeoff* model represents the utility for an outcome that has a given length of life with a quality-reducing symptom by determining an equivalent outcome with a shorter length of life without the symptom. The utility for the original outcome is the utility for that equivalent shorter symptom-free lifetime.

This section describes the quality-lifetime tradeoff model and shows a simplification based on a parametric model similar to the exponential utility model described in the previous chapter.

Using the following notation will simplify our discussion of the quality-lifetime tradeoff model. Denote a patient's utility for symptom-free life as follows:

$u(t)$ = utility for symptom-free life lasting t years

For example, Figure 10.1 showed $u(t)$ for one of the volunteers in the laryngeal cancer study. We refer to this volunteer as Patient B. The previous chapter described how to determine $u(t)$ for someone. Those methods apply in this chapter as well.

A second key relationship we will use quantifies the length-of-life tradeoffs that would be acceptable to avoid a quality-reducing symptom. This relationship will be denoted as follows:

$w_i(t)$ = Symptom-free lifetime equivalent to a lifetime of t in i^{th} quality state

The subscript i is added to this function to denote the possibility of more than one combination of symptoms and disabilities. Living with one of those combinations will be referred to as living in a quality state. The function $w_i(t)$ will be called the *quality-lifetime tradeoff function* for the ith quality state.

For example, the study reported by McNeil and her colleagues involved two quality states: life with normal speech and life with artificial speech. Figure 10.2 showed Patient B's quality-lifetime tradeoff functions for these two quality states.

If life with normal speech is thought of as quality state 1, note that by definition

$w_1(t) = t$

The more interesting case in the laryngeal cancer decision is $w_2(t)$, the quality-lifetime tradeoff function for life with artificial speech. Remember that Patient B had the following equivalences for life with and without normal speech:

- 5 years with normal artificial equivalent to 5 years with normal speech
- 10 years with normal artificial equivalent to 7 years with normal speech
- 25 years with normal artificial equivalent to 12.5 years with normal speech

Figure 10.2 showed the values for $w_2(t)$ implied by these equivalences.

Writing the mathematical expression for $w_2(t)$ is more complicated.

$$w_2(t) = \begin{cases} t & \text{if } t \leq 5 \\ 5 + 0.50 \times (t - 5) & \text{if } 5 < t \leq 10 \\ 10 + 0.37 \times (t - 10) & \text{if } t > 10 \end{cases}$$

However, $w_2(t)$ is key to how the quality-lifetime tradeoff model adjusts outcome utilities to account for quality preferences. By definition, living t years with artificial speech is equivalent to living $w_2(t)$ years with normal speech. Expressed as outcome utilities this means:

$U(w_2(t) \text{ years with normal speech}) = U(t \text{ years with artificial speech})$

Typically, the next step is to assume that

$U(w_2(t) \text{ years with normal speech}) = u(w_2(t))$

because $u(t)$ is the patient's utility for living t years and living t years with artificial speech is equivalent to living $w_2(t)$ years with normal speech. This would mean

$U(t \text{ years with artificial speech}) = u(w_2(t))$

In other words, we can combine the functions $u(t)$ and $w_2(t)$ to determine a patient's utility for any of the possible outcomes of the laryngeal cancer decision.

A key step in applying this method is to determine a patient's quality-lifetime tradeoff function for life with artificial speech $w_2(t)$. This is done using assessment questions similar to those used to determine the patient's attitudes toward risk. For example, the quality-lifetime tradeoff function for life with artificial speech might be assessed by asking questions like the following:

> *Suppose you will live another t years. For the remainder of your life you will not have normal speech. Instead, your verbal communication will be limited to what can be achieved through the artificial methods that are available after your vocal cords have been removed. How many years of life with artificial speech would you give up if doing so would mean that you could retain your normal speech?*

Let x denote the patient's answer to this question. It would follow that, for this patient

$w_2(t) = t - x$

where t is the length of life with artificial speech posed in the assessment question. In the laryngeal cancer study, this question was asked for values of t equal to 5, 10, and 25 years. The points labelled "assessed values" in Figure 10.2 showed the responses for Patient B. For example, Patient B would be willing to give up 3 years of life to retain normal speech if otherwise they would live 10 years with artificial speech. This means that

$w_2(10 \text{ years}) = 7 \text{ years}$

There is a hidden assumption in this approach that should not be overlooked. Recall that $u(t)$ is the patient's utility for a symptom-free life lasting t years. Therefore, when we write

$U(t \text{ years with artificial speech}) = u(w_2(t))$

we are assuming that the risk attitudes toward the length of life are the same for life with normal speech as they are for life with artificial speech. This may not be true for all patients. Some patients might feel very differently about risks involving the length of life if they will live without normal speech. To allow for that possibility, we should determine a different $u(t)$ for each quality state. We can denote the utility for life in the ith quality state as follows:

$u_i(t) = \text{utility for life lasting } t \text{ years in } i^{th} \text{ quality state}$

This would mean the correct expression for the utility for life with artificial speech should be written

$U(t \text{ years with artificial speech}) = u_2(w_2(t))$

where $u_2(t)$ is assessed assuming life will be lived with artificial speech.

Mathematical expression: quality-lifetime tradeoff model

A quality-lifetime tradeoff model can be expressed using the following notation:

$u_i(t) = \text{Utility for lifetime } t \text{ in } i^{th} \text{ quality state}$

$w_i(t) = \text{Equivalent lifetime } t \text{ in } i^{th} \text{ quality state}$

Then

$U(t \text{ years in } i^{th} \text{ quality state}) = u_i(w_i(t))$

Typically, the function $u_i(t)$ is assumed to be the same for all quality states.

Of course, multiple quality states each require corresponding versions of $u_i(t)$, which in turn requires multiple assessment questions. These multiple assessment questions complicate the application of the quality-lifetime tradeoff model. For this reason, quality-lifetime tradeoff analysis typically assumes

$$u_i(t) \approx u(t)$$

where $u(t)$ reflects risk attitudes for some nominal quality state, such as living without symptoms or disabilities. McNeil and her colleagues used this approximation when they determined the outcome utilities for the participants in their study of laryngeal cancer. We will return to the implications of this approximation later in the chapter.

10.3.1 Parameterizing the quality-lifetime tradeoff model

The quality-lifetime tradeoff model provides an effective representation of quality preferences. However, the mathematics used to compute an expected utility can be complicated. This section describes parameterized versions of the quality-lifetime tradeoff model that reduce that complexity.

Recall what we mean by a parametric model. These mathematical expressions can be adjusted to match something like a patient's outcome utilities by changing the values for a few elements in the expression. Those elements are the expression's parameters. In the previous chapter, we discussed the exponential utility model. This parameterized utility model can be matched to the risk attitudes of a patient by adjusting the value for what we called the risk parameter (γ). Our goal here is a similar simplification for the representation of quality preferences.

As a motivation for how we will develop a parametric quality-lifetime tradeoff model, consider the ratio $w_2(t)/t$. Referring to Figure 10.4, this ratio compares the length of life with artificial speech (t) to the equivalent length of life with normal speech ($w_2(t)$). Focusing on the three assessed values in Figure 10.2

$$\frac{w_i(5 \text{ years})}{5 \text{ years}} = \frac{5 \text{ years}}{5 \text{ years}} = 1.0$$

$$\frac{w_i(10 \text{ years})}{10 \text{ years}} = \frac{7 \text{ years}}{10 \text{ years}} = 0.7$$

$$\frac{w_i(25 \text{ years})}{25 \text{ years}} = \frac{12.5 \text{ years}}{25 \text{ years}} = 0.5$$

These ratios characterize the importance the patient places on avoiding the quality reduction with life in the ith quality state. The ratio is close to 1 if the patient places little importance on avoiding the quality reduction. The ratio is much less than 1 if the patient places great importance on avoiding the quality reduction. Notice that for Patient B, the

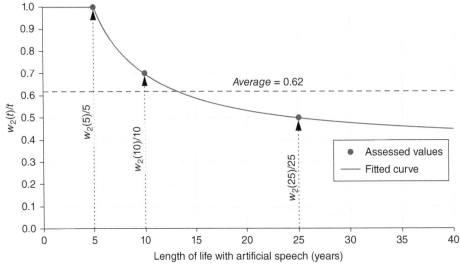

Figure 10.4 Ratio for the length of life with artificial speech ($w_2(t)$) over equivalent length of life with normal speech (t). The values for $w_2(t)$ are from Figure 10.2. The value for the ratio, averaged over a lifetime of 40 years, is shown by the dotted line.

ratios vary from 0.5–1.0. However, the parametric quality-lifetime tradeoff model we will use ignores this variation and treats the ratio $w_i(t)/t$ as a constant. In other words, the parametric quality-lifetime tradeoff model uses the approximation

$$w_i(t) \approx \phi_i \times t$$

where ϕ_i is a single value for the ratio $w_i(t)/t$.

Again, notice that the value for ϕ_i should be close to one for quality states that involve mild symptoms or disabilities. Living with these quality states is almost as good as symptom-free life. At the other extreme, ϕ_i should be close to zero for a quality state involving highly painful or disabling symptoms. For this reason, ϕ_i will be called the *quality-lifetime tradeoff parameter* for the ith quality state.

As we have already seen, the utility for outcomes with a length of life spent in a quality state can be determined by combining the utility for a length of life without symptoms ($u(t)$) and the quality-lifetime tradeoff function $w_i(t)$. That is,

$$U\left(t \text{ years in } i^{th} \text{ quality state}\right) = u\left(w_i(t)\right)$$

In other words, the utility for a life of a given length in a symptomatic outcome is the utility for its symptom-free, but shorter, equivalent lifetime. With the parametric model, $w_i(t)$ is approximated by $\phi_i \times t$. Using this approximation, we have that

$$U\left(t \text{ years in } i^{th} \text{ quality state}\right) \approx u\left(\phi_i \times t\right)$$

This expression for approximating the utilities for life in a quality state will be called the *quality-lifetime parametric utility model*.

Definition: quality-lifetime parametric utility model

Let $w_i(t)$ denote the quality-lifetime tradeoff function assessed for the ith quality state and let ϕ_i equal the value for the ratio $w_i(t)/t$ averaged over a suitable time period, such as the patient's life expectancy. The *quality-lifetime parametric utility model* uses the following approximation to determine the patient's utility for a life lasting t years on the ith quality state:

$$U\left(t \text{ years in } i^{th} \text{ quality state}\right) \approx u\left(\phi_i \times t\right)$$

The term ϕ_i is called the *quality-lifetime tradeoff parameter*.

There are several methods for choosing a value for the quality-lifetime tradeoff parameter. The method we will describe sets ϕ_i equal to the ratio $w_i(t)/t$ averaged over the patient's expected lifetime. For example, the average age for the volunteers in the laryngeal cancer was 40 years. On average, someone who is 40 years old can expect to live another 40 years. Figure 10.4 showed how the ratio $w_2(t)/t$ varies in the case of Patient B's quality-lifetime tradeoff function for life with artificial speech. As noted in Figure 10.4, the average value for the ratio $w_2(t)/t$ over a 40-year lifetime is 0.62.

Therefore, based on the average value calculation shown in Figure 10.4, we will use the following approximation to represent Patient B's quality preferences for life with artificial speech:

$$w_2(t) \approx 0.62 \times t$$

Figure 10.5 compares the values for $w_2(t)$ that were assessed for Patient B and the quality-lifetime tradeoff function approximation used in the parametric model. In effect, the parametric model approximates the curve for $w_2(t)$ by a straight line with slope equal to the value chosen for ϕ_2 (0.62).

Figure 10.6 compares (1) Patient B's utility for life with artificial speech computed using the assessed quality-lifetime tradeoff function and (2) Patient B's utility for life computed using the parametric model. The outcome utilities based on the assessed function have more credibility because they represent what Patient B actually said about their preferences. From this perspective, the parametric model underestimates the utilities for short lifetimes and overestimates the utilities for long lifetimes.

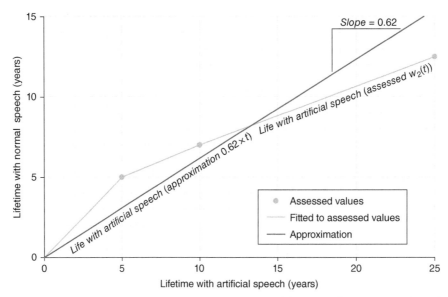

Figure 10.5 Parametric approximation of the quality-lifetime tradeoff functions for artificial speech. The grey curve shows the quality-lifetime tradeoff function fitted to the assessed values shown in Figure 10.2.

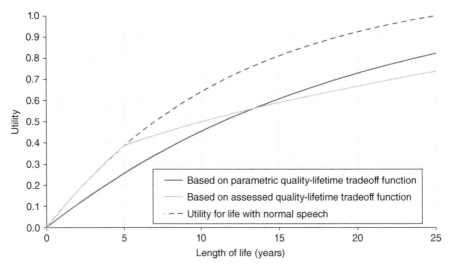

Figure 10.6 Utility for length of life with artificial speech determined using the parametric version of the quality-lifetime tradeoff function shown in Figure 10.5. The grey curve is taken from Figure 10.3 and shows the corresponding utilities based on the assessed quality-lifetime tradeoff function. For purposes of comparison, the utility for life with normal speech also is shown. All utilities have been scaled so that the utility for 25 years of life with normal speech is 1.0.

How significant are the differences between the two utility curves shown in Figure 10.6? As a starting point to answering this question, we will consider how the two curves affect the resulting expected utilities calculated for two of the laryngeal cancer treatments used in the study conducted by McNeil and her colleagues.

Of course, in order to calculate expected utilities for the two treatments, we need to have the corresponding probabilities for the possible lengths of life after treatment. McNeil and her colleagues did not publish the surgery and radiotherapy survival models they used; however, they reference an article that provides enough information to estimate the survival curves for Stage III laryngeal cancer shown in Figure 10.7 (Wang and O'Donald, 1955).

Combining the lifetime probabilities implied by the survival curves in Figure 10.7 with the assessed utility curves shown in Figure 10.3 results in the following expected utilities for the two treatments:

Expected utility for surgery $= 0.4294$
Expected utility for radiotherapy $= 0.2968$

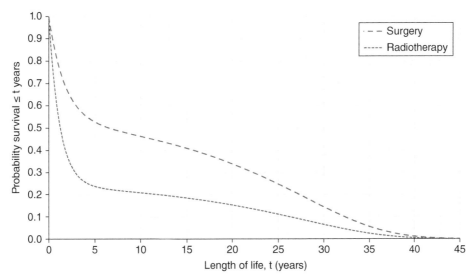

Figure 10.7 Estimated surgery and radiotherapy survival models for Stage III laryngeal cancer for a 58-year-old patient. These survival curves are derived from data reported in 1955 for a study of laryngeal cancer treatment. Adapted from Wang and O' Donald, (1955).

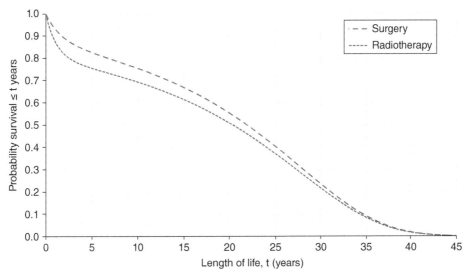

Figure 10.8 Estimated surgery and radiotherapy survival models for Stage I laryngeal cancer for a 58-year-old patient. These survival curves are derived from data reported in 1955 for a study of laryngeal cancer treatment. Adapted from Wang and O'Donald, (1955).

Therefore, assuming Patient B is a patient with Stage III laryngeal cancer who faces the survival curves shown in Figure 10.7,[1] they would prefer surgery over radiotherapy even though surgery will leave them with a life restricted to artificial speech.

For purposes of comparison, Figure 10.8 shows the survival curves for Stage I laryngeal cancer from the same study. Combining the lifetime probabilities implied by these survival curves with the assessed utility curves shown in Figure 10.3 results in the following expected utilities for the two treatments:

Expected utility for surgery = 0.6112
Expected utility for radiotherapy = 0.7409

---

[1] The survival curves shown in Figure 10.7 were derived from survival data observed in a population with an average age of 85 years consisting of 95% men and 5% women. An actual analysis of this treatment decision would adjust these survival curves to match the average age of 40 years for the population studied by McNeil and her colleagues.

Table 10.3 Comparison of surgery and radiotherapy as treatment for Stage I and Stage III laryngeal cancer based on life expectancy and expected utility calculations. Two expected utility calculations are shown. The columns labelled "Assessed" show the expected utilities calculated using the assessed outcome utilities shown in Figure 10.3. The columns labelled "Parametric" show the expected utilities calculated using the quality-lifetime parametric utility model shown in Figure 10.6.

| | | Stage I laryngeal cancer | | | Stage III laryngeal cancer | |
| | | Expected utility | | | Expected utility | |
Treatment	Life expectancy	Assessed	Parametric	Life expectancy	Assessed	Parametric
Surgery	20.2 years	0.6112	0.6538	13.0 years	0.4298	0.4362
Radiotherapy	18.6 years	0.7409	0.7409	6.5 years	0.2968	0.2968

Notice that the expected utilities have increased, which is reasonable since it is better to have Stage I cancer than Stage III cancer. However, the expected utility for radiotherapy increased more than the expected utility for surgery. Therefore, assuming Patient B is a patient with Stage I laryngeal cancer who faces the survival curves shown in Figure 10.7, Patient B now would prefer radiotherapy over surgery. That switch is because the advantage of radiotherapy – avoiding a life restricted to artificial speech – now is enough to overcome the survival advantages of surgery.

Table 10.3 shows the results of repeating these expected utility calculations using the quality-lifetime parametric utility model. Results for both Stage I and Stage III laryngeal cancer are shown. The expected utilities calculated for radiotherapy are the same for both methods because this treatment does not result in loss of normal speech. Therefore, the outcome utilities are the same with the assessed utilities and the utilities determined by the parametric model.

Table 10.3 shows that the discrepancy between the modeled utilities and the assessed utilities affects the decision analysis. The expected utilities calculated for surgery using the parametric model differ from those calculated using the assessed utilities. For example, with Stage I cancer, the expected utility for surgery is 0.6112 when calculated using the assessed utilities. This expected utility changes to 0.6538 when the parametric utility model is used. However, the change is not enough to alter that radiotherapy is preferred by Patient B for this cancer. A similar statement applies to Stage III cancer.

Therefore, at least for this example, the expected utility changes caused by use of the parametric model does not change the conclusions for how Patient B compares the two treatments.

10.3.2 Quality-lifetime parametric utility model with constant risk attitudes

So far the parametric model we have discussed has not delivered on the promise of a simplified method for computing an expected utility. The expected utilities shown in Table 10.3 were calculated by determining the probabilities for each possible length of life. Each of those probabilities were then multiplied by the corresponding outcome utilities and the products summed over all possible lifetimes to determine the patient's expected utility. In short, determining the expected utilities was not a simple calculation.

We now will turn to additional properties of the quality-lifetime parametric utility model that will fulfill the promise of simpler calculations. Those additional properties arise from the combination of the quality-lifetime parametric model we have just discussed with the exponential utility model discussed in the previous chapter.

Recall that the exponential utility model is a mathematical expression that can quantify how a patient feels about risk. When certain assumptions about how the patient views risk apply, that patient's utility for length of life can be expressed by the following mathematical expression:

Utility for life of length $t = 1 - e^{-\gamma t}$

We called γ in this expression the risk parameter because it quantified the patient's risk attitudes for the length of their life. In Chapter 9, we saw several approaches for assessing a patient's value for the parameter γ.

Assessing the value for γ in the context of symptom-free life means that the exponential utility model becomes the patient's utility for symptom-free life. That is, using the notation from earlier in this section:

$$u(t) = 1 - e^{-\gamma t}$$

As we just saw, the parametric version of quality-lifetime tradeoff function assumes

$$w_i(t) \approx \phi_i \times t$$

That is, t years in the ith quality state is equivalent to $\phi_i \times t$ years in the symptom-free quality state. Therefore, combining the exponential utility model with the quality-lifetime parametric utility model produces an expression with two parameters.

$$U\left(t \text{ years in } i^{th} \text{ quality state}\right) = u\left(w_i(t)\right) \approx u\left(\phi_i \times t\right) = 1 - e^{-\gamma \phi_i t}$$

One parameter (γ) accounts for risk attitudes and the other parameter (ϕ_i) accounts for quality preferences. The result is a simple expression for outcome utilities that can be matched to the patient's observed preferences for risk and quality by adjusting two parameters γ and ϕ_i.

For example, recall that Patient B's utilities for life with normal speech was shown in Figure 10.1 as an exponential utility model with risk parameter γ equal to 0.0815/year. Earlier, in this chapter, we determined that 0.62 was Patient B's value for the quality parameter ϕ_2. Therefore, Patient B's utilities for life with artificial speech can be expressed:

$$U\left(t \text{ years with artificial speech}\right) = 1 - e^{-\gamma \phi_2 t} = 1 - e^{-0.0815 \times 0.62 \times t} = 1 - e^{-0.0505 \times t}$$

Result: quality-lifetime parametric utility model with constant risk attitudes

Assume that utility for length of symptom-free life can be expressed as an exponential utility with risk parameter γ. Also assume that the quality-lifetime tradeoff function for the the ith quality state can be expressed by the quality parameter ϕ_i. The quality-lifetime parametric utility model can then be expressed:

Utility for life of length t in the ith quality state $= 1 - e^{-\gamma \phi_i t}$

The computational advantage of using this parametric model occurs when the uncertainty about how long the patient will live can be expressed by an exponential <u>survival</u> model. The exponential survival model will not be discussed in detail until the next chapter. However, recall that with an exponential survival model

$$P\left[\text{Alive at time } t\right] = 1 - e^{-\lambda t}$$

where the parameter λ measures the probability of death during a unit of time. In the previous chapter, we saw that with the exponential utility model, when the uncertainty about the length of life can be represented by an exponential survival model, the expected utility can be determined by the simple expression:

$$\text{Expected utility} = \frac{1}{\lambda + \gamma}$$

A similar expression can be used to determine expected utility with the quality-lifetime parametric utility model. In this case, the expected utility when the uncertainty about the length of life can be represented by the exponential survival model is

$$\text{Expected utility} = \frac{\phi_i}{\lambda + \gamma \phi_i}$$

where ϕ_i is the quality-lifetime tradeoff parameter for the ith quality state.

Result: quality-lifetime adjusted utility with exponential survival

Suppose that (1) the patient's preferences for length of life can be represented by an exponential utility model with parameter γ, (2) the patient's quality-lifetime tradeoff for life in the ith quality state can be represented by the parameter ϕ_i, and (3) the uncertainty for the length of life in an outcome can be represented by an exponential survival model with parameter λ. The patient's expected utility for that outcome is then:

$$U\left(\text{Outcome}\right) = \frac{\phi_i}{\lambda + \gamma \phi_i}$$

Therefore, when combined with the exponential utility model, the quality-lifetime parametric model can provide an efficient representation of a patient's utility for the outcomes they face in a decision problem. The resulting utility model requires one parameter to quantify risk attitudes for the length of life and one parameter for each of the possible quality states in the problem.

10.3.3 Quality-lifetime tradeoff models and risk aversion – a fly in the ointment

Recall the expression we have just derived for the quality-lifetime parametric model. This expression is:

Utility for life of length t in the ith quality state $= 1 - e^{-\gamma \phi_i t}$

where γ is the patient's risk parameter expressed in the time units of t and ϕ_i is the quality-lifetime tradeoff parameter for the ith quality state. The parameter ϕ_i quantifies how much the individual would be willing to shorten their life to avoid living with the symptom or disability that defines the quality state. Therefore, in the case of a quality-reducing symptom or disability ϕ_i always is less than one.

We also have an exponential utility model for the length of symptom-free life which can be written

Utility for symptom – free life of length $t = 1 - e^{-\gamma t}$

However, suppose that we let γ_i denotes the product $\gamma \times \phi_i$. We can then rewrite the expression that determines the utility for life in the ith quality state as follows

Utility for life of length t in the ith quality state $= 1 - e^{-\gamma_i t}$

Notice that the value of γ_i must be less than γ because ϕ_i is less than one. But then this rewritten expression can be thought of as simply an exponential utility for life spent in the ith quality state. That exponential utility model has a risk parameter value of γ_i, which is less than the risk parameter for the utility of symptom-free life.

Back in Chapter 9, we noted that the value of the risk parameter γ decreases as risk aversion decreases. Therefore, the mathematics of the quality-lifetime parametric model implies that risk aversion for life in a quality state must decrease as the importance of avoiding that quality state decreases. Perhaps it is true that for some patients, risk aversion decreases when the quality of their lives decrease. But risk aversion is innate in how we perceive risk. It is troubling to have that change in risk aversion dictated by the mathematical structure of the utility model.

This problematic mathematical property is one reason for considering the alternative to the quality-lifetime tradeoff model that will be discussed after we first consider a nontechnical controversy involving the use of these analytic tools.

Result: quality-lifetime tradeoff model and risk aversion

The quality-lifetime tradeoff model implies that risk aversion decreases as the quality of life decreases. With the quality-lifetime parametric model, an individual's risk aversion for life with a symptom or disability is $\gamma \phi_i$ where γ is the individual's risk parameter and ϕ_i is the quality-lifetime tradeoff parameter, which must be less than 1.

10.3.4 Quality-lifetime tradeoff modelling and healthcare policy analysis

Before considering an alternative to the quality-lifetime tradeoff model, a comment should be made about the widespread use of life length adjustment techniques in health care policy analysis. Starting in the late 1960s, healthcare policy analysis began using a concept known by the acronym QALY to incorporate quality of life concerns. QALY stands for *quality-adjusted life years*. As the name suggests, QALY analysis adjusts the number of years an individual might live according to the quality of life experienced during those years. Therefore, mathematically a QALY is equivalent to the quality-lifetime tradeoff model described in this chapter. In recent years, QALY-based analysis has generated considerable controversy.

The idea behind the use of QALYs is that healthcare programs should promote the quality of life as well as the length of life. Using QALYs to adjust the total number of years lived by the members of a population reflects this idea. For example, consider an analysis of two programs, Program A and Program B. Suppose that both programs will result in similar life expectancies for the targeted population. Also suppose that Program A increases the time people spend in a preferable quality state. Adjusting length of life calculations to account for this quality difference provides a way to understand the differences between the two programs.

In particular, suppose Program A helps prevent the development of diabetes whereas Program B improves survival after the onset of diabetes. Recall the assumption that both programs result in similar life expectancies. But Program A also increases the time spent without the treatment burden and disability associated with diabetes once it occurs. When choosing between these two programs QALY-based analysis would favor Program A over Program B.

However, consider the impact of choosing between these two programs from the perspective of individuals with diabetes. Choosing Program A might make sense based on the total resulting QALYs. But that choice puts individuals with diabetes at a disadvantage since Program A provides no benefits for this subpopulation. Resolving the inegalitarian implications of policy choices like this remains an important controversy in the field of healthcare policy analysis.

10.4 Quality-survival tradeoff models

This chapter focuses on measuring a patient's concerns about the symptoms and disabilities they might face. A meaningful analysis of a patient's decision must account for those concerns. The previous section described an approach that measures how the patient feels about the quality of their life by asking how much the patient would be willing to shorten their lifetime to avoid a loss of quality. The greater the importance the patient places on avoiding that quality loss, the greater the length-of-life tradeoff they would accept to avoid that reduction. Accordingly, that approach was called the *quality-lifetime tradeoff model*.

The quality-lifetime tradeoff model works reasonably well except for distortions caused by an implied assumption that risk aversion changes when the quality of life is reduced. Those distortions increase as the quality reduction caused by a symptom or disability worsens. The current section describes an alternative approach to analyzing quality preferences that avoid this problematic assumption. The alternative that will be described has a parametric model that retains the computational simplicity of the quality-lifetime parametric model but can more closely match the patient's actual outcome utilities.

Once again, consider a disability such as the loss of normal speech. Another measure of how the patient feels about the loss of normal speech is to propose a hypothetical treatment that could restore normal speech but could also cause immediate death. A patient who places great importance on having normal speech would choose the hypothetical treatment even if the probability of survival is low. A patient who places less importance on normal speech would require a higher survival probability for that hypothetical treatment.

The minimum acceptable survival probability for avoiding a quality-of-life reduction is the key concept in this second approach to measuring quality preferences. The greater the importance placed on avoiding the reduction the lower the acceptable survival probability. In other words, this approach measures quality preferences by the survival tradeoff that would be acceptable to the patient. Therefore, we will call this survival-based approach to measuring quality preferences the *quality-survival tradeoff model*.

The quality-survival tradeoff model can be represented by the following standard gamble assessment question:

The gamble on the right is preferred if the probability of surviving is greater than $s(t)$. The guaranteed outcome on the left is preferred if the probability of surviving the gamble is less than $s(t)$. Note that length of life (t) is included because the acceptable survival probability may depend on how long the patient will live.

Scaling outcome utilities so that the utility for immediate death is zero, the equivalence in this standard gamble assessment question leads to the following mathematical expression for the utility for life with the disability:

$$U\left(\begin{array}{c}\text{Live } t \text{ years with}\\ \text{quality of life loss}\end{array}\right) = s(t) \times U\left(\begin{array}{c}\text{Live } t \text{ years without}\\ \text{quality of life loss}\end{array}\right) + \left(1 - s(t)\right) \times U\left(\text{Live 0 years}\right)$$

$$= s(t) \times U\left(\begin{array}{c}\text{Live } t \text{ years without}\\ \text{quality of life loss}\end{array}\right) + \left(1 - s(t)\right) \times 0$$

$$= s(t) \times U\left(\begin{array}{c}\text{Live } t \text{ years without}\\ \text{quality of life loss}\end{array}\right)$$

How does this expression compare to the corresponding expression used with the quality-lifetime tradeoff model? Recall that with the quality-lifetime tradeoff model, the corresponding expression for living t years with a quality-of-life loss is

$$U\left(\begin{array}{c}\text{Live } t \text{ years with}\\ \text{quality of life loss}\end{array}\right) = U\left(\begin{array}{c}\text{Live } w(t) \text{ years without}\\ \text{quality of life loss}\end{array}\right)$$

The term $w(t)$ is a value less than t representing how much the patient would be willing to shorten their life in order to avoid the loss in quality.

In other words, the quality-lifetime tradeoff model adjusts for quality by reducing the length of life. In contrast, the quality-survival tradeoff model adjusts for living with a quality loss by directly reducing the utility for the length of life. This difference may seem subtle; however, we will see that it avoids the fly-in-the-ointment mentioned for the quality-lifetime tradeoff model.

Definition: quality-survival tradeoff model

A *quality-survival tradeoff* model represents the utility for an outcome that has a given length of life, and a quality-reducing disability, by determining the minimum probability of survival, without the disability, the patient would accept in order to avoid the disability. The utility for the original outcome with the disability is that minimum survival probability multiplied by the utility for living the same length of life free of the disability.

10.4.1 Assessing quality preferences with the quality-survival tradeoff model

Consider life without normal speech. The following question can be used to assess $s_2(t)$, which measures a patient's quality preference for loss of normal speech in the quality-survival tradeoff model.

Suppose you will live another t years. For the remainder of your life you will not have normal speech. Instead, your verbal communication will be limited to what can be achieved through the artificial methods that are available after your vocal cords have been removed. What survival probability would you require for a risky treatment that could restore normal speech but could also cause your immediate death?

The answer to this question is the value for $s_2(t)$. This question can be represented by the following standard gamble assessment question:

Once again, we call $s_2(t)$ the minimum acceptable survival probability for avoiding life with artificial speech. If we scale utility so that a life of 0 years has the utility of 0.0, notice that the equivalence in this diagram can be expressed mathematically as

$$U\left(\text{Live } t \text{ years with artificial speech}\right) = s(t) \times U\left(\text{Live } t \text{ years with normal speech}\right)$$

Suppose the assessment question was asked with t equal to 10 years and assume Patient B answered with a probability of 0.78. This means that for Patient B

$$s_2(10 \text{ years}) = 0.78$$

Similarly, suppose that Patient B answered with a probability of 0.73 when t is equal to 25 years. Then

$$s_2(25 \text{ years}) = 0.73$$

Finally, if faced with a lifetime of 5 years or less, we will assume Patient B would require that survival be certain for a treatment that would preserve normal speech. This means

$$s_2(5 \text{ years}) = 1.00$$

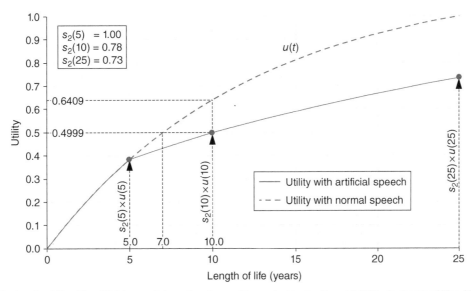

Figure 10.9 Utility for length of life with artificial speech based on the quality-survival tradeoff model. Utility for length of life with normal speech is shown as a dotted curve. The former ($u(t)$) is derived from the latter by multiplying $u(t)$ by the corresponding survival probabilities ($s_2(t)$). All utilities have been scaled so that the utility for 25 years of life with normal speech is 1.0.

Figure 10.9 shows Patient B's utility for life with artificial speech, given these three answers to the assessment question.

The outcome utilities plotted for 5, 10, and 25 years in Figure 10.9 were determined directly from the expression

$$U\left(\text{Live } t \text{ years with artificial speech}\right) = s(t) \times U\left(\text{Live } t \text{ years with normal speech}\right)$$

For example, Patient B's value for $s_2(10 \text{ years})$ is 0.78 and according to the dotted curve in Figure 10.9, the utility for a 10-year length of life with normal speech is 0.6409. Therefore,

$$U\left(\text{Live 10 years with artificial speech}\right) = s(t) \times U\left(\text{Live 10 years with normal speech}\right)$$
$$U\left(\text{Live 10 years with artificial speech}\right) = 0.78 \times 0.6409 = 0.4999$$

Similar calculations determine the utilities for living 5 and 25 years with artificial speech. The remainder of the utility curve shown in Figure 10.9 was drawn by interpolating between these three assessed values.

At first glance, the quality-survival tradeoff model appears to require a different assessment process. However, a quality-survival tradeoff model also can be inferred from the same questions used by the quality-lifetime tradeoff model. More specifically, the minimum acceptable survival probabilities used by the quality-survival tradeoff model can be determined from the length-of-life tradeoffs, the patient would accept to avoid a quality reduction. This equivalence would be important for patients who find it easier to think about the quality of their life in terms of lifetime reductions rather than survival probabilities.

For example, recall that the following are the lifetime reductions Patient B would accept in order to avoid the loss of normal speech:
- 5 years with normal artificial equivalent to 5 years with normal speech
- 10 years with normal artificial equivalent to 7 years with normal speech
- 25 years with normal artificial equivalent to 12.5 years with normal speech

These three assessments mean that for Patient B

$$U\left(\text{Live 5 years with artificial speech}\right) = U\left(\text{Live 5 years with normal speech}\right)$$
$$U\left(\text{Live 10 years with artificial speech}\right) = U\left(\text{Live 7 years with normal speech}\right)$$
$$U\left(\text{Live 25 years with artificial speech}\right) = U\left(\text{Live 12.5 years with normal speech}\right)$$

Consider the minimum acceptable survival probability with a lifetime of 10 years, which is denoted $s_2(10)$. We just saw that

$$U\left(\text{Live 10 years without normal speech}\right) = s_2(10) \times U\left(\text{Live 10 years with normal speech}\right)$$

But

$U(\text{Live 10 years with artificial speech}) = U(\text{Live 7 years with normal speech})$

This means

$U(\text{Live 7 years with normal speech}) = s_2(10) \times U(\text{Live 10 years with normal speech})$

We can rearrange this expression as follows:

$$s_2(10) = \frac{U(\text{Live 7 years with normal speech})}{U(\text{Live 10 years with normal speech})}$$

The dotted curve in Figure 10.9 shows Patient B's utilities for length of life with normal speech:

$U(\text{Live 7 years and normal speech}) = 0.4999$
$U(\text{Live 10 years and normal speech}) = 0.6409$

Inserting these values into the expression for $s_2(10)$ yields

$$s_2(10) = \frac{U(\text{Live 7 years and normal speech})}{U(\text{Live 10 years and normal speech})} = \frac{0.4999}{0.6409} = 0.7800$$

We can repeat this process to determine the values for $s_2(5)$ and $s_2(25)$. In other words, Patient B's answers to the quality-lifetime tradeoff questions told us the minimum survival probabilities needed to use the quality-survival tradeoff model to represent Patient B's preferences.

The opposite also is true. Answers to the quality-survival tradeoff assessment questions imply the information required to represent Patient B's preferences with the quality-lifetime tradeoff model.

Therefore, the quality-survival tradeoff model has the same assessment process as the quality-lifetime tradeoff model. This means that both assessment processes produce the same outcome utilities. This raises the question, why consider the quality-survival tradeoff model in the first place? The answer is found in the corresponding parametric model for representing quality preferences by survival tradeoffs.

10.4.2 Parameterized quality-survival tradeoff model

The quality-lifetime tradeoff model discussed in the previous section adjusts for the quality of life by first reducing the length of life. Utility is then determined for that reduced lifetime. In contrast, the quality-survival tradeoff model starts by determining the utility for the length of life, without the loss in quality. That utility is then adjusted to account for the quality reduction caused by the symptoms or disabilities that are part of the outcome.

Given this comparison of the two models, recall that the parametric version of the quality-lifetime tradeoff model uses a fixed value ϕ_i to quantify the length of life adjustment. That is, the utility for life in the ith quality state is approximated as follows

$U(\text{Live } t \text{ years in } i^{th} \text{ quality state}) \approx U(\text{Live } \phi_i \times t \text{ years in symptom free quality state})$

where ϕ_i is the average value for the ratio of the length of life in the ith quality state over the equivalent length of life in a symptom-free quality state. Figure 10.4 showed how this average was calculated.

On the other hand, the parametric version of the quality-survival tradeoff model uses a fixed value θ_i to quantify the utility adjustment. Recall that with the quality-survival tradeoff model the utility for life in the ith quality state is

$U(\text{Live } t \text{ years in } i^{th} \text{ quality state}) = s_i(t) \times U(\text{Live } t \text{ years in symptom free quality state})$

The parametric version of the quality-survival parametric model is the approximation:

$U(\text{Live } t \text{ years in } i^{th} \text{ quality state}) \approx \theta_i \times U(\text{Live } t \text{ years in symptom} - \text{free quality state})$

In other words, the parameter θ_i approximates $s_i(t)$ by a constant.

Figure 10.10 shows how the minimum acceptable survival probability for life with artificial speech varies with the length of life. We denote these probabilities by $s_2(t)$. The curve in Figure 10.10 is based on Patient B's assessed values for $s_2(t)$.

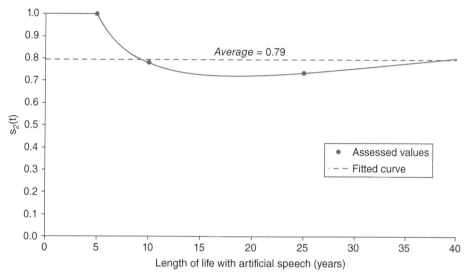

Figure 10.10 Patient B's minimum survival probabilities for avoiding loss of normal speech ($s_2(t)$). The curve for lifetimes past 25 years are determined by extrapolating the quality-lifetime tradeoff function values shown in Figure 10.2.

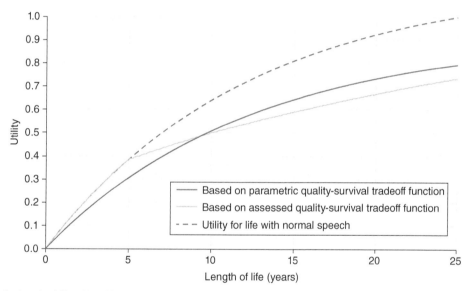

Figure 10.11 Utility for length of life with artificial speech determined using the parametric version of the quality-survival parametric model. The grey curve is taken from Figure 10.9 and shows the corresponding utilities based on the assessed quality-lifetime tradeoff function. For purposes of comparison, the utility for life with normal speech also is shown. All utilities have been scaled so that the utility for 25 years of life with normal speech is 1.0.

Assuming Patient B can expect to live at most another 40 years, the average value for $s_2(t)$ has been calculated over a 40-year period. The result is value of 0.79 for θ_2. Figure 10.11 compares the resulting parametric model to the quality-survival tradeoff model based on the assessment of Patient B's quality preferences. That is, the parametric version of the quality-survival tradeoff model for Patient B is

$$U\left(\text{Live } t \text{ years in } i^{th} \text{ with artificial speech}\right) \approx 0.79 \times u(t)$$

Figure 10.11 compares the values for this approximation to the utility model assessed for Patient B.

Figure 10.12 compares the parametric utility model shown in Figure 10.11 to the corresponding parametric model based on the quality-lifetime tradeoff model. Both parametric utility models also are compared to the utility model assessed for Patient B. Note that the quality-survival tradeoff model more closely matches the assessed utility for this patient. This closer match is typical for comparisons of the two parametric models.

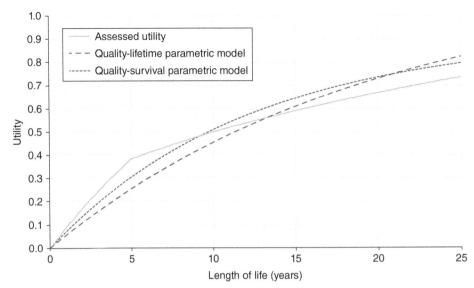

Figure 10.12 Patient B's assessed utilities for length of life with artificial speech compared with utilities determined by the quality-lifetime parametric model and the quality-survival parametric model. All utilities have been scaled so that the utility for 25 years of life with normal speech is 1.0.

As before, the utility for symptom-free life can be represented by the exponential utility model described in Chapter 9. This leads to the following definition of the quality-survival parametric utility model:

Utility for the life of length t in the ith quality state $= \theta_i \times \left(1 - e^{-\gamma t}\right)$

Notice that this utility model does not adjust for a loss in the quality of life by changing how the patient's risk attitudes are represented. The risk parameter γ is not changed. Instead, the quality reduction is represented by an overall reduction in the utility for the outcome. Therefore, the problematic distortion of risk attitudes is avoided.

Definition: quality-survival parametric model

The *quality-survival parametric model* represents the utility for an outcome in which the patient will live for time t in the ith quality state as follows:

Utility for the life of length t in the ith quality state $= \theta_i \times \left(1 - e^{-\gamma t}\right)$

where γ is the patient's risk parameter expressed in the time units of t and θ_i is the quality-survival tradeoff parameter for the ith quality state.

10.4.3 Parameterized quality-survival tradeoff model and exponential survival

As we did in the previous section, suppose that the uncertainty for the length of life is such that:

$$P\left(\text{Survival} \leq t\right) = 1 - e^{-\lambda t}$$

where t is the length of life and λ is the death rate expressed in the time units of t. With the quality-survival parametric model, the expected utility for the outcome is:

Expected utility with exponential survival in the ith quality state $= \dfrac{\theta_i}{\gamma + \lambda}$

where the term θ_i is the patient's quality-survival tradeoff parameter for the ith quality state and γ is the patient's risk parameter. As with the other quality tradeoff model, the complicated mathematics required to prove this result are not shown here.

Result: quality-survival adjusted utility with exponential survival

Suppose that (1) the patient's preferences for length of life can be represented by an exponential utility model with parameter γ, (2) the patient's quality-survival tradeoff for life in the ith quality state can be represented by the parameter θ_i, and (3) the uncertainty for the length of life in an outcome can be represented by an exponential survival model with parameter λ. The patient's expected utility for that outcome is then:

$$U(\text{Outcome}) = \frac{\theta_i}{\gamma + \lambda}$$

This means the quality-survival parametric model, when combined with the exponential utility model, provides a simple expression for determining the expected utility for an outcome. As with the quality-lifetime parametric model, determining the expected utility requires one parameter for risk attitudes and one parameter for the quality state. The discussion will now turn to how to determine values for those quality parameters.

10.5   What does it all mean? – an extended example

This chapter concludes the discussion of outcome utilities. Chapter 8 introduced the concept of risk aversion and showed how to represent this inevitable part of how patients view uncertainty by a von Neumann–Morgenstern utility model. That chapter introduced utility models as mathematical expressions that measure the importance the patient places on an outcome when there is uncertainty about the patient experiencing that outcome. We called those measures the outcome utilities.

Chapter 9 and the current chapter extended the theoretical concept of an outcome utility to establish a more practical framework for analyzing clinical decision problems. Those extensions used parametric models to simplify the process required to measure patient preferences by outcome utilities. To see the importance of parametric models, consider the alternative of directly assessing the patient's utilities for possible outcomes in a decision problem.

10.5.1   Direct approach to outcome utility assessment

For example, suppose that a decision problem can be summarized as the choice between treatment or no treatment when disease is either present or absent. The corresponding decision tree is shown in Figure 10.13. Note that this simple problem has only four possible outcomes:

- No treatment and no disease
- Treatment and no disease
- Treatment and disease
- No treatment and disease

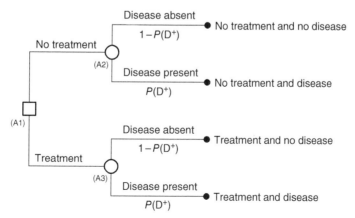

Figure 10.13 Tree for decision between treatment or no treatment when disease is either present or absent. This decision tree is used to illustrate direct approach to utility assessment.

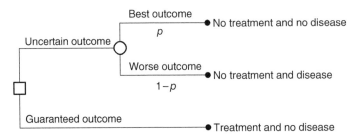

Figure 10.14 Decision tree for the standard gamble assessment question that determines the utility for the outcome **Treatment and no disease**. The value for *p* such that the uncertain outcome and the guaranteed outcome are equivalent is the patient's utility for **Treatment and no disease**.

Note that we have listed these outcomes in order of decreasing preference. For example, the treatment has no value unless **Treatment and disease** is preferred to **No treatment and disease**. Similarly, this would not be an interesting problem unless **No treatment and no disease** is preferred to **Treatment and no disease**. Otherwise, treatment would always be chosen, regardless of the presence or absence of disease. Finally, we assume **Treatment and no disease** is preferred to **Treatment and disease** because it usually is.

Given the order of preference, we can start the direct approach to utility assessment with the following reference values:

U(No treatment and no disease) = 1.0

U(Treatment and no disease)　　= 0.0

Direct utility assessment then uses the standard gamble question to determine the patient's utilities for the remaining two outcomes. Figure 10.14 shows the decision tree for this assessment question when applied to the outcome **Treatment and no disease**.

Of course, a patient's utility for the intermediate outcomes only can be assessed in the context of an actual disease and an actual treatment. Therefore, suppose the disease is a myocardial infarction and the treatment is hospitalization. Given this context, the patient's utility for the outcome **Treatment and no disease** might be assessed using the following question:

Suppose that you must choose between two alternatives. One alternative is to spend a few days in a hospital but to otherwise be healthy. The other alternative is to stay out of the hospital but there is a probability that you are experiencing a myocardial infarction. How large must the probability of a myocardial infarction be for you to choose the second alternative and be admitted to a hospital?

A similar question would be used to determine the utility for the outcome **Treatment and disease**.

The decision presented in the standard gamble assessment question (Figure 10.14) looks almost as complicated as the decision presented in the original decision (Figure 10.13). The only difference is that the standard gamble question involves three outcomes whereas the original problem involves four outcomes. Utility assessment only makes sense if the patient can resolve the decision presented in Figure 10.14 but not the decision presented in Figure 10.13.

The one advantage of the direct approach to utility assessment is that the complexity of the standard gamble assessment remains the same even when the number of possible outcomes in the original problem grows. In other words, directly assessing the utilities for a decision problem with hundreds of possible outcomes still only requires an assessment question involving three of the possible outcomes. Of course, this advantage is offset by the proliferation of assessment questions the patient must answer. A decision problem with a dozen possible outcomes requires that the patient remain focused during a dozen standard gamble assessment questions. Direct utility assessment quickly becomes impractical when the complexity of the decision tree starts to match the complexity of an actual clinical decision.

Moreover, direct utility assessment questions present the patient with a cognitive challenge. Think about the question posed by the standard gamble assessment question in Figure 10.14. Answering this question requires the patient to balance how they feel about unnecessary treatment with how they feel about not treating a disease they might have. Moreover, the patient must express how they balance these two concerns by providing a single value for a probability *p*. This cognitive challenge increases as more treatments and possible disease states are included in the analysis. In other words, the direct approach to utility assessment requires the patient to give meaningful answers to a large number of hard-to-answer questions.

> **Definition: direct approach to utility assessment**
>
> The direct approach to utility assessment starts by identifying the best and worst possible outcome, which are assigned the utility of 1.0 and 0.0, respectively. Separate standard gamble assessment questions are used to determine the utilities for each remaining outcome. The disadvantages of direct assessment are:
> * Large number of assessment questions required for a complex decision problem.
> * Cognitive challenge of comparing outcomes that combine multiple issue, such as the length of life and the quality of life.

McNeil and her colleagues addressed these challenges by using a different approach in both of their two studies of patient preferences. Consider their study of laryngeal cancer treatment. A patient with this treatment decision faces a range of possible outcomes that differ according to the length of life and the quality of life. Direct utility assessment would have required separate assessment questions for each possible length of life combined with each possible quality state.

Instead, McNeil and her colleagues characterized each outcome as a combination of two dimensions: (1) how long the patient lives and (2) whether the patient would live that life with natural speech. They measured their volunteers' preferences for each dimension separately. One set of assessment questions determined a volunteer's utility for the length of life in a quality state. Another set of questions determined the adjustments needed to those utilities to reflect how the patient felt about the quality of life that would be experienced in a quality state.

Separating the assessment process according to the length of life and the quality of life reduced the cognitive challenge of answering the questions. The parametric models described in this chapter, and the preceding chapter, greatly reduced the number of required questions. We saw that two approaches can then be used to combine the results of the two assessment processes into a single expression for determining a patient's outcome utilities for this decision problem.

This chapter concludes with a demonstration. We will apply the concepts in this chapter and the preceding chapter to the treatment decision faced by patients suspected of having a pulmonary embolism. The results will be used in a later chapter that discusses the important concept of threshold probabilities.

> **Definition: outcome separation approach to utility assessment**
>
> Utility assessment by outcome separation represents each possible outcome as combination of dimensions, such as the length of life and the quality of life. The patient's preferences for each dimension are measured separately. The outcome utilities are determined by combining the preference measures for each of the dimensions comprising an outcome. The disadvantages of direct assessment are the validity of the assumptions used to
> * Simplify how preferences are assessed for an outcome dimension.
> * Combine the preferences assessed for the outcome dimensions into an overall outcome utility.

10.5.2   Outcome utility assessment based on outcome decomposition

A threshold probability marks the point where the possibility of a treatable disease justifies starting treatment. The discussion of threshold probabilities in that later chapter will show how the potential harms and benefits of a treatment interact to determine when the treatment should be started. In turn, outcome utilities play a central role in quantifying those potential harms and benefits. The following discussion demonstrates how the decomposition approach can determine the outcome utilities needed to establish a threshold probability.

The example of how to treat suspected pulmonary embolism illustrates the discussion in that later chapter. Timely treatment with anticoagulants can save the patient's life by dissolving the blood clot. Anticoagulants also can cause intracranial hemorrhaging, which can lead to significant disability or death. Figure 10.15 shows a decision tree representing this clinical dilemma.

The dilemma starts with the uncertainty about actual presence of the pulmonary embolism. That uncertainty is represented by chance nodes **B2** and **B4** in the decision tree. Without treatment, the patient can survive either because there was no pulmonary embolism or because the body's own clot-dissolving mechanisms have been successful. The probability of death from untreated pulmonary embolism is assumed to be 0.5000 (node **B3**).

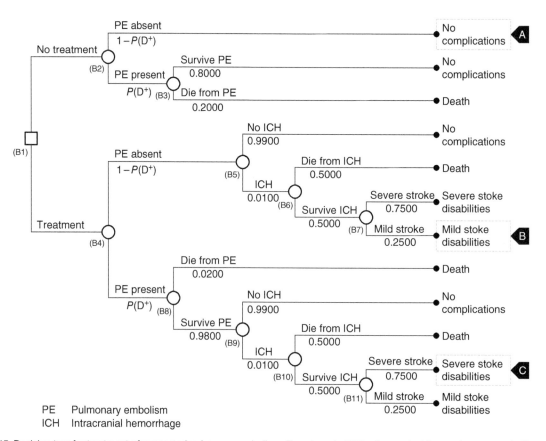

PE   Pulmonary embolism
ICH   Intracranial hemorrhage

Figure 10.15 Decision tree for treatment of suspected pulmonary embolism. Branch probabilities for survival from pulmonary embolism and central nervous system bleed are from published literature. Branch probabilities for death from central nervous system bleed and severity of stroke were estimated by the author. The letters A, B, and C designate outcomes discussed in the narrative.

Note that the decision tree ignores the possibility of residual damage after surviving an untreated pulmonary embolism. Therefore, survival after an untreated pulmonary embolism is assumed to be equivalent to not having a pulmonary embolism.

Treatment of a pulmonary embolism reduces the probability of death from the disease to 0.5000 (node **B8**). However, the probability that treatment will cause a hemorrhagic stroke is 0.0100 (nodes **B5** and **B9**). The probability of dying from a hemorrhagic stroke from excessive anticoagulation is 0.5000 (nodes **B6** and **B10**). Surviving a hemorrhagic stroke will lead to either mild or severe disability (nodes **B7** and **B11**). The probability of a mild stroke is 0.25 and a severe stroke is 0.75. We assume here that the probabilities of treatment complications are the same regardless of whether the patient had a pulmonary embolism.

The patient who survives faces life in the following three quality states:

1. No complications
2. Mild stroke disabilities
3. Severe stroke disabilities

The patient also faces the uncertainty of how long they will live if they survive the episode and uncertainty about possible complications of treatment. Quantifying that uncertainty requires different survival models for the following possibilities:

- The patient has no residual complications from the disease or treatment. For this case, the example will assume an exponential survival model with the life expectancy of a 55-year-old woman (35 years).
- The patient spends the remainder of their life with mild disability from a stroke. Life expectancies between 30 and 32 years were reported for 50-year-old women with post-stroke disabilities classified on the modified Rankin Scale as 0 or 1 (Shavelle *et al.*, 2019). Therefore, this example will assume an exponential survival model with a life expectancy of 30 years for this case.

- The patient spends the remainder of their life with severe disabilities from a hemorrhage stroke. Life expectancies between 7 and 25 years were reported for 50-year-old women with post-stroke disabilities classified on the modified Rankin Scale as 2 or greater (Shavelle *et al.*, 2019). Therefore, this example will assume an exponential survival model with a life expectancy of 15 years for this case.

Determining the outcome utilities for this decision problem starts with assessing the patient's utility for life with no complications. This example assumes that an exponential utility model represents the patient's utility for the length of life. Recalling from the discussion in Chapter 9, this assumption means the utility for a life of length t can be represented as follows:

$$u(t) = \frac{1 - e^{-\gamma t}}{\gamma}$$

The value for γ, which we call the risk parameter, can be determined by asking a question like the following:

Suppose that you have a disease that will cause your death, on average, in 15 years. Also suppose that if this disease were cured you could expect to live, on average, another 35 years. If there is a risky treatment that will either cure your disease or cause your immediate death, how large would probability of surviving have to be for you to choose this treatment?

The choice of 15 and 35 years used in this wording of the question is arbitrary. The length of these average outcomes can be adjusted to describe a scenario that fits the patient's circumstances. The values used in the sample wording shown earlier are based on a 55-year-old woman's life expectancy without complications (35 years) and their life expectancy after surviving a severe stroke (15 years).

In general, this assessment question can be represented as the decision tree shown in Figure 10.16.

As explained in Chapter 9, the following expression determines the value for the risk parameter γ (see Subsection 9.2.6):

$$\gamma = \frac{p/X_A - 1/X_B}{1 - p}$$

where p is the answer to the assessment question shown in Figure 10.16.

The example will assume that 0.13/year is the resulting value for γ. Given this assumption, the following expression determines the utility for life of t years without complications:

$$U(\text{Life of } t \text{ years without complications}) = \frac{1 - e^{-0.1300 \times t}}{0.1300}$$

The usual assumption is that the value for the risk parameter is independent of the patient's quality state. In other words, we assume the patient would provide the same answer to the assessment question if their remaining life would be lived in any of the quality states for the problem.

In order to determine the patient's utility for life with those disabilities, we must adjust the expression to represent the quality-of-life reduction. How to make this adjustment depends on the quality tradeoff model we decide to use. For the reasons discussed in the preceding section, we will use the quality-survival tradeoff model. This model adjusts for living with a disability by determining the minimum survival probability, the patient would be required to undergo a hypothetical treatment that would either eliminate the disability or cause sudden death.

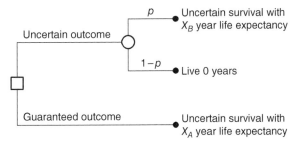

Figure 10.16 Decision tree for the assessment question that determines the patient's utility for the length of life.

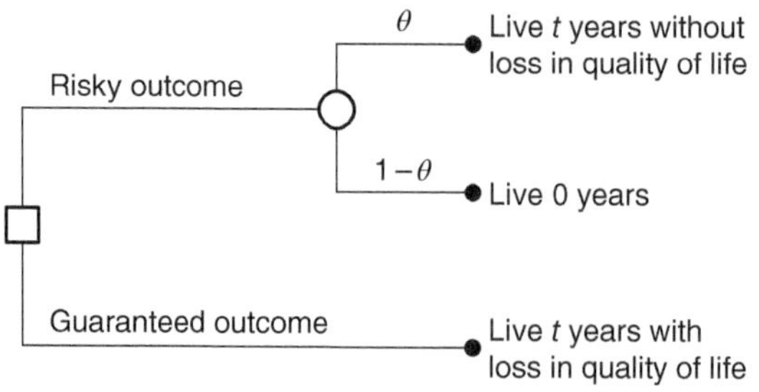

Figure 10.17 Decision tree for the assessment question that determines the patient's quality parameter for a given length of life.

Living with the disabilities of a mild stroke is one of the possible quality states faced by a patient with suspected pulmonary embolism. The different ways a mild stroke can affect a patient's life complicates the assessment of the quality parameter for living in this quality state. The corresponding assessment question must describe a representative level of disability for a mild stroke. The following wording of the assessment question is based on the definition of disabilities classified as level 1 – or mild stroke – on the modified Rankin Scale:

Suppose that you will live the remainder of your life with some difficulties speaking and minor reductions in your mobility. Suppose there is a risky treatment that could cause your immediate death. If this treatment is successful it will not change how long you will live. However, you will no longer have difficulties with speaking and mobility. How large with the probability of surviving the hypothetical treatment have to be for you to choose the treatment?

Figure 10.17 shows the general form for this assessment question expressed as a decision tree. The patient's answer is what we called the minimum acceptable survival probability and is represented by the probability θ in Figure 10.17. In this example, we assume that the patient would require at least an 80% chance of surviving. Therefore, the answer to this assessment question implies a value of 0.8 for the quality parameter θ.

Recall that the quality-survival parametric model determines the utility for a lifetime of t years in a health state by the expression

$$U(\text{Live } t \text{ years in quality state}) = \theta \times U(\text{Live } t \text{ years without complications})$$

So far we have determined that

$$U(\text{Life of } t \text{ years without complications}) = \frac{1 - e^{-0.1300 \times t}}{0.1300}$$

and that when the quality state is living with a mild stroke

$$\theta = 0.80$$

Therefore,

$$U(\text{Life of } t \text{ years with mild stroke disabilities}) = 0.8000 \times \frac{1 - e^{-0.1300 \times t}}{0.1300}$$

A similar process determines the quality adjustments needed to express the patient's utility for life with the severe stroke disabilities. The parameter θ for this quality state is determined using the answer to an assessment question like the following:

Suppose that you will live the remainder of your life with significant difficulties speaking as well as very limited mobility. These disabilities will keep you from caring for yourself. Suppose there is a risky treatment that could cause your immediate death. If this treatment is successful it will not change how long you will live. However, you will no longer have difficulties with speaking and mobility. Independent living would again become a possibility. How large with the probability of surviving the hypothetical treatment have to be for you to choose the treatment?

This example supposes that the patient's answer to these questions imply a value of 0.3 for the quality parameter θ. It would follow that

$$U(\text{Life of } t \text{ years with severe stroke disabilities}) = 0.3000 \times \frac{1 - e^{-0.1300 \times t}}{0.1300}$$

We now know enough to determine the utilities for each of the outcomes in the decision tree for this problem. The last step is to combine the utility model for length of life, adjusted by the appropriate quality parameter, with the corresponding survival model.

For example, consider the outcome labelled "A" in Figure 10.15. The patient experiences this outcome if there is no treatment and there is no pulmonary embolism. The following parametric utility model determines the utility for a life of length t years with this outcome:

$$U\left(\text{Life of } t \text{ years without complications}\right) = \frac{1 - e^{-0.1300 \times t}}{0.1300}$$

The probability the patient will live t years during this outcome is derived from the exponential survival model with parameter $1/35$ years, or 0.0286/year. That is

$$P\left[\text{Alive in } t \text{ years without complications}\right] = 1 - e^{-0.0286 \times t}$$

Recall from the discussion earlier in this chapter that if the quality-adjusted utility for life can be represented by the parametric model

$$U\left(\text{Life of } t \text{ years in } i^{\text{th}} \text{ quality state}\right) = \theta_i \times \frac{1 - e^{-\gamma \times t}}{\gamma}$$

and the length of life is determined by the exponential survival model

$$P\left[\text{Alive in } t \text{ years}\right] = 1 - e^{-\lambda \times t}$$

Then the expected utility is given by the expression:

$$\text{Expected utility} = \frac{\theta_i}{\lambda + \gamma}$$

For the outcome labeled A in the decision tree, the risk parameter θ_i is 1 since this is life without complications. Therefore, using the other parameter values for this outcome, we have that

$$\text{Expected utility for no complications} = \frac{\theta_i}{\lambda + \gamma} = \frac{1}{0.0286 + 0.1300} = 6.3063$$

What we have determined is the utility for any of the outcomes in the decision tree that follows from (1) the absence of a pulmonary embolism and no treatment, (2) unnecessary treatment without intracranial hemorrhaging when there is no pulmonary embolism, or (3) successful treatment of a pulmonary embolism without intracranial hemorrhaging.

Now consider the outcome labelled "B" in Figure 10.15. The patient experiences this outcome if they survive a mild stroke caused by treatment. The following parametric model utility determines the utility for a life of length t years during this outcome:

$$U\left(\text{Life of } t \text{ years with mild stroke disabilities}\right) = 0.8000 \times \frac{1 - e^{-0.1300 \times t}}{0.1300}$$

The corresponding survival model is

$$P\left[\text{Alive in } t \text{ years with mild stroke disabilities}\right] = 1 - e^{-0.0333 \times t}$$

It follows that

$$\text{Expected utility for mild stroke disabilities} = \frac{\theta_i}{\lambda + \gamma} = \frac{0.8000}{0.0333 + 0.1300} = 4.8980$$

Repeating the same process for the outcome labelled "C" in Figure 10.15 yields

$$\text{Expected utility for severe stroke disabilities} = \frac{\theta_i}{\lambda + \gamma} = \frac{0.3000}{0.0667 + 0.1300} = 1.5254$$

Table 10.4 Utilities for the possible outcomes of the pulmonary embolism treatment decision.

Outcome	Utility derived in narrative	Rescaled utility
No complications	6.3063	1.0000
Mild stroke disabilities	4.8980	0.7767
Severe stroke disabilities	1.5254	0.2419
Death	0.0000	0.0000

Finally, Table 10.4 lists the utilities for the possible outcomes of the pulmonary embolism treatment decision. Notice that this table also contains a column labelled "Rescaled utilities." This column contains the outcome utilities rescaled so that utility for life with no complications is 1.0. The values for the rescaled outcome utilities are interesting because they are the utilities that should have been determined by the direct approach to utility assessment described earlier.

The outcome utilities shown in this table will be used in a later chapter to demonstrate how the threshold for starting treatment balances the possible benefits and harms of treatment.

Summary

- A *quality-lifetime tradeoff* model represents the utility for an outcome that has a given length of life, and a quality-reducing symptom, by determining an equivalent outcome with a shorter length of life, but without the symptom. The utility for the original outcome is the utility for that equivalent shorter symptom-free lifetime.
- A quality-lifetime tradeoff model can be expressed using the following notation:

$u_i(t)$ = Utility for lifetime t in i^{th} quality state

$w_i(t)$ = Equivalent life time t in i^{th} quality state

Then

$$U(t \text{ years in } i^{th} \text{ quality state}) = u_i(w_i(t))$$

Typically, the function $u_i(t)$ is assumed to be the same for all quality states.
- Let $w_i(t)$ denote the quality-lifetime tradeoff function assessed for the ith quality state and let ϕ_i equal the value for the ratio $w_i(t)/t$ averaged over a suitable time period, such as the patient's life expectancy. The *quality-lifetime parametric utility model* uses the following approximation to determine the patient's utility for a life lasting t years on the ith quality state:

$$U(t \text{ years in } i^{th} \text{ quality state}) \approx u(\phi_i \times t)$$

The term ϕ_i is called the *quality-lifetime tradeoff parameter*.
- Assume that utility for length of symptom-free life can be expressed as an exponential utility with risk parameter γ. Also assume that the quality-lifetime tradeoff function for the ith quality state can be expressed by the quality parameter ϕ_i. The quality-lifetime parametric utility model can then be expressed:

Utility for life of length t in the ith quality state $= 1 - e^{-\gamma\phi_i t}$
- Suppose that (1) the patient's preferences for length of life can be represented by an exponential utility model with parameter γ, (2) the patient's quality-lifetime tradeoff for life in the ith quality state can be represented by the parameter ϕ_i, and (3) the uncertainty for the length of life in an outcome can be represented by an exponential survival model with parameter λ. The patient's expected utility for that outcome is then:

$$U(\text{Outcome}) = \frac{\phi_i}{\lambda + \gamma\phi_i}$$

- The quality-lifetime tradeoff model implies that risk aversion decreases as the quality of life decreases. With the quality-lifetime parametric model, an individual's risk aversion for life with a symptom or disability is $\gamma\phi_i$ where ϕ_i is the quality-lifetime tradeoff parameter and γ is the individual's risk parameter.
- A *quality-survival tradeoff* model represents the utility for an outcome that has a given length of life, and a quality-reducing symptom or disability, by determining the minimum probability of survival the patient would accept in order to avoid the symptom or disability. The utility for the original outcome is that minimum survival probability multiplied by the utility for living the same length of life free of the symptom or disability.
- The *quality-survival parametric* model represents the utility for an outcome in which the patient will live for time t in the ith quality state as follows:

Utility for life of length t in the ith quality state $= \theta_i \times \left(1 - e^{-\gamma t}\right)$

where γ is the patient's risk parameter expressed in the time units of t and θ_i is the quality-survival tradeoff parameter for the ith quality state.

- Suppose that (1) the patient's preferences for length of life can be represented by an exponential utility model with parameter γ, (2) the patient's quality-survival tradeoff for life in the ith quality state can be represented by the parameter θ_i, and (3) the uncertainty for the length of life in an outcome can be represented by an exponential survival model with parameter λ. The patient's expected utility for that outcome is then:

$$U(\text{Outcome}) = \frac{\theta_i}{\lambda + \gamma}$$

Epilogue

Chapters 8, 9, and 10 have established a method for quantifying the patient's preferences for the possible outcomes of a decision. This method starts with the theoretical foundation established by von Neumann and Morgenstern. From that foundation, these chapters built a framework for assessing a patient's utilities for possible outcomes based on risk attitudes for length of life and preferences for quality of life. Simple parametric models were developed that approximate outcome utilities in a manner that lends itself to use in a clinical setting. Those approximations require assumptions about how patients view the uncertainty in their lives.

What remains to be done is the establishment of survival models that provide the outcome probabilities needed to complete the analysis. These survival models represent the uncertainty for the different lengths of life possible with an outcome. The resulting probabilities can be combined with the corresponding outcome utilities to compute the expected utility for each alternative in a clinical decision problem. The nature of the approach guarantees that the alternative with the greatest expected utility is the alternative that best matches the preferences of the patient.

The next chapter will start the discussion of survival models. That discussion will describe the exponential survival model, which has already been mentioned, as well as what will be called an actuarial survival model. These two models can be combined to produce a general representation of the uncertainty faced by patients in many decision problems.

Bibliography

McNeil, B.J., Weichselbaum, R., and Pauker, S.G. (1978) Fallacy of the five-year survival in lung cancer. *New England Journal of Medicine*, **299**, 1397–401.

McNeil, B.J., Weichselbaum, R., and Pauker, S.G. (1981) Speech and survival. Tradeoffs between quality and quantity of life in laryngeal cancer. *New England Journal of Medicine*, **304**, 982–7.

Shavelle, R.M., Brooks, J.C., Strauss, D.J., and Turner-Stokes, L. (2019) Life expectancy after stroke based on age, sex, and Rankin grade of disability: a synthesis. *Journal of Stroke and Cerebrovascular Diseases*, **28**(12), 104450.

Wang, C.C. and O'Donald, A.R. (1955) Cancer of the larynx: five-year results with emphasis on radiotherapy. *New England Journal of Medicine*, **252**, 743–7.

CHAPTER 11

Survival models: representing uncertainty about the length of life

11.1 Introduction

Time plays critical roles in most medical outcomes. Those roles include measuring how long life lasts and marking when events occur. This chapter focuses on the first of these roles – time as a measure of a patient's lifetime.

Uncertainty is part of what complicates time's role as an outcome measure. The range of possible lifetimes almost always is known only as a set of probabilities for how long the patient might live. Those probabilities are represented by what we call a survival model.

Earlier chapters already used survival models. In Chapter 8, we saw how a survival model provided the length of life probabilities needed to compute the expected utility for an outcome. In general, survival models usually are needed to represent risk attitudes in the analysis of a decision. The relationship between a survival model and the corresponding length of life probabilities will be a central focus of this chapter.

The methods to be discussed typically combine two basic survival models. One of these is the exponential survival model. We often used this parametric model in earlier chapters to represent the uncertainty of how long a patient's life will last. The mathematical expression representing the exponential survival model has computational advantages when combined with an exponential *utility* model, as was discussed in Chapter 9. This chapter explores the validity of assuming that mathematical expression. Particular attention will be paid to cases where the length of a life is controlled by a disease or injury. We will see that this simple survival model is more than a computational convenience in these cases.

However, the purpose of medicine can be seen as lessening the control those diseases and injuries have on a patient's life. An alternative to the exponential survival model will be needed when a threat to a patient's life has been successfully addressed. This need will be addressed by a second basic survival model – the actuarial survival model.

Curing a disease or successfully treating an injury does not mean the patient will live forever. Instead, the survival of these fortunate patients usually resembles the survival of similar members of the general population. The observed survival probabilities in the general population constitute what we will call an actuarial survival model. This chapter will show how to combine exponential survival models and actuarial survival models to establish a credible representation of long life will last for a patient.

Mention should be made about what this chapter will not cover. Survival model analysis plays a central role in the important field of predictive modelling. Statistical regression techniques, founded on the seminal work of David Cox

Medical Decision Making, Third Edition. Harold C. Sox, Michael C. Higgins, Douglas K. Owens, and Gillian Sanders Schmidler.
© 2024 John Wiley & Sons Ltd. Published 2024 by John Wiley & Sons Ltd.

(Cox, 1972), have discovered important relationships between how long patients will live and the diseases and treatments they experience. This chapter will not attempt to summarize this important but complex field. Instead, the goals of this chapter are mathematical expressions that provide a creditable approximation for the uncertainty faced by a patient after a decision. Combining those approximations with the utility models described in the preceding three chapters will determine the expected utilities for the options available to that patient. The option with the greatest expected utility will be the option the patient should choose.

Returning to what will be covered in this chapter, the discussion starts with the common properties of all survival models. This will lead to the Kaplan–Meyer survival model, which provides a general framework for estimating survival models from survival observations. Next, this chapter will discuss the two basic survival models: the exponential survival model and the actuarial survival model. The final section describes how to combine those two basic survival models to establish a mathematical expression that quantifies the uncertainty of how long a patient will live.

11.2 Survival model basics

A survival model quantifies the probability that the patient will remain alive as time passes. Time typically is measured relative to where the period of interest begins, such as the start of a chosen treatment. For example, Figure 11.1 shows the survival models for radiotherapy and surgery used by McNeil and her colleagues in their study of patient preferences for lung cancer treatments (McNeil, 1978). For a patient whose lifetime uncertainties are represented by one of these two survival models, time zero is when the treatment began.

Focusing for a moment on the survival model for radiotherapy, labelled $S_{Rad}(t)$ in Figure 11.1, notice that

$$S_{Rad}(t) = \text{Probability alive at time } t \text{ with radiotherapy}$$

where t is measured relative to the start of treatment. The maximum value for a survival model always occurs at time zero and decreases as time advances. The curve for $S_{Rad}(t)$ equals 1.0 at time zero because there is no immediate risk of death for patients undergoing radiotherapy.

On the other hand, consider the survival curve for patients undergoing surgery in Figure 11.1. That survival curve is labelled $S_{Surg}(t)$. Notice that $S_{Surg}(0)$ is less than 1.0 in order to account for the perioperative risk with lung cancer surgery. The analysis performed by McNeil and her colleagues assumed a 5% operative mortality rate. This operative risk is represented by setting $S_{Surg}(0)$ equal to 0.95.

Of course, after time zero, the survival probabilities always decrease as time advances since the probability of being alive at some time in the future is never more than the probability of being alive today.

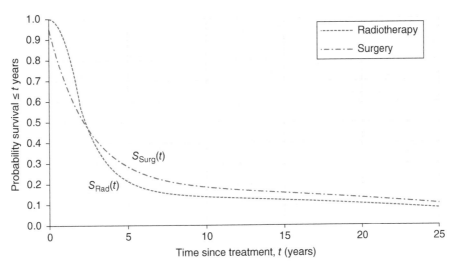

Figure 11.1 Survival probabilities for survival curves use in comparison of radiotherapy and surgical treatment for lung cancer. Adapted from McNeil (1978).

The two curves in Figure 11.1 only show the patient's survival probabilities out to 25 years after the start of treatment. With either treatment, the probability of still being alive at 25 years is approximately 10% for the 60-year-old man represented in the analysis discussed back in Chapter 8. Being alive in 25 years means that the patient is no longer likely to die from lung cancer. However, they will not live forever. This means that if the survival models shown in Figure 11.1 were extended far enough into the future, the curves ultimately would reach zero. How those extensions are made will be covered later in this chapter.

11.2.1 Survival probabilities

Three groups of values are associated with a survival model. The first of these are the values of the survival model itself. These are called the *survival probabilities* and will be denoted by $S(t)$. That is

$$S(t) = P[\text{Death after time } t]$$

For example, Figure 11.1 shows the patient's survival probabilities for surgery and radiotherapy. Survival probabilities usually are determined from observations of how long patients live in clinical situations that match that of the patient of interest.

11.2.2 Lifetime probabilities

The second important group of values associated with a survival model are the probabilities that the patient's life will last exactly a specific length of time, such as 5 years. These probabilities will be called the *lifetime probabilities* and will be denoted by $L(t)$. That is

$$L(t) = P[\text{Length of life} = t]$$

Lifetime probabilities are important because they have a key role in expected utility analysis. Recall that we need to know the lifetime probabilities for an outcome to determine the expected utility for that outcome. For example, these were the probabilities listed in Table 8.1 when we calculated the expected utility for the lung cancer treatments. The uncertainty about the length of the patient's life with an outcome is expressed by the lifetime probabilities. The expected utility for that outcome is the sum of the lifetime probabilities multiplied by the patient's corresponding utilities for those lifetimes. Recall that Chapters 8 and 9 showed how to determine those utilities for the patient's lifetimes.

11.2.3 Lifetime probabilities and the representation of time

There is a subtlety in how time is represented that must be understood in order to work with lifetime probabilities. A lifetime probability only is meaningful if time has a granularity, such as days, months, or years. That granularity represents the inexactness in how time is represented. For example, when we say that the patient lived for 1 year, we do not mean that the patient's life lasted exactly 12 months or 52 weeks or 365 days. Instead, saying that the patient's lifetime was 1 year means that the patient lived *approximately* 1 year. In other words, granularity means that time is expressed in terms of time intervals. For example, using a 1-year granularity, saying that life lasted 5 years means that death occurred after 5 years but before 6 years.

With this convention, the probability that death occurs during an interval is easily computed from a survival model. Suppose that a time interval runs between times t_A and t_B. Then

$$P[\text{Death during time interval}] = P[\text{Dead at } t_B \mid \text{Alive at } t_A] = S(t_A) - S(t_B)$$

Giving time a granularity means that time can only have discrete values such as 0, 1, and 2 years. The uncertainty for discrete values is expressed by what statisticians call a *probability mass function*. A probability mass function expresses the probability that a variable has a particular value. Without time granularity, the uncertainty about the length of life would be expressed by something called a *probability density function*. Working with probability density functions requires mathematics that is beyond the scope of this book. On the other hand, working with probability mass functions only requires simple arithmetic.

For example, how do we determine the probability that a lung cancer patient's life will last exactly 5 years after radiotherapy in an analysis based on years? Figure 11.2 shows an expanded view of the survival probability curve for radiotherapy. Note that the survival probability for 5 years is 0.2143 and the survival probability for 6 years is 0.1811.

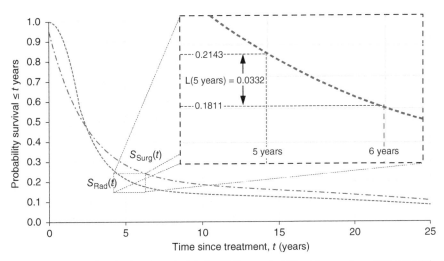

Figure 11.2 Expanded view of Figure 11.1 showing how to calculate the lifetime probability at 5 years for radiotherapy (L(5 years)).

Therefore, the probability that the patient's life will last more than 5 years but less than 6 years is the difference between 0.2143 and 0.1811, or 0.0332.

Figure 11.3 shows the lifetime probabilities derived by repeating this calculation for the survival models for radiotherapy and surgery shown in Figure 11.1.

In general, if $L(t)$ denotes the lifetime probability at time t and $S(t)$ is the corresponding survival model, then $L(t)$ can be determined by the following relationship:

$$L(t) = S(t) - S(t+1)$$

The reader may wonder why the value for $L(t)$ was not computed using a time interval centered on t. Remember that $L(t)$ is the probability that death occurs *during* an interval rather than at a specific point in time. Whether we associate that probability with the midpoint of the interval or one of the endpoints is arbitrary. The lifetime probability measures the likelihood of the outcome that death falls within the interval, whose length is the granularity of the time representation. On the other hand, we must designate a specific time point in order to pair that lifetime probability with its corresponding utility. That pairing will be required to compute an expected utility. How to choose that specific point in the interval will be discussed later in this chapter.

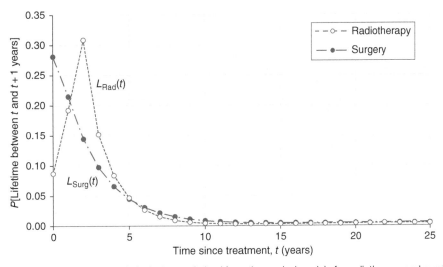

Figure 11.3 Lifetime probabilities when time granularity is 1 year, derived from the survival models for radiotherapy and surgical treatment shown in Figure 11.1.

11.2.4 Hazard rates

The third important value associated with a survival model is called the *hazard rate* and will be denoted by $H(t)$. The hazard rate quantifies how the risk of death varies as the patient reaches different lifetimes by aging. For example, if the patient survives 5 years, what is the probability the patient will die before year 6? The hazard rate quantifies this risk of death.

Therefore, time granularity chosen for the analysis also is critical to the hazard rate. The hazard rate at time t is the probability of death before time $t+1$ if the patient lives until time t. Sometimes the hazard rate also is called the *mortality rate*.

The hazard rate can be expressed as a conditional probability:

$$H(t) = P[\text{Die before } t+1 \mid \text{Alive at time } t]$$

From the definition of conditional probability

$$P[\text{Die before } t+1 \mid \text{Alive at time } t] = \frac{P[\text{Die before } t+1 \text{ and Alive at time } t]}{P[\text{Alive at time } t]}$$

But numerator in the ratio on the right is the probability that death falls within a specific time period. In order for death to fall within a time period, the patient must be alive at the beginning of the time period and dead at the end of the time period. That is

$$P[\text{Die before } t+1 \text{ and Alive at time } t] = S(t) - S(t+1)$$

The denominator in the ratio is

$$P[\text{Alive at time } t] = S(t)$$

Therefore

$$H(t) = \frac{S(t) - S(t+1)}{S(t)} = \frac{L(t)}{S(t)}$$

Figure 11.4 shows the hazard rates for radiography and surgery derived from the survival curves shown in Figure 11.1. In other words, the curves in Figure 11.1 show how the probability that death will occur within a year will change over time for the two treatments.

Notice in Figure 11.4 that at time zero, the hazard rate is higher for surgery than it is for radiotherapy. The high hazard rate for surgery at time zero includes the operative risk associated with surgical treatment for lung cancer as well

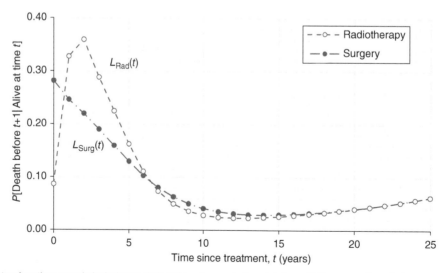

Figure 11.4 Hazard rate when time granularity is 1 year, derived from the survival models for radiotherapy and surgical treatment shown in Figure 11.1.

as the other risks faced by the patient during the first year. Also notice that, after the third year, the hazard rate drops rapidly for both treatment options. The longer the patient survives, the more likely it is that their cancer has been cured. This means the risk of death from lung cancer drops, which decreases the overall risk of death faced by the patient.

Figure 11.4 shows that 20 years after treatment, the hazard rates for the two treatments are nearly identical. The patient is virtually certain to be free of lung cancer 20 years after treatment if they are still alive. By that age, the risks now faced by the patient are the same risks any 80-year-old person faces. The slow increase in the hazard rate after 15 years reflects the increasing risk of death that we all face as we age.

We will now see that hazard rates play a central role in determining a survival model from observations of patient survival.

Key concepts: Survival model values

Survival probability:

$$S(t) = P[Die\ after\ time\ t]$$

Lifetime probability:

$$L(t) = P[\text{Die at time } t] = S(t) - S(t+1)$$

Hazard rate:

$$H(t) = P[\text{Die before } t+1 \,|\, \text{Alive at time } t] = \frac{S(t) - S(t+1)}{S(t)} = \frac{L(t)}{S(t)}$$

11.2.5   Estimating a survival model from observations

Several approaches can be used to estimate a survival model from a series of observations. For example, Table 11.1 shows a hypothetical study that started with 100 patients. In this study, at the end of each month, the patients were contacted to see if they were still alive. There are three possibilities:

1. Patient found to be still alive
2. Patient found to have died
3. Patient lost to follow up

Note that 93 of the original 100 patients were located at the end of the first month and found to be alive. Five patients were located and found to have died. Two patients were lost to follow up. Therefore, the second month began with the 93 patients who were still alive and reachable by the study.

At the end of the second month, the number of patients who still could be tracked had dropped to 92 patients. Among the 92 patients found, 88 were found to be alive and 4 were found to have died. The remaining 1 patient could no longer be reached.

By the end of the tenth month, the total number of patients being tracked had dropped to 52 patients. Fifty of those patients were still alive at 10 months, 2 had died and 4 more were lost to follow up. Therefore, by the end of the 10-month study, a total of 34 patients were found to have died and 16 were lost to follow up during the study. Those 16 lost patients complicate how we would estimate the survival curve implied by this hypothetical follow-up study.

One approach to determining the survival model is to simply divide the total number of patients (100) into 100 minus the reported deaths (34). For example, 5 deaths were reported by the end of Month 1. This suggests that the survival probability at the end of the first month is 95 divided by 100, or 0.95. By the end of Month 10, the total number of reported deaths is 34. Continuing the same line of reasoning, the survival probability at the end of the tenth month is 66 divided by 100, or 0.66.

The survival model generated by this approach might be called the *optimistic survival model* since it assumes that patients lost to follow up are still alive. Sixteen patients were lost to follow up by the end of the tenth month. Not counting those lost patients as dead means we are assuming they are still alive. Of course, some of the 16 patients lost to follow up may have died and those patients were lost to follow up because their families had more pressing concerns than answering queries from a research team. Therefore, the optimistic survival function probably overestimates the probability of survival because some of the deaths may have been missed.

Table 11.1 Hypothetical follow-up study of 100 patients.

Month	Found alive	Found dead	Lost to follow up	Estimated hazard rate
1	93	5	2	0.0510
2	88	4	1	0.0435
3	84	4	0	0.0455
4	80	3	1	0.0361
5	74	4	2	0.0513
6	70	3	1	0.0411
7	64	4	2	0.0588
8	60	3	1	0.0476
9	56	2	2	0.0345
10	50	2	4	0.0385
		Total: 34	Total: 16	Average: 0.0448

A *pessimistic survival model* assumes that all patients lost to follow have died. Under this assumption, the total number of deaths for the end of Month 10 would be the 34 patients known to have died and the 16 patients lost to follow up, for a total of 50 deaths. This would imply a survival probability of 0.50 for Month 10. But a patient lost to follow up might have moved and not notified the research team. Therefore, the pessimistic survival model is likely to underestimate the probability of survival since some of the patients assumed to have died may still be alive.

11.2.6 Kaplan–Meier survival model

A third alternative is called the *Kaplan–Meier survival model*, after the two statisticians who independently discovered this approach (Kaplan and Meier, 1958). Recall that a hazard rate is the probability of death during the next time interval. A Kaplan–Meier survival model interprets survival data as estimates of the hazard rate faced by members of the study population. In turn, those estimated hazard rates imply a survival model.

Consider the number of patients located during a given month. These patients are at risk of dying during that month. For example, 100 patients were at risk of dying during the first month in the hypothetical study shown in Table 11.1. However, two of those patients were lost to follow up. The 98 patients whose outcome is known are used to estimate the hazard rate during the first month. Five of those 98 patients died during Month 1. Therefore, the probability of dying – the hazard rate – for those 98 patients can be estimated by dividing 5 by 98, or 0.0510.

The Kaplan–Meier survival model assumes that patients lost to follow up faced the same hazard rate as patients who were found during follow up. Under this key assumption, the probability of surviving until the end of Month 1 would be

$$P[\text{Survive until the end of Month 1}] = 1 - 5/98 = 0.9490$$

Now consider Month 2. The research team found 92 of the patients at the end of Month 2. Four of those patients were reported to have died during Month 2. It follows that the hazard rate for the second month is estimated to be 4 over 92, or 0.0435. Once again the hazard rate measures the probability of dying during the second month implying

$$P[\text{Survive until the end of Month 2}]$$
$$= P[\text{Surviving to end of Month 1}] \times (1 - \text{Month 2 hazard rate})$$
$$= 0.9490 \times (1 - 0.0435)$$
$$= 0.9077$$

Similarly, 4 of the 88 patients located at the end of Month 3 were alive for a hazard rate of 4 over 88, or 0.0455. So,

$$P[\text{Survive until the end of Month 3}]$$
$$= P[\text{Surviving to end of Month 2}] \times (1 - \text{Month 3 hazard rate})$$
$$= 0.9077 \times (1 - 0.0455)$$
$$= 0.8665$$

Continuing this recursive calculation until the end of Month 10 generates the survival probabilities shown in Figure 11.5. These survival probabilities constitute the Kaplan–Meier survival model for the observations in Table 11.1. Figure 11.5 also shows the optimistic and pessimistic survival models for the hypothetical study. Notice that optimistic and pessimistic survival models provide an upper and lower bound for the Kaplan–Meier survival model.

The general process used to generate a Kaplan–Meier survival model can be summarized as follows. Let n_i denote the number of patients tracked at the end of the ith month and d_i denote the number of patients found to have died during the ith month. The ratio d_i / n_i estimates the hazard rate faced by patients during the ith month and $S(k)$, the value of the Kaplan–Meier survival model for month k, is given by

$$S(k) = (1 - d_1 / n_1) \times (1 - d_2 / n_2) \times \cdots \times (1 - d_k / n_k)$$

Definition: Kaplan–Meier survival model

If n_i is the number of patients tracked at the end of the ith month and d_i is the number of patients found to have died during the ith month, then $S(k)$, the value of the Kaplan–Meier survival model for month k, is given by

$$S(k) = (1 - d_1 / n_1) \times (1 - d_2 / n_2) \times \cdots \times (1 - d_k / n_k)$$

The ratio d_i / n_i estimates the hazard rate faced by patients during the ith month.

Clearly, hazard rates play a central role in the Kaplan–Meier survival model. Note that the curve for the Kaplan–Meier survival model is shown in Figure 11.5 as a series of horizontal line segments. Each line segment depicts the assumption that the hazard rate is constant between observations. Perhaps this is a dubious assumption but it is traditionally made in depictions of Kaplan–Meier survival curves.

Also, note that the hazard rate estimate is 0.0510 for the first month and 0.0435 for the second month. Do these changes represent actual changes in the medical condition that determines the hazards faced by the patient or are these changes simply the chance variations in the data? Given the lack of a clear trend in the hazard rates shown in Table 11.1, it might be reasonable to assume the latter explanation and average the hazard rates for the first 2 months. Extending this reasoning across the entire study implies the average hazard rate of 0.0448 for patients in the study.

This suggests what will be called the *constant hazard rate survival model*. Let ρ denote the average hazard rate observed in a follow-up study. The constant hazard rate survival model denoted by $S^*(t)$ is defined as follows:

$$S^*(t) = \rho \times S^*(t-1)$$

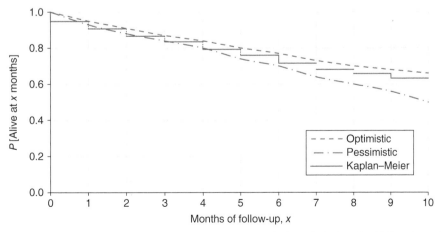

Figure 11.5 Optimistic, Pessimistic, and Kaplan–Meier survival curves for data from the hypothetical study of 100 patients shown in Table 11.1.

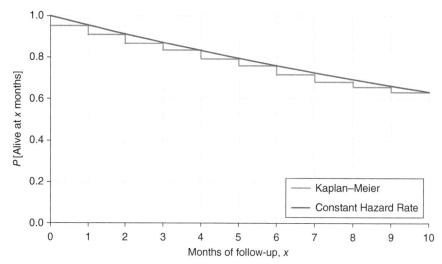

Figure 11.6 Constant hazard rate model based on average hazard rate observed in data.

Based on the observations in Table 11.1, Figure 11.6 compares the Kaplan–Meier survival model to the constant hazard rate survival model with ρ equal to the average value of 0.0448 for the study. Note that the alignment between the two models is very good.

> **Definition: Constant hazard rate survival model**
>
> With a constant hazard rate survival model, the probability that death will occur during the next time interval, given that the patient has survived until the start of the interval, is constant.

11.3 Medical example – survival after breast cancer recurrence

We now will move the discussion to representing a patient's survival after discovery of a breast cancer recurrence. We will focus on survival after discovery of a recurrence that is distant from the site of the original tumor. The data used was obtained from the National Cancer Institute's Surveillance Epidemiology and End Results (SEER) registry (Stokes *et al.*, 2008). Our analysis will focus on women who were over 65 years of age at the time of diagnosis. The average age of the women in this subgroup was 76 years, which included 622 women.

Figure 11.7 shows the Kaplan–Meier survival curve derived from this dataset. We will consider this curve as the basis for determining the survival model for a woman who was 75 years old at the time of diagnosis of a distant recurrence of breast cancer. Notice in Figure 11.7 that the probability this 75-year-old woman will survive until the age of 77 is less than 25%. The survival curve in Figure 11.7 only shows the uncertainty for the survival probabilities during the first 10 years following diagnosis because that was the length of follow-up period reported in the study.

Not all of the deaths represented in Figure 11.7 were caused by breast cancer. These were older women who faced numerous other risks that could have caused their deaths. We might call those deaths from other causes the *expected deaths* in the study population.

Therefore, the survival curve shown in Figure 11.7 can be thought of as a combination of survival curves for two different groups. One group consists of women dying from breast cancer. The other group consists of women dying from other causes. What we will see is that the breast cancer deaths mostly occur during the first years of the follow-up period. Deaths from other causes occurred through the follow-up period but dominate the deaths in the later part of the follow-up period.

Later in this chapter, we will see how to estimate the number of deaths from other causes – the expected deaths – based on what is called the actuarial survival model. For now, think of the actuarial model as representing the survival

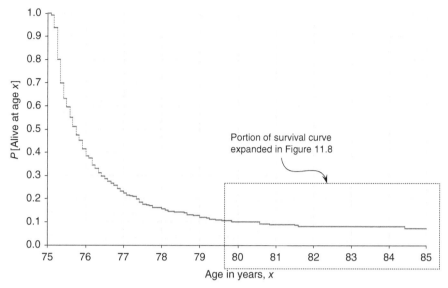

Figure 11.7 Kaplan–Meier survival curve observed in 622 women with distant recurrences of breast cancer. Data is from a study of women treated for metastatic cancer. Adapted from Stokes *et al.* (2008).

of a woman in the general population. In other words, for our patient, the actuarial survival model would provide her survival probabilities if she no longer had the elevated risk of dying from breast cancer she faced back when she was diagnosed with a recurrence at age 75.

Figure 11.8 shows the overlap between the observed survival probabilities in Figure 11.7 and the corresponding actuarial survival model for a 75-year-old woman. This second depiction of the survival curve has been restricted to ages starting at 80 and ending at 85. Notice the close overlap between the two curves for this age range.

The number of patients represented by the Kaplan–Meier survival curve shown in Figure 11.8 is small. Only about 10% of the original 622 patients survived beyond the first 5 years of follow-up. However, the overlap shown in Figure 11.8 suggests that the uncertainty about the patient's remaining lifetimes can be represented by the actuarial survival model after the age of 80. From a medical perspective, this makes sense. 5-year post-treatment survival typically is taken as evidence that a cancer has been fully managed. In other words, after reaching 80 years of age, the patient's survival model approximates that of any 80-year-old woman.

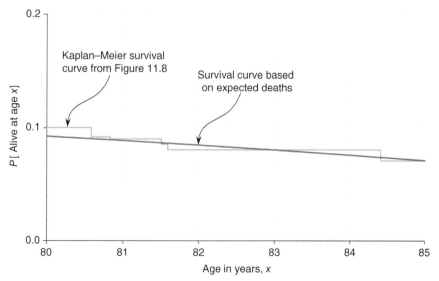

Figure 11.8 Comparison of the expected deaths for women between the ages of 80 and 85 and the Kaplan–Meier survival curve shown in Figure 11.7.

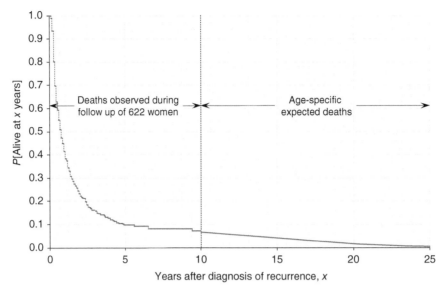

Figure 11.9 Survival curve for 75-year-old woman with distant recurrence of breast cancer. Based on a 10-year follow-up of 622 women and the age-specific expected deaths. We call this an observation-based survival model.

This alignment of survival models after age 80 leads to the composite survival model shown in Figure 11.9. The details in how the survival model in Figure 11.9 is assembled will be discussed later in this chapter. However, the central idea is that the patient's survival for the first 10 years following diagnosis is what was observed in the 622 patients. After 10 years, the patient's survival matches that of any comparably aged woman. In the following discussion, this will be called the *observation-based survival model*.

In principle, an observation-based survival model, like the one shown in Figure 11.9, achieves our goal of a credible representation of the uncertainty about a patient's length of life. Indeed, McNeil and her colleagues used this approach to generate the survival models used in their studies of lung cancer and laryngeal cancer treatment. However, for computational purposes, reducing the observation-based survival model to a simpler parametric form would be useful. How this is done starts with a discussion of the exponential survival model, which is the topic of the next section.

Definition: Observation-based survival model

An observation-based survival model uses an age-adjusted actuarial survival model to extend the estimated survival probabilities beyond the follow-up period for a study of survival in a population that matches the characteristics of the patient.

11.4 Exponential survival model

As said in earlier chapters, the exponential survival model provides a convenient representation of the uncertainty about how long a patient will live. Like all parametric models, the validity of the exponential survival model rests on an assumption. In this case, that assumption is that the hazard rate is constant. The exponential survival model assumes the probability of death during a given period of time, such as a year, remains constant for the remainder of the patient's life.

The mathematical expression for the exponential survival model is:

$$P[\text{Alive at time } t] = e^{-\lambda t}$$

where e is that constant known in mathematics as Euler's number and λ is the probability of death, or hazard rate, during the unit of time used to express t. For example, if t is expressed in years then λ is the probability of death during the next year. In other words, λ is the hazard rate for the patient facing the uncertainty representing by the exponential survival model. The exponential survival model is a constant hazard rate survival model because the parameter λ is itself a constant.

One of the convenient features of the exponential survival model is that life expectancy is the reciprocal of the model parameter ($1/\lambda$). This feature attracted considerable interest and became known by the acronym DEALE (Declining Exponential Approximation of Life Expectancy) when the usefulness of the exponential survival model was recognized by the medical decision analysis community (Beck *et al.*, 1982).

Definition: Exponential survival model

The exponential survival model is expressed:

$$P\left[\text{Alive at time } t\right] = e^{-\lambda t}$$

where the parameter λ is the probability of death during the next unit of time, as measured by t. The hazard rate for the exponential survival model is the constant λ. Life expectancy with the exponential survival model is $1/\lambda$.

This section will discuss how the exponential survival model can be adjusted to represent the possible outcomes faced by a patient. However, first some technical details about the exponential survival model will be discussed.

11.4.1   Lifetime probabilities with the exponential survival model

Figure 11.10 shows the lifetime probabilities for an exponential survival model that has a life expectancy of 10 years. Recalling the earlier discussion of time granularity, the lifetime probabilities shown in this figure are based on a time granularity of 1 year. That discussion of granularity left unanswered the important question about how to determine a patient's expected utility given that probability has been determine for a range of lifetimes rather than a specific number of years.

For example, consider a patient whose length of life is represented by the exponential survival model in Figure 11.10. According to this survival model, the probability is 0.0577 that the patient's length of life is between 5 and 6 years. What is the corresponding utility if the patient's lifetime falls in this time interval?

Chapter 8 described utility models for length of life; however, those models apply to specific lifetimes, not a range of lifetimes. What specific length of life should be chosen to represent the range of lifetimes from 5 to 6 years? Selecting 5 years would undervalue most of the possible lifetimes in this range. Conversely, selecting 6 years would overvalue the possible lifetimes. So, now the question becomes "what is the corresponding utility if the patient's lifetime is 5.5 years?".

What happens with an exponential survival model when the patient's preferences also can be represented by an exponential *utility* model? In Chapter 9, we saw that with an exponential utility model, the patient's preferences for different lifetimes can be calculated by the expression

$$\text{Utility for life of } t \text{ years} = \frac{1 - e^{-t\gamma}}{\gamma}$$

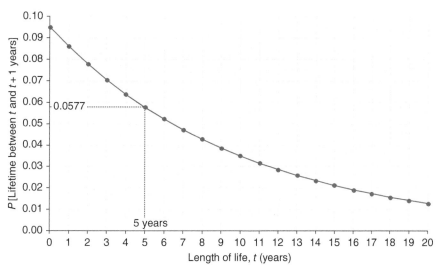

Figure 11.10 Lifetime probabilities for exponential survival model when life expectancy is 10 years and time granularity is 1 year.

where γ is the parameter for the exponential utility model and t is the length of life measured in years. One feature of this utility model is that the parameter γ quantifies the patient's risk aversion. The stronger the patient's risk aversion, the larger the value of γ.

Normally, in order to calculate the expected utility, we would determine the expected utility by determining the utility for each possible length of life, multiplying that utility by the corresponding probability for that length of life, and summing the results. This would be a complicated calculation. However, the discussion in Chapter 9 also noted that if the patient's survival with an outcome can be represented by an exponential survival model with a life expectancy of $1/\lambda$, then

$$\text{Expected utility} = \frac{1}{\gamma + \lambda}$$

This means that with the exponential utility model, the expected utility for an outcome can be determined without that complicated calculation. Instead, the expected utility can be calculated directly from the parameters for the survival model and the utility model.

Therefore, approximating the observation-based survival curve shown in Figure 11.9 by an exponential survival model would be convenient. This approximation would greatly simplify how we calculate the expected utility for a patient faced with that survival model. Instead of adding up a lot of term, the expected utility could be calculated using the simple formula shown earlier.

11.4.2 Fitting an exponential survival model to observations – first attempt

We have just seen that assuming an exponential survival model represents the uncertainty for the length of life simplifies how we incorporate risk attitudes into a decision analysis. However, is this assumption justified?

We will answer this important question in two stages. First, we will show that directly fitting an exponential survival model to observations, like those shown in Figure 11.9, can lead to misleading results. In other words, the assumption is not strictly true. Observed survival probabilities often depart significantly from the probabilities implied by an exponential survival model. Nevertheless, we will start with this direct approach to fitting an exponential survival model in order to demonstrate how this is done. We also will establish a meaningful metric for quantifying the mismatch.

The second stage will examine how to combine the exponential and actuarial models to compose a survival model that matches the observation-based survival model. This more complicated model is based on the earlier observation that patients with a medical condition, like a breast cancer recurrence, actually face two possible causes of death. The first of these is the medical condition itself. Distant recurrence of breast cancer often is a fatal condition for the patient. We will see that survival for patients with distant recurrences often does align with an exponential survival model. The second cause of death are all the other reasons why people die. Ideally, the threat from these other causes of death should be represented by the age-adjusted actuarial model as was demonstrated in Figure 11.9.

There are several ways to directly fit an exponential survival model to an observation-based survival model. Perhaps the simplest approach is to match the life expectancies for the exponential survival model and the observation-based survival model.

Computing the life expectancy for the observation-based survival model in Figure 11.9 is time consuming but straightforward. First, the lifetime probabilities are calculated from the survival probabilities. The lifetime probabilities are multiplied by the corresponding lifetimes and the products are summed to calculate the life expectancy implied by the survival model. For the survival model in Figure 11.9, the result is a calculated life expectancy of 27.2 months or 2.27 years.

Computing the life expectancy for an exponential survival model is far easier. Recall that for this survival model, the life expectancy is one over the hazard rate (λ). Therefore, the exponential survival model fitted to the observation-based survival model for distant recurrences of breast cancer would have a hazard rate of 1 over 2.72 years or 0.4407/year.

Figure 11.11 compares the resulting exponential survival curve with the original observation-based survival model. There are similarities between the shape of the two survival curves but also some big differences. How significant are those differences?

Recall how we answered this type of question in Chapter 9 when we compared the survival curves for two lung cancer treatments (see Subsection 9.3.3). Those two treatments resulted in different survival curves for the patient. A utility function representing the patient's risk attitudes provided the outcome utilities for the possible lengths of

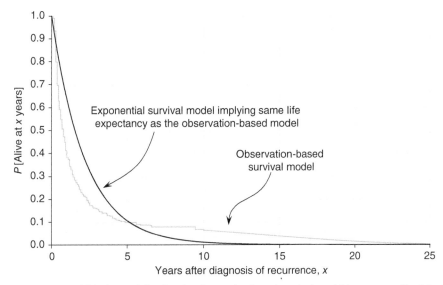

Figure 11.11 Exponential survival model (black curve) fitted to the observation-based survival model for women with distant recurrence shown in Figure 11.10 (grey curve) by matching life expectancies.

life after treatment. Combining those outcome utilities with the corresponding survival probabilities determined an expected utility for each of the two treatments. The differences between the resulting expected utilities meant one treatment was preferred to the other for ranges of risk attitudes.

However, the significance of the difference between the two calculated expected utilities was difficult to decide. We simply knew there was a difference between two abstract numbers determined by complicated calculations. Therefore, we translated the expected utilities into certainty equivalents. Recall that a certainty equivalent for a gamble is a guaranteed outcome that has the same utility as the expected utility for the gamble. When we compared the certainty equivalents for the two treatments we found that for a patient with a given level of risk aversion ($\gamma = 0.15/\text{year}$), undergoing surgery was equivalent to a guaranteed 3.26 years whereas undergoing radiotherapy was equivalent to a guaranteed 2.97 years (see Figure 9.9). In other words, switching from surgery to radiotherapy would be equivalent to adding roughly 3 months to a 3-year lifetime for this patient.

Figure 11.12 shows the results of using the same approach to compare the two survival models in Figure 11.11. As usual, an exponential utility model is assumed to represent the patient's risk attitudes. We adjusted that utility model to represent different risk attitudes by changing the value for a term in the model we call the risk parameter (γ). A risk parameter value of zero implies risk indifference. Increasing the value of the risk parameter increases the level of risk aversion represented by the model.

According to Figure 11.12, a patient with a risk parameter value of 0.15/year would consider facing the uncertainty of the observation-based survival model shown in Figure 11.9 to be equivalent to a guaranteed lifetime of 1.93 years. On the other hand, that same patient would consider living a guaranteed 1.46 years to be equivalent to facing the uncertainty represented by the exponential survival model shown in Figure 11.11. This means that for this level of risk aversion, there is roughly a half-year difference between the exponential survival model and the observation-based survival model.

Notice in Figure 11.12 that the difference between the two survival models decreases as the level of risk aversion decreases. When the patient is risk indifferent – in other words, they have a risk parameter value of 0 – the two survival models imply the same certainty equivalents. This result is to be expected. As we discussed in Chapter 8, risk indifference means the two survival models are equivalent to their respective life equivalents. By design, the two survival models have the same life expectancies. Therefore, the two survival models would be equivalent to a patient who is risk indifferent.

As noted at the beginning of this subsection, there is more than one way to directly fit an exponential survival model to an observation-based survival model. However, the results are roughly the same for these alternative approaches. The essential conclusion is that a simple exponential survival model does not always provide a good approximation for the lifetime uncertainties faced by patients.

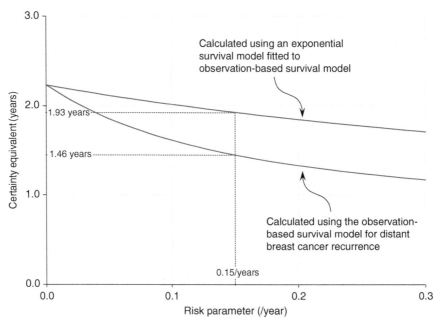

Figure 11.12 Comparison of the certainty equivalents for experiencing the observation-based survival model shown in Figure 11.10 and the corresponding exponential survival model shown in Figure 11.11.

11.5 Actuarial survival models

The previous section described the exponential survival model, which is one of the two survival models often used to represent the uncertainty faced by a patient in an outcome. As we have just seen, by itself, the exponential survival model does not always align well with survival observations. This section describes a second survival model that can be combined with the exponential survival model to more closely matched survival observations. This second model is called the *actuarial survival* model.

The actuarial survival models used in this book are derived from the life tables published by the US Social Security Administration (SSA). Each year these life tables report the number of deaths occurring in various age groups. The SSA uses the life tables to determine the current age-specific annual mortality rates for the US population. We will use these annual mortality rates as the hazard rates for a member of the general population.

Definition: Actuarial survival model

An actuarial survival model uses the annual mortality rates derived from the life tables published by the United States. SSA as estimates for the hazard rates for members of the general population.

Figure 11.13 shows the annual mortality rates reported by the SSA in 2017. Notice that the vertical dimension in this graph shows the logarithm of the mortality rates for various age groups. This is what data scientists call a semilogarithmic graph. Using a semilogarithmic graph allows the dramatic changes that occur in hazard rates over a lifetime to be displayed on a single page. Starting at approximately one chance in 10 000 for young children, the chance of dying within a year climbs one thousand times to over one chance in 10 for centurions. Clearly, the survival model representing these hazard rates departs significantly from the exponential survival model, with its assumption of a constant hazard rate.

What we mean by "general population" is that the mortality rates shown in Figure 11.13 combine the risks from all of the possible causes of death. When considering the survival of a patient with a potentially fatal disease, we recognize the patient faces a risk of dying from that fatal disease. The patient also faces the risk from all of the other possible causes of death. We will assume the mortality rates, observed in the entire population, quantify the risk of death from those other causes.

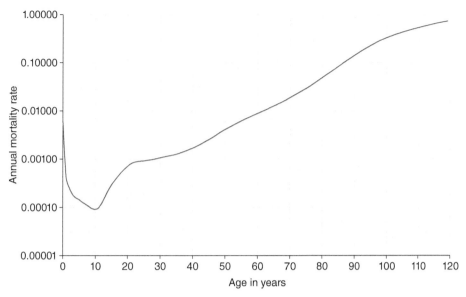

Figure 11.13 Age-specific annual mortality rates reported by the Social Security Administration for 2017.

11.5.1   Age- and gender-specific actuarial survival models

Another perspective on the actuarial survival model is that it represents the survival of a patient based solely on their age. Of course, age is seldom the only fact known about a patient. Earlier in this chapter we determined the survival model for breast cancer patients. Almost all breast cancer patients are women. Therefore, the actuarial model we used was limited to members of the general population who are women.

Figure 11.14 compares the annual mortality rates for men and women. Notice the striking differences between the annual mortality rates for young men and women. While the annual mortality rates are low for 20-year-olds, the probability of death during the next year for young men in this age group (0.0011/year) is almost 3 times as high as it is for young women of a similar age (0.0004/year). This difference between men and women shrinks as we age, but it continues throughout our lifetimes.

We have been discussing a 75-year-old patient with a distant recurrence of breast cancer. We can use the curve for women in Figure 11.14 as the actuarial survival curve for this patient. Back in the discussion of Kaplan–Meier survival curves we saw how this was done. The process starts with the patient alive at age 75. Therefore, the survival

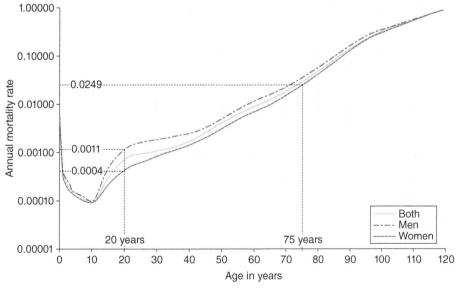

Figure 11.14 Age-specific annual mortality rates for men and women reported by the Social Security Administration for 2017.

probability at age 75 is 1. From the annual mortality rates (a.k.a., hazard rates) in Figure 11.14 we know the probability is 0.0249 that this woman will die from all causes before reaching 76 years of age. Therefore,

$$P[\text{Alive at 76}] = P[\text{Alive at 75}] \times P[\text{Not die before 76} \mid \text{Alive at 75}]$$
$$= P[\text{Alive at 75}] \times \left(1 - P[\text{Die before 76} \mid \text{Alive at 75}]\right)$$
$$= 1.0000 \times (1 - 0.0249) = 0.9751$$

Figure 11.15 shows the results of repeating this calculation to the end of life for a 75-year-old woman. The result is the age-specific actuarial survival curve used back in Figure 11.9 to extend the survival model for our 75-year-old patient.

Figure 11.16 repeats the analysis we have just seen for men and women over a range of ages.

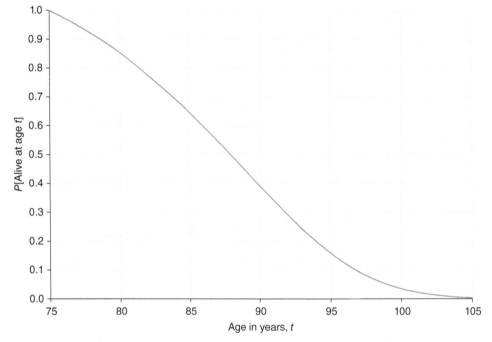

Figure 11.15 Actuarial survival model for 75-year-old woman based on life tables reported by the Social Security Administration for 2017.

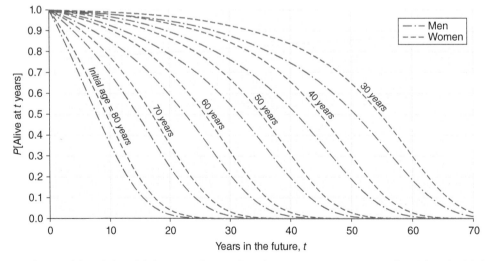

Figure 11.16 Age-specific actuarial survival models for men and women based on life tables reported by the Social Security Administration for 2017. Adapted from Social Security Administration for 2017.

11.5.2   Further adjustments of the actuarial survival model

Often the patient's age and sex are not the only reason for adjusting the actuarial survival model. Typically, the patient of interest has a medical condition that threatens the patient's survival. In some cases, the patient continues to face an increased residual risk even after successful treatment. That residual risk implies greater annual mortality rates than are represented in the life tables for the general population.

For example, recall the study of lung cancer treatment conducted by McNeil and her colleagues (McNeil, 1978). The lung cancer treatments in their analysis had 10-year survival probabilities of between 0.1 and 0.2 (see Figure 8.2). They used an adjusted actuarial survival model to determine the survival probabilities for a patient successfully treated for lung cancer. They reasoned that survival probabilities for a patient with lung cancer, even after 10 years, would still be less than what are found in the general population, if only because 90% of patients with lung cancer have a history of smoking. In turn, a history of smoking increases the risk of death from heart disease. Successful treatment of lung cancer would not reduce the additional risk from heart disease.

They accounted for this additional risk by assuming a 50% increase in the actuarial mortality rates. These higher mortality rates were used to extrapolate a patient's survival model after 10 years. For example, the average age of a patient in their study was 67 years. Referring to Figure 11.17, based on the life tables for the general population, the annual mortality rate for someone who is 67 is 0.0146. Therefore, McNeil and her colleagues assumed the probability that this 67-year-old patient would live until age 68 is 1.5 times 0.0146 or 0.0219.

Changing the annual mortality rates changes the corresponding survival model. The same methods described in the discussion of Kaplan–Meier survival models can be used to calculate the adjusted actuarial survival model shown in Figure 11.18 for a 67-year-old patient who survives lung cancer.

11.6   Two-part survival models

After the discussions in the previous sections, an overview of this chapter's goal would be timely. For most outcomes that follow a decision, the patient will face uncertainty about the length of their subsequent life. Decision analysis depends on a comparison of the patient's utilities for these possible outcomes. Determining an outcome utility requires knowing the probabilities for the possible lengths of life. Those length-of-life probabilities constitute a survival model. This chapter describes representations for survival models.

Once the preliminary survival model concepts were covered, the discussion in this chapter turned to what we called the observation-based survival model. Determining these two-part representations of how long a patient will live typically starts with observations of survival for similar patients during a follow-up period. What is learned from those observations is extended beyond the follow-up period using versions of what we called the actuarial survival model. Those extensions make up the second part of the observation-based survival model.

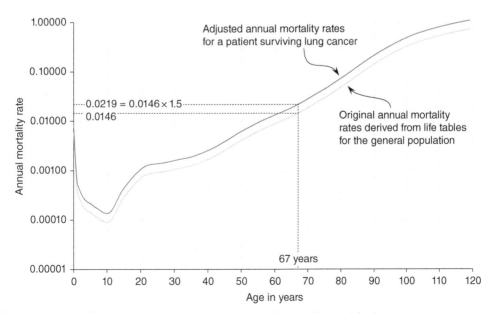

Figure 11.17 Adjusted annual mortality rates used to extend the survival model for a patient surviving lung cancer.

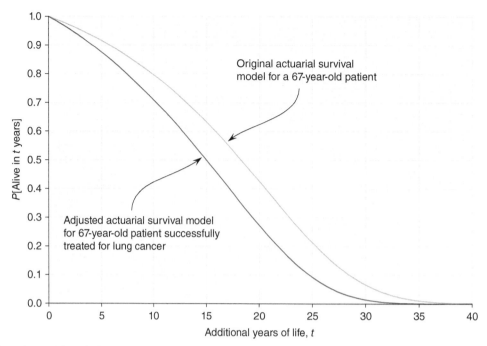

Figure 11.18 Adjusted actuarial survival model for a 67-year-old patient who survived lung cancer.

In principle, the observation-based survival models achieve this chapter's goal. Using published life tables to extend the survival rates observed during a follow-up study produces a survival model for the patients represented by the study population. The problem is that a specific patient seldom fully matches the patients in populations used in follow-up studies. Therefore, a method is needed for adjusting an observation-based survival model to the characteristic of that specific patient.

Another shortcoming of the observation-based survival model is how this representation of the probabilities for the patient's length of life complicates calculating expected utility. Expected utility is calculated by multiplying the outcome utilities by the corresponding probabilities from the survival model and summing the results. As we saw earlier in this chapter, that complicated calculation is replaced by a much simpler arithmetic calculation when the exponential survival model can be used. But then, we also saw that an exponential survival model does not always align with the observation-based survival model it is approximating.

The two-part survival models described in this section address these two shortcomings by combining an exponential survival model with an actuarial survival model. The exponential survival model will represent the uncertainty for the near-term portion of the patient's life. The properties of an exponential survival model usually provide a good match to the risks faced by the patient during this period. The actuarial survival model will represent the uncertainty for the balance of the patient's life. The result of combining an exponential survival model with an actuarial survival model is a mathematical expression that can be adjusted to a given patient's characteristics and retains the computational advantages that have been discussed.

11.6.1 Representing observed survival with an exponential survival model – second attempt

Recall that the observation-based survival model for breast cancer recurrence started with follow-up data for 622 patients. Figure 11.19 shows the survival probabilities for the patients among those 622 patients who died apparently from breast cancer during the follow-up period. These survival probabilities were determined by subtracting the number of deaths that would have been expected during the follow-up period. The average age for the 622 patients was 75 years. Therefore, the expected number of deaths was determined using the actuarial survival model for 75-year-old women (see Figure 11.15). The result shown in Figure 11.9 is the observed survival curve for a patient who will eventually die because of the breast cancer recurrence.

The survival curve shown in Figure 11.19 implies a life expectancy of 1.01 years. Figure 11.20 shows an exponential survival model based on this life expectancy. That is, the exponential survival model shown in Figure 11.19 has an annual mortality rate of 1 over 1.01 years or 0.9924/year. Notice that Figure 11.20 superimposes the curve for the exponential survival model (black curve) over the observed survival curve for these patients (grey curve). Except for a few

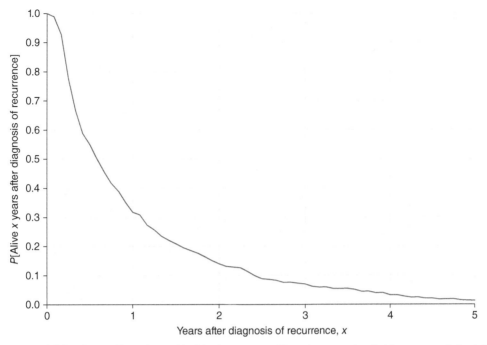

Figure 11.19 Survival probabilities observed in patients with distant recurrence of breast cancer, who died from cancer during follow-up period.

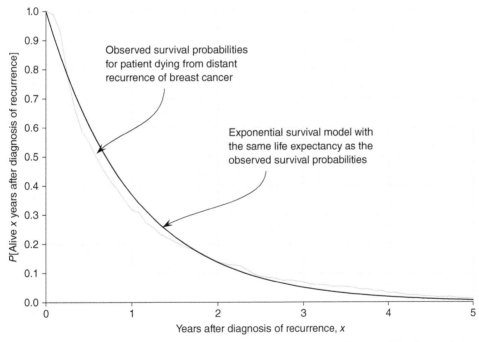

Figure 11.20 Exponential survival model for patients with a distant recurrence of breast cancer (black curve) fitted to survival probabilities shown in Figure 11.19 (grey curve).

small deviations, the two curves are closely matched. Therefore, the exponential survival curve shown in Figure 11.20 provides a good representation of the patient's survival if breast cancer ends their life.

What is the probability breast cancer will cause the patient's death? Subtracting the expected deaths from the 622 patients implies that 550 patients died from cancer during the follow-up period. This suggests that the probability our 75-year-old patient will die from cancer is 550 over 622, or 88%. Figure 11.20 showed what their survival model would be if this were true. Otherwise, the patient has a 12% probability of dying from other causes. The survival model for this second possibility is the age-specific actuarial survival model described in the previous section.

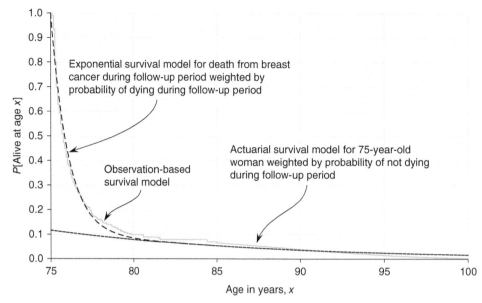

Figure 11.21 Two-part survival model for 75-year-old woman with distant recurrence of breast cancer. This model is the sum of the exponential survival model for patients dying from cancer in Figure 11.20, weighted by the probability of dying from cancer, and actuarial survival model for a 75-year-old woman, weighted by the probability of dying from other causes. The original observation-based survival model from Figure 11.9 is shown in grey.

Therefore, given the agreement shown in Figure 11.20, the survival probabilities for the 75-year-old patient with a distant recurrence of breast cancer can be approximated by the expression

$$P[\text{Alive in } t \text{ years}] = 0.88 \times e^{-0.9924t} + 0.12 \times A_{75, \text{Woman}}(t)$$

Note that we are using $A_{75, \text{Woman}}(t)$ to denote the actuarial survival model for 75-year-old woman. Figure 11.21 shows the excellent alignment between this two-part survival model and original observation-based survival model. The observation-based survival model is barely visible as the grey curve in this figure. It is barely visible because of the close alignment between the two models.

In general, we have demonstrated a two-part survival model for a patient faced with a life-threatening medical condition. The survival model for a patient is:

$$P[\text{Alive in } t \text{ years}] = \rho e^{-\lambda t} + (1 - \rho)A(t)$$

where

ρ is the probability the patient will die because of the medical condition
λ is the patient's mortality rate if they die because of the medical condition
$A(t)$ is the corresponding age-specific actuarial survival model

We will call this the *parametric two-part survival model*.

Definition: Parametric two-part survival model

The *parametric two-part survival model* uses the following expression to determine the survival probabilities for a patient with a life-threatening condition:

$$P[\text{Alive in } t \text{ years}] = \rho e^{-\lambda t} + (1 - \rho)A(t)$$

where
ρ is the probability the patient dies because of the condition
λ is the patient's mortality rate if they die because of the condition
$A(t)$ is the corresponding age-specific actuarial survival model

---

11.6.2   Age adjusting a survival model

The discussion earlier in this chapter showed how McNeil and her colleagues adjusted the mortality rates for their patients to represent the residual risk faced because of lung cancer. This was a judgment-based adjustment that demonstrated the inevitable role for subjective judgment in survival models. Age adjustment provides another example of how subjectivity applies to survival model development. The example used in this chapter involves a 75-year-old patient. That age was chosen because it matched the average age of the patients in the study that provided the data. How would the survival model differ for a 50-year-old patient with distant recurrence of breast cancer?

We will answer this question using the two-part survival model that has just been described. Recall that this parametric model states:

$$P[\text{Alive in } t \text{ years}] = \rho e^{-\lambda t} + (1 - \rho)A(t)$$

The parameter ρ is the probability the patient will die from cancer and the parameter λ is the patient's mortality rate if death is caused by cancer. The changes required to represent the survival for the 50-year-old patient will be described in terms of these two parameters, as well as the actuarial survival model $A(t)$.

The obvious change is to the patient's actuarial survival model $A(t)$. Figure 11.22 shows the actuarial model for a 50-year-old woman ($A_{50,\text{Woman}}(t)$). The probabilities for the survival model would replace the probabilities for the corresponding model for a 75-year-old woman ($A_{75,\text{Woman}}(t)$).

The survival probabilities shown in Figure 11.22 are derived from the life tables reported by the SSA. However, what about the other two model parameters ρ and λ? These parameters characterize the patient's experience if she does die because of breast cancer. The current parameter values were derived from a population of patients who, on the average were considerably older than a 50-year-old woman.

The published data about the effects of age on cancer treatment survival does not perfectly match a 50-year-old patient with breast cancer. However, there are published findings that can inform how the survival model parameters should be adjusted. A 2017 study of treatment survival for all types of cancers in Asia reported a 27.8% survival rate in patients between the ages of 50 and 59 years (Lu *et al.*, 2017). The same study reported a 16.9% survival rate for patients between the ages of 70 and 79 years. An older Finish study reported similar age group survival rates for patients with breast cancer (Holli and Isola, 1997). This suggests that the ratio for the probability of dying from breast cancer (ρ) in a 50-year-old patient is 16.9%/27.8% or about 60% of what it is for a 75-year-old patient. Therefore, a reasonable adjustment for ρ would be to change its value from 0.88 to 0.50.

What about λ, which is the mortality rate for death from breast cancer? The Asian study of cancer treatment survival also reported that the 12-month mortality rate for patients between 50 and 59 years was 7.7%. The 12-month mortality rate for between 70 and 79 years was 14.5%. This suggests the mortality rate for a 50-year-old patient who dies from

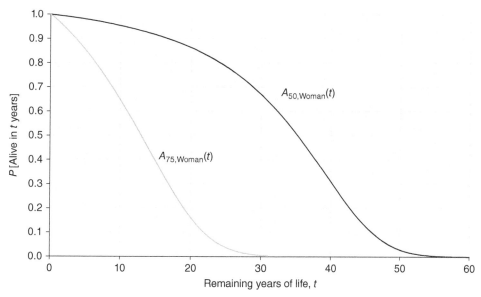

Figure 11.22 Actuarial survival model for 50-year-old woman (black curve) compared to actuarial survival curve for 75-year-old woman (grey curve).

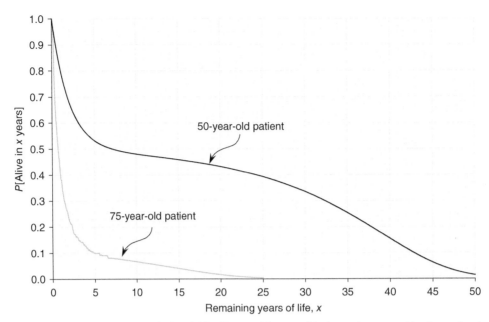

Figure 11.23 Age-adjusted parametric two-part survival model for 50-year-old woman (black curve) compared to observation-based survival model for 75-year-old woman (grey curve).

cancer is approximately half of what it is for the 75-year-old patient. Therefore, the value for λ will be changed from 0.9924/year to 0.5000/year.

In summary, the parametric two-part survival model for a 50-year-old patient with a distant recurrence of breast cancer would be

$$P\left[\text{Alive in } t \text{ years}\right] = 0.50 \times e^{-0.5t} + 0.50 \times A_{50,\text{Woman}}\left(t\right)$$

Figure 11.23 compares this survival model to the observation-based survival model that was developed for the 75-year-old patient.

This demonstration of age adjustment based on the two-part exponential survival model could have incorporated other factors that might alter the patient's survival, such as the effectiveness of treatment. Treatment differences would be captured by the values for ρ, the probability the treatment fails to eliminate the disease, and λ the patient's subsequent hazard rates if the treatment fails. The values for these parameters typically would be based on subjective opinions. However, those subjective opinions would be visible statements of the assumptions that have been made. Sensitivity analyses would be used to explore the consequences of uncertainty due to these subjective judgments about the model parameters.

11.6.3 Computing outcome utilities with the parametric two-part survival model

We have called the two-part survival model discussed in this section a "parameterized" model. However, this is only partially true. Only the part of the survival model that is parametric is what happens to the patient if they die because of the medical condition. As we saw in Figure 11.20, at least for distant recurrence of breast cancer, that part of the patient's survival can be represented by an exponential model.

The uncertainty about the patient's life if they do not die because of the medical condition is represented by an actuarial survival model. Unfortunately, unlike the exponential survival model, there is no simple expression that can be used to calculate the expected utility with an actuarial survival model.

Nevertheless, the following relatively simple expression can be used to determine the outcome utility when the patient's survival is represented by a parameterized two-part survival model:

$$\text{Outcome Utility} = \frac{\rho}{\gamma + \lambda} + \left(1 - \rho\right) \times \text{Expected utility with actuarial model}$$

where

γ measures the patient's risk attitudes in an exponential utility model
ρ is the probability the patient will die because of the condition
λ is the patient's life expectancy if they die because of the condition

---

Result: Computing outcome utilities with the parametric two-part survival model

The following expression can be used to calculate the outcome utility when the uncertainty about the length of life can be expressed as a parametric two-part survival model:

$$\text{Outcome Utility} = \frac{\rho}{\gamma + \lambda} + (1 - \rho) \times \text{Expected utility with actuarial model}$$

where
γ measures the patient's risk attitudes in an exponential utility model
ρ is the probability the patient will die because of the condition
λ is the patient's life expectancy if they die because of the condition

---

Evaluating the first part of this expression only requires simple arithmetic. The challenging part is determining the value for the expected utility with the actuarial model.

The only way to calculate the expected utility with an actuarial model is to add up the utilities for each possible length of life, weighted by the corresponding lifetime probability. We have seen several examples of this time-consuming but straightforward process in this chapter. In this case, those outcome probabilities are determined by the actuarial model for the patient.

As we saw in Figure 11.16, the probabilities for an actuarial model depend on the patient's age at time zero. The semilogarithmic graph in Figure 11.24 shows how those age-specific changes affect the resulting outcome utility calculations. Note that outcome utilities were calculated using actuarial models that combined the life tables for men and women. This was done to simplify the resulting figure.

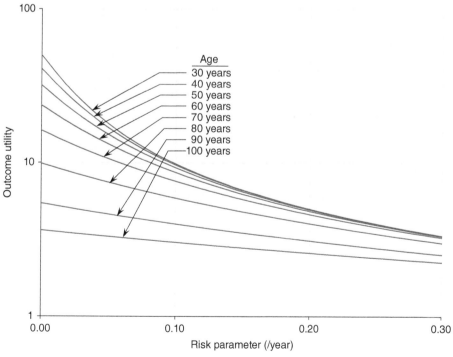

Figure 11.24 Calculated outcome utility when length of life is represented by actuarial survival model for combined men and women. An exponential utility model determined the length of life utilities for these calculations. The horizontal axis shows the risk parameter value used in the utility model.

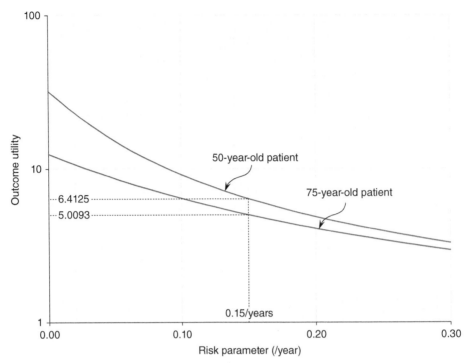

Figure 11.25 Outcome utilities when uncertainty about length of life is represented by the actuarial survival model for a 50-year-old woman and a 75-year-old woman.

On the other hand, Figure 11.25 shows the same outcome utilities based on two actuarial survival models for women. One curve shows the outcome utilities calculated for a 75-year-old woman. The other curve shows the outcome utilities calculated for a 50-year-old woman. We can use the calculated utilities shown in Figure 11.25 to determine the outcome utilities for the two women with breast cancer recurrences we have used as examples in this chapter.

For example, suppose that the risk attitudes for these women can be represented by a risk parameter value of 0.15/year. That is, γ equals the nominal value of 0.15/year for both women we have been using in this chapter. In the case of the 75-year-old woman, her outcome utility, given the survival model we have determined for her, can be calculated by the following expression:

$$\text{Outcome Utility} = \frac{\rho}{\gamma + \lambda} + (1 - \rho) \times \text{Expected utility with actuarial model}$$

$$= \frac{0.8800}{0.1500 + 0.9925} + 0.1200 \times \text{Expected utility with actuarial model}$$

$$= 0.7702 + 0.1200 \times \text{Expected utility with actuarial model}$$

From Figure 11.25, we see that for this patient her expected utility would be 5.0093 if she faced the uncertainty implied by the actuarial survival model for a 75-year-old woman. Therefore, her outcome utility for experiencing a distant recurrence of breast cancer is

$$\text{Outcome Utility} = 0.7702 + 0.1200 \times \text{Expected utility with actuarial model}$$

$$= 0.7702 + 0.1200 \times 5.0093 = 1.3714$$

Performing the same calculation for the 50-year-old woman, we have that

$$\text{Outcome Utility} = \frac{\rho}{\gamma + \lambda} + (1 - \rho) \times \text{Expected utility with actuarial model}$$

$$= \frac{0.5000}{0.1500 + 0.5000} + 0.5000 \times 6.4125 = 3.9755$$

These two calculations demonstrate an interesting feature of how age changes outcome utilities. Both women in these examples have the same medical conditions – the distant recurrence of breast cancer. Both women also have the same level of risk aversion. However, because of age, these two women have different utilities for the outcomes they face. Those differences should be reflected in how decisions are made about their care.

For example, suppose that both women were offered a highly risky treatment that could eliminate the breast cancer that has reappeared. In particular, suppose that the risk of perioperative death for both women is 50% for this hypothetical treatment. If the women survive this risky treatment, they will face the survival of any other similarly aged woman. In other words, their survival would match what is described by their age-specific actuarial survival model. Their alternative is to face the uncertainty represented by the survival models we have described for these two women.

According to Figure 11.25, for the 50-year-old woman, the risky treatment has a 0.50 probability of resulting in an outcome that has a utility of 6.4125. This means the expected utility for the risky treatment is 0.5 times 6.4125 or 3.2062. Recall that we calculate the certainty equivalent for a gamble by finding the guaranteed outcome that has the same utility as the gamble. The 50-year-old woman's certainty equivalent for the same risky treatment, which is a gamble that has the utility of 3.2062, is 4.37 years. On the other hand, we just determined this 50-year-old woman's utility for living with the uncertainty of the breast cancer recurrence has a utility of 3.9755. For this patient, this utility has a certainty equivalent of 6.05 years. Therefore, the 50-year-old would not choose the risky treatment. The woman views this decision as a choice between 6.05 and 4.37 years. So, the difference is significant.

The same calculation would lead to a different decision for the older woman. For her, the risky treatment has the expected utility of 0.5 times 5.0093 or 2.5046, which corresponds to a certainty equivalent of 3.14 years. The alternative of forgoing the treatment would leave her with an outcome that has a utility of 1.3714, which corresponds to a certainty equivalent of 1.54 years. Neither option is as good as what the younger woman faces. However, for this woman, the risky treatment has a higher certainty equivalent (3.14 years versus 1.54 years), meaning it would be the preferred alternative. This woman views this decision as a choice between 3.14 and 1.54 years. So, her choice is clear as well.

11.6.4 Limitations

The parametric two-part survival model described in this chapter is an approximation and like all approximations, the validity of this convenient expression has its limits. Those limits should be understood.

Recall the first step in developing this model. That step started by identifying what we called the expected deaths in the study population. We used the actuarial survival model to estimate those expected deaths. The key assumption is that what we might call the *unexpected deaths* are caused by the breast cancer. Therefore, we used the survival observations for the expected deaths to determine the survival model for patients who eventually die because of breast cancer recurrence.

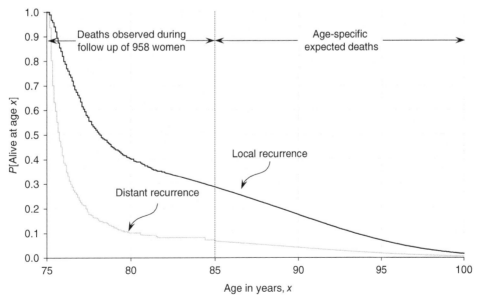

Figure 11.26 Observation-based survival curve for a 75-year-old woman with local recurrence of breast cancer. The observation-based survival model for a 75-year-old woman with distant recurrence of breast cancer, from Figure 11.9, is shown as a grey curve.

The next step was to fit an exponential survival model to the survival observations for patients dying because of their cancer recurrence. We used this exponential survival model to represent the survival probabilities for the 75-year-old patient if she were to die from cancer. The agreement between the exponential survival model and observed survival model was good. Therefore, as was shown in Figure 11.21, replacing the observed survival rates with the exponential survival model resulted in model that closely matched the observation-based survival model.

The reason why the parametric two-part model works for this example is the close match shown in Figure 11.20. This same match can be found with other medical conditions; however, what if the patient's survival does not match an exponential model when the medical condition causes the patient's death? The same study that provided the data for the example of distant breast cancer recurrence also provided follow-up data for 958 patients with local recurrences (Stokes *et al.*, 2008). We will use this second data set to explore the answer to this important question.

Figure 11.26 shows the observation-based survival model for a 75-year-old woman with a *local* recurrence of breast cancer. As before, this survival model was developed from the observations of the 958 patients and the corresponding age-specific actuarial survival model. For the purposes of comparison, this figure also shows the observation-based survival model for distant recurrence (grey curve). Notice that with the local recurrence, the probability of being alive after 10 years is far greater than it was for distant recurrence. Once the expected deaths are accounted for in the 958 patients, 474 were left as patients who probably died from the local recurrence. This implies the probability of dying from a local recurrence is 474 over 958 or 0.50. Recall that the same logic implied the probability of dying from a distant recurrence was 0.88.

Figure 11.27 shows the survival probabilities for the patient if they die because of the local recurrence (grey curve). This figure also shows the exponential survival model fitted to this observation-based survival model (black curve). As with the example of distant recurrences, the exponential survival model was fitted by matching life expectancies. A life expectancy of 1.9 years for the exponential survival model implies an annual hazard rate of 0.5361/year. Notice that the fit between the exponential survival model and the observed survival model is not as good as it was with a distant recurrence.

Therefore, the parametric two-part survival model fitted to the observation-based survival curve shown in Figure 11.26 is

$$P[\text{Alive in } t \text{ years}] = 0.50 \times e^{-0.5361t} + 0.5 \times \text{Expected utility with actuarial model}$$

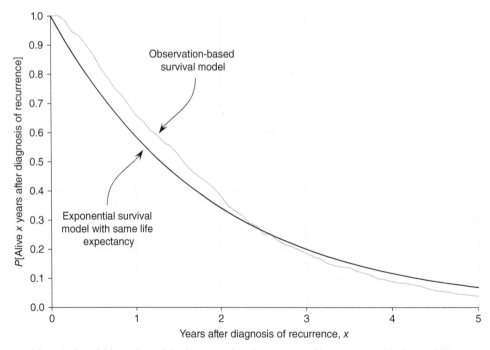

Figure 11.27 Exponential survival model for patients dying because of local recurrence of breast cancer (black curve) fitted to survival probabilities fitted to survival observations (grey curve).

Figure 11.28 compares this two-part exponential survival model to the observation-based survival model for local recurrence of breast cancer.

There are differences between the two survival curves shown in Figure 11.28, but those are not large. Figure 11.29 uses certainty equivalents to measure the importance of these differences. Recall that a similar curve (Figure 11.12) was used earlier in this chapter to compare the agreement between the simple exponential survival model and the observation-based survival model. In that earlier comparison, the differences were very large – roughly half a year. On the other hand, Figure 11.29 shows that the deviations for the two-part exponential model are reduced to less than a single month for a wide range of risk attitudes.

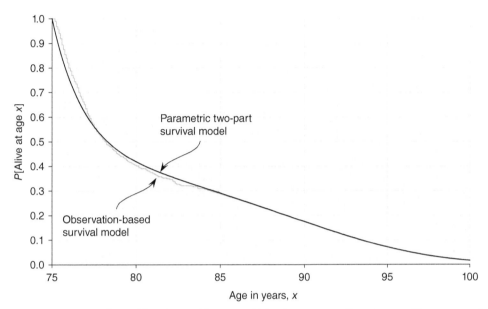

Figure 11.28 Parametric two-part survival model for 75-year-old woman with local recurrence of breast cancer. The corresponding observation-based survival model is shown in grey.

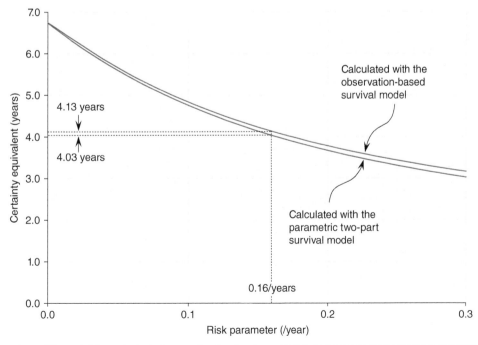

Figure 11.29 Comparison of the certainty equivalents for experiencing the observation-based survival model shown in Figure 11.26 and the parametric two-part survival model shown in Figure 11.28. The outcome utilities were calculated assuming an exponential utility model. The outcome utilities were converted to the patient's certainty equivalents. The utility model parameter is shown on the horizontal axis.

Summary

- Three key values characterize a survival model:

  Survival probability:

  $$S(t) = P[Die\ after\ time\ t]$$

  Lifetime probability:

  $$L(t) = P[\text{Die at time } t] = S(t) - S(t+1)$$

  Hazard rate:

  $$H(t) = P[\text{Die before } t+1 \mid \text{Alive at time } t] = \frac{S(t) - S(t+1)}{S(t)} = \frac{L(t)}{S(t)}$$

- If n_i is the number of patients tracked at the end of the ith month and d_i is the number of patients found to have died during the ith month, then $S(k)$, the value of the Kaplan–Meier survival model for month k, is given by

  $$S(k) = (1 - d_1/n_1) \times (1 - d_2/n_2) \times \cdots \times (1 - d_k/n_k)$$

  The ratio d_i/n_i estimates the hazard rate faced by patients during the ith month.
- With a constant hazard rate survival model the probability that death will occur during the next time interval, given that the patient has survived until the start of the interval, is constant.
- An observation-based survival model uses an age-adjusted actuarial survival model to extend the estimated survival probabilities beyond the follow-up period for a study of survival in a population that matches the characteristics of the patient.
- The exponential survival model is expressed:

  $$P[\text{Alive at time } t] = e^{-\lambda t}$$

  where the parameter λ is the probability of death during the next unit of time, as measured by t. The hazard rate for the exponential survival model is the constant λ. Life expectancy with the exponential survival model is $1/\lambda$.
- An actuarial survival model uses the annual mortality rates derived from the life tables published by the United States. SSA as estimates for the hazard rates for members of the general population.
- The *parametric two-part survival model* uses the following expression to determine the survival probabilities for a patient with a life-threatening condition:

  $$P[\text{Alive in } t \text{ years}] = \rho e^{-\lambda t} + (1 - \rho) A(t)$$

  where

  ρ is the probability the patient dies because of the condition
  λ is the patient's mortality rate if they die because of the condition
  $A(t)$ is the corresponding age-specific actuarial survival model
- The following expression can be used to calculate the outcome utility when the uncertainty about the length of life can be expressed as a parametric two-part survival model:

  $$\text{Outcome Utility} = \frac{\rho}{\gamma + \lambda} + (1 - \rho) \times \text{Expected utility with actuarial model}$$

  where

  γ measures the patient's risk attitudes in an exponential utility model
  ρ is the probability the patient will die because of the condition
  λ is the patient's life expectancy if they die because of the condition

Epilogue

This chapter began with the two roles time plays in medical outcomes. The discussion in this chapter focused on one of these roles – time as a measure of how long the patient will live. The survival models that were described quantify the uncertainty a patient faces about the length of their life. The structure of these survival models can be adjusted to match the patient's age and gender as well as other factors affecting survival.

The other role for time in a medical outcome is representing when events will occur in the patient's life. Those events can affect the quality of the patient's life as new symptoms and disabilities appear. Events also can affect the patient's survival by marking the onset of life-threatening disease processes. The next chapter will show a representation of an outcome that captures how these events unfold.

Bibliography

Beck, J.R., Kassirer, J.P., and Pauker, S.G. (1982) A convenient approximation of life expectancy (The "DEALE"). *The American Journal of Medicine*, **73**, 883–8.

Cox, D.R. (1972) Regression models and life-tables. *Journal of the Royal Statistical Society Series B (Methodological)*, **34**(2), 187–220.

Holli, K and Isola, J. (1997) Effect of age on the survival of breast cancer patients. *European Journal of Cancer*, **33**(3), 425–8.

Kaplan, E.L. and Meier, P. (1958) Nonparametric estimation form incomplete observations. *Journal of the American Statistical Association*, **53**(282), 457–81.

Lu, C.H., Lee, S.H., Liu, K.H. *et al.* (2017) Older age impacts on survival outcome in patients receiving curative surgery for solid cancer. *Asian Journal of Surgery*, **41**, 333–40.

Stokes, M.E., Thompson, D., Montoya, E.L. *et al.* (2008) Ten-year survival and cost following breast cancer recurrence: estimates from SEER-Medicare data. *Value in Health*, **11**(2), 213–20.

CHAPTER 12

Markov models

12.1 Introduction

The survival models described in the previous chapter quantify much of the uncertainty faced by a patient following a decision. The exact number of remaining years of life is never certain for any patient. In many cases, relatively simple mathematical expressions can represent that uncertainty.

However, the survival models that have been described are themselves static structures since they do not change as time passes. In contrast, the effects of an illness or an injury on a patient's survival often can change over time. Illnesses and injuries can progress or heal, which can alter the mortality rates faced by the patient. This means that static models, like the two-part survival models, sometimes are unable to fully represent the dynamics of how medical conditions can evolve to change their effects on a patient's survival.

With medical conditions that greatly shorten a patient's remaining lifetime, the distortions caused by using a static survival model usually are insignificant. That is why the two-part survival model worked well for examples involving breast cancer in the previous chapter. Recall that patients dying from a breast cancer recurrence usually do so in 5 years or less. The mortality rates faced by those unfortunate patients can change during their few remaining years. But the size of those changes will be small when compared to the high mortality rates causing those shortened lifetimes.

On the other hand, with chronic diseases and behaviors that cause injury over long periods, the dynamics of how a medical condition affects survival can be more pronounced. Consider smoking as an example. The increase in the annual mortality rate faced by a first-time smoker is negligible. However, after a few decades that same behavior often leads to illnesses that have very high annual mortality rates. Using a single average value to represent the mortality rates associated with smoking greatly overestimates the risks faced by the first-time smoker and greatly underestimates the risk faced when one of those life-threatening conditions has developed.

Moreover, the length of life implied by a survival model is not the only important property of the corresponding outcomes. Outcomes often include future changes in the symptoms and disabilities experienced by patients. The timings of those changes, and their durations, also affect how patients view the outcomes they face following a decision because those symptoms and disabilities affect the quality of the patient's life. As we saw in Chapter 10, the quality of life can be an important consideration in a clinical decision.

This chapter describes mathematical models that capture the dynamic nature of the uncertainty in outcomes, both with regard to the length of life as well as the quality of life. These are called *Markov models*. The Russian mathematician Andrey Andreyevich Markov first described the models that bear his name in the late nineteenth century. A full description of Markovian analysis requires more mathematics than is appropriate for this book. Instead, this chapter will follow a narrow path through this complex topic, touching only on the features of Markov models needed to represent medical outcomes in the analysis of a decision.

Medical Decision Making, Third Edition. Harold C. Sox, Michael C. Higgins, Douglas K. Owens, and Gillian Sanders Schmidler.
© 2024 John Wiley & Sons Ltd. Published 2024 by John Wiley & Sons Ltd.

The discussion in this chapter further focuses on how to develop a Markov model. This focused discussion begins with the key concepts used in a Markov model, including the assumptions made about applying those concepts to represent a patient's possible outcomes. The second section provides examples of how to determine the probabilities required by a Markov model. A short third section will conclude the chapter by outlining how Markov models can be analyzed.

12.2 Markov model basics

12.2.1 Health states and transition probabilities

Markov models use two fundamental concepts to represent the uncertainty in a medical outcome. Health states are the first of these concepts. The unfolding of a medical outcome typically involves a sequence of stages during which the patient experiences various symptoms, disabilities, and risks. For example, the reappearance of a cancer often starts close to the site of the original diagnosis. As the returning cancer spreads the patient will experience changing symptoms and disabilities as different organs and tissue are affected. A Markov model of this progression uses health states corresponding to the stages marking the spread of the disease.

Inevitably the definition of the health states in a Markov model requires the approximation of a continuous process by a set of discrete stages. With the example of cancer recurrence, those stages typically are defined by a set of landmarks encountered during the progression of the disease. The analyst adjusts the definition of the stages according to the goals of the analysis. The only requirements are that (1) all of the possibilities are represented, and (2) the patient's condition fits into exactly one of the stages. In other words, recalling the terminology used in the discussion of decision trees, the set of health states used in a Markov model must be collectively exhaustive and mutually disjoint.

We used a concept similar to health states when we discussed the utility for the quality of life in Chapter 10. A quality state represents a possible combination of symptoms and disabilities experienced by a patient. Typically those symptoms and disability reduce the quality of the patient's life. The quality adjustments made to outcome utilities were based on the tradeoffs the patient would accept to avoid a less desirable quality state. Similarly, symptoms and disabilities experienced by the patient at various stages in the progression of their medical condition define a health state. However, the definition of a health state also includes changes in how the patient's condition might progress to other health states. This brings us to the second key concept in Markov models.

Transition probabilities are the second fundamental concept used in Markov models. The dynamic nature of an outcome corresponds to changes between the health states. Transition probabilities quantify the uncertainty about when those changes happen. More specifically, a transition probability quantifies the likelihood that a change takes place during a time interval of a given length, such as a month or a year.

> **Definition: health state**
>
> A health state is a collection of symptoms and levels of disability a patient will experience during the unfolding of an outcome. The health states used in a Markov model are collectively exhaustive and mutually disjoint. This means that at any point in the unfolding of an outcome, the patient's condition must be represented by exactly one of the health states in the Markov model.

For example, suppose that a Markov model based on a 1-year time interval includes health states A and B. That Markov model would include a transition probability quantifying the likelihood that at the end of a year, the patient is in health state B if they began the year in health state A.

> **Definition: transition probability**
>
> Suppose that a Markov model includes health states A and B. The *transition probability* from health state A to health state B is the probability that the patient is in B at the end of a time interval if the patient had been in health state A at the beginning of the time interval.

Note that the use of a common time interval length is central to expressing a transition probability. All transition probabilities used in a Markov model are expressed relative to the same length time interval. In effect, using a common time interval length partitions the continuum of time into fixed-length time intervals in much the same way as health states partition the progression of the patient's condition into mutually exclusive stages.

12.2.2 Markov model diagrams and notation

Figure 12.1 shows a diagram for the simplest of all possible Markov models. This model consists of two health states: (1) **Alive** and (2) **Dead**. The diagram uses circles to represent the two health states, each containing the corresponding name and an index number, enclosed in paratheses. The possible transitions between health states are depicted by arcs and labelled by the corresponding transition probabilities. For example, the transition probability p_{12}, and the corresponding arc, denotes a transition from the **Alive** health state to the **Dead** health state. Note that the first subscript "1" for the transition probability p_{12} indicates the starting health state (**Alive**). The second subscript "2" indicates the destination health state (**Dead**).

The Markov model diagram in Figure 12.1 also contains two arcs, each ending in the health state where they began. These are called the *survival transitions* because they represent the continuation of the patient in the same health state. For example, the survival transition with the probability p_{11} represents the possibility that the patient will remain alive at the end of the time interval if they were alive at the beginning of the time interval. The transition probability p_{11} is called the *survival probability* for the **Alive** health state.

Definition: survival probability

The *survival probability* for health state A is the probability that the patient is in A at the end of a time interval if the patient was in health state A at the beginning of the time interval.

Applying the survival probability terminology to the transition probability labelled p_{22} in Figure 12.1 may seem peculiar because this transition represents the likelihood that a patient who has died will remain dead. However, stepping away from the grim reality of the **Dead** health state, notice that the underlying mathematical concept still applies. The transition probability p_{22} measures the likelihood of remaining in the corresponding health state during a time interval. For the **Dead** health state, that survival probability is one.

The **Dead** health state in Figure 12.1 is called a *trapping state* because it has no exiting transitions. Once the patient enters this health state, they never move to another health state. The Markov models we will consider always have at least one trapping state. When modeling survival, that trapping state will correspond to the end of life.

Markov models also can be built with less grim trapping states. Consider the analysis of a decision that affects the length of recovery for a patient with a non-fatal medical condition, meaning the probability of death is not an issue. The trapping state in this model might be the **Recovered** health state. Assuming relapse is not an issue, entering the **Recovered** health state would mark the end of an outcome.

Definition: trapping state

A health state is a trapping state if there are no possible transitions to other health states in the Markov model.

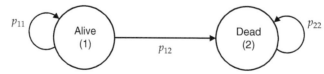

Figure 12.1 Two-state Markov model of survival.

Returning to health states in general, recall that health states defining a Markov model must be collectively exhaustive and mutually exclusive. This means that at any moment, the patient's condition must match exactly one of the health states in the model. It follows that the probabilities for the transitions originating from any health state must sum to one because the patient must either stay in that health state or change to one of the other health states. Referring to the two-state Markov model in Figure 12.1, notice that this means:

$p_{11} = 1 - p_{12}$ and $p_{22} = 1$

In general, for a Markov model with n possible heath states, the requirement that transition probabilities from any health state must add up to one can be expressed as follows:

For any health state $j : p_{j1} + p_{j2} + \ldots + p_{jj} + \ldots + p_{jn} = 1$

Transition probability requirement

Let n equal the total number of health states in a Markov model. Then:

For any health state $j : p_{j1} + p_{j2} + \ldots + p_{jj} + \ldots + p_{jn} = 1$

Figure 12.2 shows a slightly more complicated Markov model, involving three possible health states. The outcomes represented by this model are for a patient who has been successfully treated for breast cancer but faces the possibility of a future recurrence. The three health states in this second Markov model are: (1) **Disease-free**, (2) **Breast cancer recurrence**, and (3) **Dead**.

The two health states **Disease-free** and **Breast cancer recurrence** both have possible transitions to the third health state **Dead**. In other words, the patient can die either while they are free of disease or after the cancer has recurred. Presumably, death would be more likely during a time interval once there has been a recurrence. This change in the probability of dying would be represented by the differences in the transition probabilities p_{13} and p_{23}. That is, p_{23} would be greater than p_{13}.

The difference between the probability of dying for the **Disease-free** and **Breast cancer recurrence** health states illustrates how Markov models represent the changes in the uncertainties involved with an outcome. Referring to the discussion of dynamic processes in the introduction, Markov models provide a dynamic representation of what happens to a patient during an outcome.

The health states **Disease-free** and **Breast cancer recurrence** in Figure 12.2 also illustrate how Markov models can represent the quality-of-life differences possible with an outcome. Consider the two possible outcomes for the Markov model in Figure 12.2, both lasting exactly 5 years.

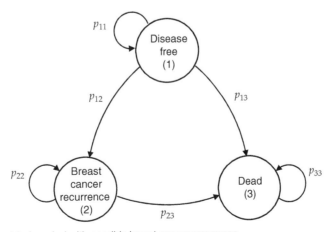

Figure 12.2 Three-state Markov model of survival with possible breast cancer recurrence.

The first outcome is spent entirely in the **Disease-free** health state. Assume a time interval of 1 month is used to express the transition probabilities. This first outcome, lasting 5 years, would consist of 60 time intervals, all spent in the **Disease-free** health state. The outcome ends after 60 time intervals because the patient died from some cause other than the recurrence of the cancer.

Because the second outcome also lasts 5 years, it also would consist of 60 time intervals. However, suppose with this second outcome the patient is in the **Disease-free** health state only for the first 12 months. At the end of a year, the patient finds themselves in the **Breast cancer recurrence** health state. They stay in this less desirable health state for the remaining 48 time intervals. At the end of 5 years, the patient succumbs to the recurrent breast cancer.

Both of these two outcomes mean the same length of life for the patient. However, one is spent free of symptoms while the other is mostly spent living with the pain and anxiety of breast cancer recurrence. The relative likelihood of these two outcomes depends on the value for the transition probability p_{12}. If p_{12} is small, the first more desirable outcome is more likely. As the value for p_{12} increases, the likelihood of the second outcome grows.

12.2.3 Markov independence

So far, no mention has been made of the assumption that is defining property of Markov models. This key assumption – called *Markov Independence* – is that transitions from any health state are independent of the health states that were encountered prior to reaching the health state.

The Markov model in Figure 12.3 illustrates the implications of Markov independence. Note that recurrence of breast cancer is now represented by two health states: **Local recurrence** and **Distant recurrence**. This refinement of the Markov model in Figure 12.2 represents how the risk of death changes with progression of the cancer. The discomfort and anxiety will increase for most patients as their health state changes from the **Local recurrence** health state to the **Distant recurrence** health state. Therefore, these two health states also represent how quality of life can change for the patient.

Markov independence

Markov independence means that the transition probabilities from any health state are independent of how the health state is reached.

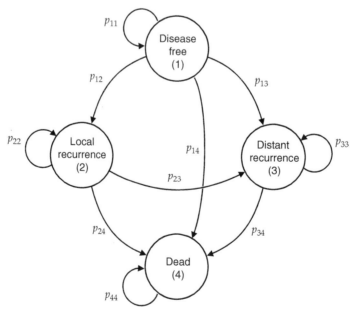

Figure 12.3 Four-state Markov model of breast cancer, using separate health states for different stages of recurrence.

However, notice in Figure 12.3 that there are two possible paths from the **Disease-free** health state to the **Distant recurrence** health state. These two paths are highlighted in Figure 12.4. With Path 1, the patient's health state proceeds first to the **Local recurrence** health state before reaching the **Distant recurrence** health state. Therefore, the change from the **Disease-free** health state to the **Distant recurrence** health state requires at least 2 time intervals. With Path 2, the change from the **Disease-free** health state to the **Distant recurrence** health state requires only 1 time interval.

There are at least two medical explanations for the second path. One explanation is that Path 2 represents a scenario in which the physician treating the original breast cancer treatment overlooked a distant recurrence that was present when breast cancer was first diagnosed. This would mean the untreated distant recurrence has had more time to affect the organ or tissue where it resides. Another explanation is that the distant recurrence did first appear after the original treatment but is the result of a transition from a local recurrence to a distant recurrence, all within a single time interval. In other words, this is a very fast-growing cancer.

Either explanation suggests that the breast cancer recurrence indicated by Path 2 is more aggressive than the breast cancer recurrence indicated by Path 1. Therefore, arriving at the **Distant recurrence** health state by way of Path 2 should mean a greater value for mortality rate p_{34}. In other words, the path to the **Distant recurrence** health state changes the probabilities for a subsequent transition. This contradicts the Markov independence assumption, which requires that the transition probabilities for a health state are independent of how the health state is reached.

Figure 12.5 shows how to modify the Markov model for breast cancer recurrence to avoid contradicting the Markov independence assumption. Notice in Figure 12.5 that the possibility of a distant recurrence is represented by two health states: **Slow distant recurrence** and **Fast distant recurrence**. The values for the transition probabilities p_{35} and p_{45} represent the difference in the risk of death for the two paths to a distant recurrence. Path 1 in Figure 12.4 would be represented in Figure 12.5 by a transition from **Disease-free** to **Local recurrence**, followed by a second transition from **Local recurrence** to **Slow distant recurrence**. On the other hand, Path 2 in Figure 12.4 would be represented in Figure 12.5 by a single transition from **Disease-free** to **Fast distant recurrence**. Differences between the transition probabilities p_{35} and p_{45} would represent the difference between the mortality rates for slow and fast distant recurrences.

In short, Markov independence can be interpreted as assuming history does not matter, which often is not the case with medical outcomes. The approach demonstrated in Figure 12.5 addresses the problem with assuming history does not matter by including the relevant history in the definition of the health states. If the speed with which distant recurrence appears matters, then the health states are modified to incorporate this relevant feature of how a cancer recurrence progresses.

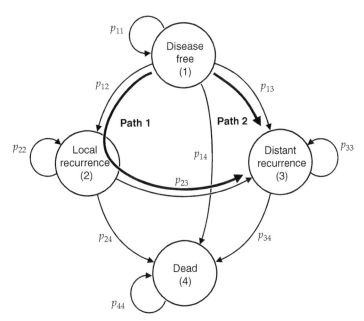

Figure 12.4 Copy of the Markov model in Figure 12.3 showing two alternate paths to the **Distant recurrence** health state.

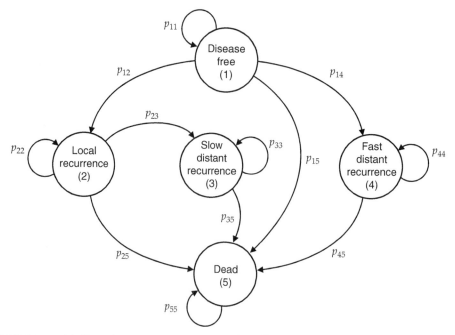

Figure 12.5 Five-state Markov model of breast cancer recurrence representing different paths to distant recurrence.

12.2.4 Stationarity assumption

Markovian analysis is often based on a second, closely related assumption, called the *stationarity assumption*. In the context of a Markov model, stationarity means that the values for the transition probabilities do not change with time. We will see that assuming stationarity often is problematic, particularly when the typical length of life is long. A long length of life means the patient's underlying health has a chance to change as it always does for all humans.

> **Stationarity**
>
> A Markov model has stationarity if the values for the transition probabilities are constant.

For example, the Markov model shown in Figure 12.6 is a copy of the four-state model first shown in Figure 12.3. Consider the transition probability p_{34}, which measures the mortality rate for patients with a distant recurrence of breast cancer. These patients have a life expectancy of a little over 12 months, which is not enough time for significant changes due to aging. Therefore, it would be reasonable to assume that p_{34} does not change much during the time this probability represents the patient's mortality rate.

Figure 12.7 provides empirical support for the assertion that the mortality rate is constant for the **Distant recurrence** health state. The curves in this figure are for women dying after diagnosis of a distant recurrence of breast cancer (Stokes *et al.*, 2008). The grey curve in Figure 12.7 is the Kaplan–Meier survival curve fitted to observations from the same dataset discussed in the previous chapter. The life expectancy for those patients was 12.6 months. The black curve is an exponential survival model fitted to the observations represented by the Kaplan–Meier survival curve. This exponential survival model has the same life expectancy as the observed survival curve.

Recall that an exponential survival model, like a stationary Markov model, assumes that the risk of death is constant. Therefore, the close agreement between the two survival curves supports the assumption of stationarity, at least for the transition probability from the **Distant recurrence** health state to the **Dead** health state.

However, returning to the Markov model in Figure 12.6, consider the transition probability p_{14}. This probability is the risk of death if the patient appears to be free of breast cancer. As depicted in the Markov model, this patient can experience a cancer recurrence in the future. However, until that happens, a patient in the **Disease-free** health state faces the same risk of death as any similarly aged person.

As we saw in the discussion of the actuarial survival model in Chapter 11, the survival model for individuals without a known fatal disease differs greatly from an exponential survival model with its constant hazard rate. Therefore,

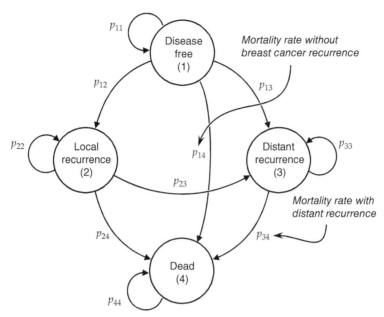

Figure 12.6 Copy of the Markov model shown in Figure 12.3.

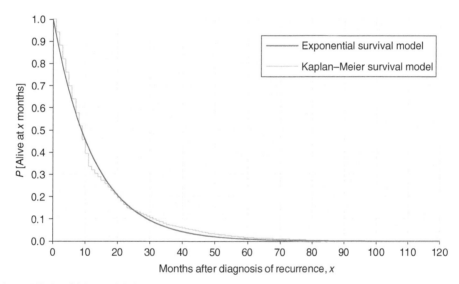

Figure 12.7 Comparison of Kaplan–Meier model of survival and exponential survival model for patients with a breast cancer distant recurrence. Adapted from Stokes *et al.* (2008).

stationarity cannot be assumed for p_{14}. Instead, the value for p_{14} should match the actuarial hazard rates described in Chapter 11. Those actuarial hazard rates grow as the patient ages, which means the transition probability p_{14} should change over time. Changing values for p_{14} contradicts the stationarity assumption.

Possible changes in p_{14} matter less if the time spent in the **Disease-free** health state is short. In turn, the time spent in the **Disease-free** health state will be short if transitions to either the **Local recurrence** or **Distant recurrence** health states are highly likely. In other words, if the transition probabilities p_{12} or p_{13} are large, the patient's health state is **Disease-free** for only a few time intervals. In this case, the changes in p_{14} will be insignificant during the short time the patient is free of disease.

In general, the validity of the stationarity assumption decreases as the time spent in health states increases. Therefore, stationary Markov models for medical conditions in which the patient has a high likelihood of remaining disease free are problematic. The mortality rates for a disease-free patient increase as the patient ages. The longer the patient remains disease free, the more the mortality rate faced by the patient departs from any assumed constant value.

Three different approaches are used to address problems with the stationarity assumption. Perhaps the simplest approach is to use average values for transition probabilities that change with time.

For example, the breast cancer recurrence Markov model shown in Figure 12.6 includes a **Disease-free** health state. Under the stationarity assumption, as long as the patient remains in this health state, they face an exponential survival model because the mortality rate (p_{14}) is constant. According to the life table analysis discussed in Chapter 11, the life expectancy is 12.4 years for a 75-year-old woman who is free of disease. Therefore, with an exponential survival model the mortality rate should result in a life expectancy of 12.4 years for a 75-year-old woman who remains free of disease. Recall that with an exponential survival model the mortality rate is one over the life expectancy, or for a 75-year-old woman:

$$\text{Mortality rate} = \frac{1}{12.4 \text{ years}} = 0.0804/\text{year}$$

This suggests an average value of 0.0804/year for the mortality rate represented by p_{14}. Later, when we discuss the estimation of transition probabilities we will find this first approach to dealing with the stationarity assumption to be useful.

The second more complicated approach to addressing problems with the stationarity assumption is to use additional health states to represent changes in transition probabilities as the patient ages. Figure 12.8 shows a portion of a Markov model that demonstrates how this would be done with the breast cancer problem we have been discussing.

Once again, the breast cancer recurrence Markov model, shown in Figure 12.6, includes a **Disease-free** health state. Mortality rates for the patient in this health state are represented by the transition probability p_{14}, which must be constant under the stationarity assumption. Therefore, if the patient is a 75-year-old woman at the start of the analysis, the logical value for p_{14} would be annual mortality rate for 75-year-old woman. According to the actuarial survival model discussed in Chapter 11, the mortality rate for a 75-year-old woman is 0.0249/year. However, the mortality rate for women increases to 0.0743/year by the time the patient reaches the age of 85 years. In other words, using the morality rate for a 75-year-old woman as the value for p_{14} greatly underestimates the probability the patient will die if she survives to the age of 85 years.

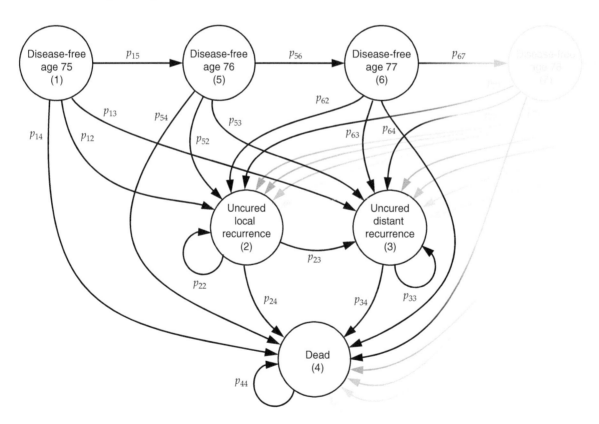

Figure 12.8 Breast cancer Markov model that accounts for changes in actuarial mortality rates.

The Markov model shown in Figure 12.8 avoids this underestimation by adding age-specific disease-free health states. Starting in the **Disease-free age 75** health state, after 1 year, the patient changes to the **Disease-free age 76** health state, assuming the patient neither dies nor experiences a breast cancer recurrence. During the first year, the probability of advancing 1 year is p_{15} in Figure 12.8. Since the transition probabilities add up to one for any health state

$$p_{12} + p_{13} + p_{14} + p_{15} = 1 \text{ or } p_{15} = 1 - p_{12} - p_{13} - p_{14}$$

The transition probability p_{14} equals the annual mortality rate for a 75-year-old woman. Similarly, the transition probability p_{54} equals the annual mortality rate for a 76-year-old woman, and so forth. The Markov model would be extended to include age-specific disease-free health states for all of the ages the patient might expect to reach.

The Markov model shown in Figure 12.8 also can represent how the probabilities for the occurrence of local or distance recurrences change with the passing of time. Often, the probability of a recurrence decreases as a patient continues to be disease free. The transition probabilities originating from the corresponding age-specific disease-free health state would represent this change in the uncertainty faced by the patient. Therefore, p_{52} would be less than p_{12} and p_{53} would be less than p_{13}.

This second approach to dealing with the stationarity assumption fully avoids any distortions caused by how transition probabilities change overtime. However, this approach complicates analyzing the resulting Markov model because of the large number of required health states.

Finally, the third approach is to use a stationary Markov model that allows for changes in the transition probabilities. This approaches fundamentally changes how Markov models are analyzed. However, this approach is often used in the analysis of complex policy questions, as will be discussed later.

Methods for representing nonstationary transition probabilities

1. Use an average value to represent the range of values for a transition probability that changes over time.
2. Add health states that represent the different values for a transition probability that changes over time.
3. Use a nonstationary Markov model.

12.2.5 Acyclic graph assumption

Some readers might notice that all of the Markov models described so far in this chapter are acyclic. By "acyclic" we mean that the possible transitions in the model are such that once a health state has been left, there is no sequence of transitions that return back to that same health state.

Acyclic

A Markov model is acyclic if, for every health state, there is no possible sequence of transitions that return to health state once it has been left.

In case of cancer recurrence, the lack of a return to the **Disease-free** health state in Figure 12.6 would appear to exclude the possibility of successful salvage treatments. Of course, salvage treatment often can return the patient to a disease-free condition after a recurrence. An arc from the corresponding recurrence state to the **Disease-free** health state would represent the possibility of a return to the disease-free condition.

One answer to this apparent gap in the Markov models we have discussed is that the definitions of the **Local recurrence** and **Distant recurrence** health states contain the possibility of a salvage treatment. Presumably, a patient with a recurrence would undergo further treatment. The possible effects of additional treatments would be reflected in the mortality rates for the corresponding health states. In other words, the Markov models that have been discussed imply the existence of salvage treatments in the definition of the corresponding health state.

On the other hand, the Markov model shown in Figure 12.9 makes the existence of salvage treatments explicit in the case of a local recurrence.[1] This Markov model has the same health states as the four-state models that have been discussed. However, notice that an arc has been added showing the possibility of a transition from the **Local**

---

[1] In order to simplify the Markov model diagrams, the discussion will focus only on the **Local recurrence** health state.

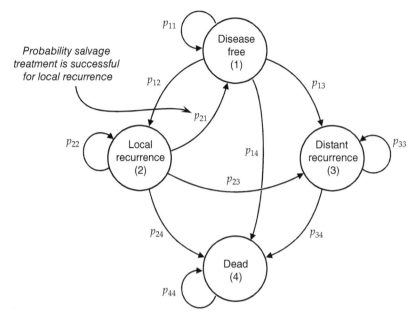

Figure 12.9 Cyclic version of four-state Markov model for breast cancer survival with explicit representation of salvage treatment for local recurrence.

recurrence health state back to the **Disease-free** health state. The corresponding transition probability p_{21} quantifies the likelihood that salvage treatment will be successful.

However, what does it mean to return to the **Disease-free** health state? Most likely, the chance of another local recurrence in the future has changed. This means the transition probability p_{12} is not the same, which contradicts the Markov independence assumption. Moreover, for many patients recovering from a recurrence is not the same as remaining disease free because of the psychological trauma of having breast cancer return.

Figure 12.10 shows an acyclic Markov model that represents salvage treatment for a local recurrence. In this alternative model, the **Local recurrence** health state has been replaced by a **Local recurrence treatment** health state. This new

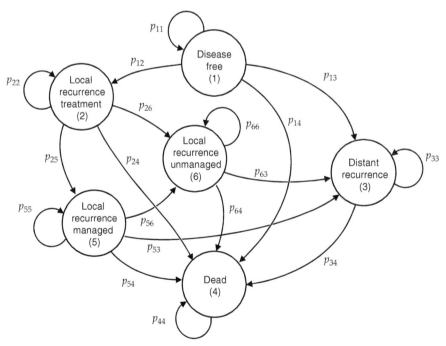

Figure 12.10 Markov model representing possible recovery from a local recurrence of breast cancer.

health state represents the salvage treatment that is started when a local recurrence is found. The patient remains in this health state for one or more time intervals.

Assuming the patient does not die during salvage treatment, they face two possibilities. One possibility is the patient moves into the **Local recurrence unmanaged** health state if the salvage treatment fails. In this health state, the local recurrence continues, and the patient faces the increased likelihood of progressing to a distant recurrence. The other possibility is the patient moves into the **Local recurrence managed** health state if the salvage treatment is successful. This health state is much like the **Disease-free** health state, except that the patient continues to experience whatever residual anxiety they feel because of the recurrence. Also, in the **Local recurrence managed** health state, there is the possibility of proceeding to a distant recurrence. However, that possibility is less than it would be if the salvage treatment had failed. That is p_{53} would be less than p_{63}.

The uncertainty about the time spent enduring salvage treatment is represented by the survival probability p_{22}. If the salvage treatment lasts exactly 1 time interval p_{22} would be zero. Larger values for p_{22} would represent longer times for the salvage treatment. The relative size of the transition probabilities p_{25} and p_{26} represents the relative likelihood that salvage treatment will succeed.

The Markov model in Figure 12.10 also represents the possibility that salvage treatment, which initially appears to be successful, can later be followed by a subsequent appearance of a local recurrence. The transition probability p_{56} measure the likelihood of that possibility.

The reason for discussing the Markov model in Figure 12.10 is to demonstrate how these models can be extended to capture the details in a medical decision without reverting to models that are not acyclic. Avoiding returns to health states avoids the medical contradictions that have been discussed. Acyclic Markov models also are easier to analyze.

12.3   Determining transition probabilities

The previous section shows that Markov models provide structures that represent the dynamics, as well as the uncertainty, for the outcomes that can follow a decision. Those structures are collections of health states that are linked by transitions representing changes in the patient's condition over time. The probabilities for those transitions quantify the uncertainty in how an outcome will unfold.

This section shows how to determine the transition probabilities used in a Markov model. The process that will be described is complicated in places and may be challenging for some readers. Moreover, understanding this process is not needed to appreciate the role for Markov models in analyzing medical decisions. Therefore, this section can be skipped. However, transition probabilities are essential to the definition of a Markov model. Readers involved in the use of Markov models should understand how values are determined for transition probabilities.

A transition probability is, of course, a probability. Any of the methods discussed elsewhere in this book for assigning a value to a probability could be used. This includes subjective probability assessment. However, this section focuses on empirical methods for determining the value of a transition probability.

It should be noted that the work involved in determining the transition probabilities typically requires more effort than selecting the states and transitions that define a Markov model. The work required to determine the transition probability values usually must bridge the gap between the medical concepts embodied in a Markov model and what is available from well-documented studies. The paucity of credible studies can force the restructuring of a model. This means the processes that will be described in this section are a critical part of Markovian analysis.

12.3.1   Markov model used to illustrate how transition probabilities are determined

The five-state Markov model, shown in Figure 12.11, will be used to illustrate how transition probabilities are determined. This model represents the survival of a 75-year-old woman who has been diagnosed with a breast cancer recurrence. This patient's survival can follow two possible paths. One path is successful salvage treatment that completely eliminates the breast cancer that has reappeared. In this case, the patient's survival matches that of any similarly aged woman. This possibility is represented by the **Successful treatment** health state in Figure 12.11.

The other possibility is the breast cancer recurrence does not respond to treatment. In this case, the patient will still face the same survival risks that are faced by anyone of their age. However, unsuccessful treatment also means the patient faces an additional risk of breast cancer that has reappeared. The amount of that additional risk depends on the stage of the recurrence. The possibility of unsuccessful salvage treatment is represented in Figure 12.11 by the health states **Local recurrence** and **Distant recurrence**.

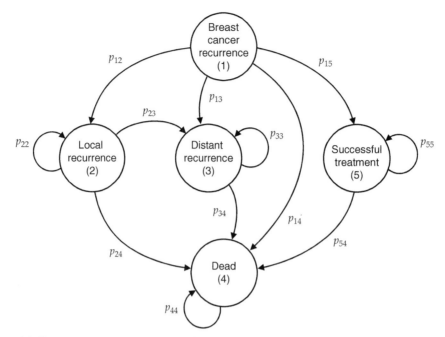

Figure 12.11 Markov model of breast cancer recurrence used to demonstrate how transition probabilities are determined.

Notice that the Markov model shows a transition from the **Local recurrence** health state to the **Distant recurrence** health state. This transition represents the increased risk that comes with a local recurrence. A patient with a local recurrence that cannot be controlled faces a different survival model than a patient without a recurrence. However, the increased risk faced by this patient is not because of the local recurrence itself. A tumor that exists only at the site of the original breast cancer usually does not become life threatening until it spreads to a vital organ, in other words, until it metastasizes and becomes a distant recurrence. The probability p_{23} measures the speed of that transition.

Finally, notice that the Markov model in Figure 12.11 does not show a survival transition for the initial **Breast cancer recurrence** health state. This means the patient remains in the initial health state for exactly 1 time interval, which will be 1 month in this example. The time spent in the **Breast cancer recurrence** health state represents the duration of the salvage treatment. In order to simplify the discussion this example will assume treatment lasts exactly 1 month.

12.3.2 Determining mortality rates

We will start by determining values for the mortality rates in the Markov model. These are the transition probabilities for the arcs leading to the **Dead** health state (see Figure 12.12). As already noted, the mortality rate for the **Successful treatment** health state is the mortality rate for a 75-year-old woman. If we were constructing a nonstationary Markov model this transition probability (p_{54}) would change, as the patient aged, to match the actuarial hazard rates for a 75-year-old woman. However, we will focus on stationary Markov models and use an average value for p_{54}.

Mortality rates in Markov models

In a Markov model, a mortality rate is the transition probability for an arc connecting a health state to a trapping state representing death.

The life expectancy for a 75-year-old woman is 12.4 years or 149 months. This means the value for p_{54} is the constant mortality rate that results in a life expectancy of 149 months. The discussion of exponential survival models in Chapter 11 noted that when the mortality rate is constant, the patient's life expectancy is one over the patient's mortality rate. In a stationary Markov model, all of the mortality rates are constant. Therefore, the patient's life expectancy of 149 months means they face the following mortality rate in the **Successful treatment** health state:

$$p_{54} = \frac{1}{149 \text{ months}} = 0.0067 / \text{month}$$

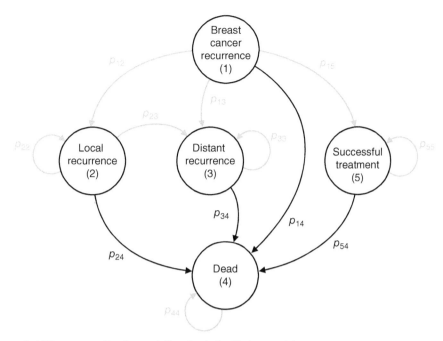

Figure 12.12 Transition probabilities representing the mortality rates in the Markov model.

It follows that

$$p_{55} = 1 - p_{54} = 1 - 0.0067/\text{month} = 0.9933/\text{month}$$

Next, we will consider the mortality rate for the **Distant recurrence** health state (p_{34}). This transition probability measures the likelihood of death during a 1-month time interval if the patient has metastatic breast cancer that has not been treated successfully.

The survival curve in Figure 12.13 can be used to determine the risk of dying, each month, faced by a patient with metastatic cancer. We first saw this survival curve in the discussion of the two-part survival model back in Chapter 11. The patients represented in this curve are from a group of 622 women with distant recurrence of breast cancer (Stokes *et al.*, 2008).

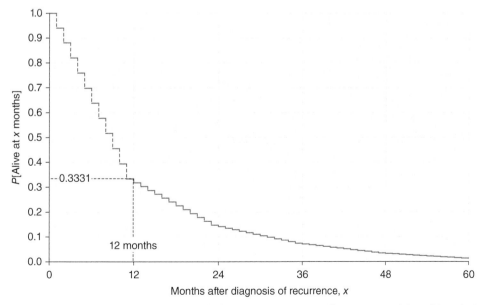

Figure 12.13 Kaplan–Meier survival model for patients diagnosed with a distant recurrence of breast cancer. Adapted from Stokes *et al.* (2008).

Table 12.1 Monthly mortality rates for distant recurrence of breast cancer.

	Months since first detection of distant recurrence					
	12	24	36	48	60	Average
Observed survival probability	0.3331	0.1477	0.0743	0.0349	0.0142	
Implied 1-month survival probability	0.9125	0.9234	0.9303	0.9325	0.9316	0.9260

The top row in Table 12.1 contains the values for the survival probabilities, shown in Figure 12.13, for various follow-up times. For example, 12 months after the first detection of the recurrence, the probability that a patient was alive is 0.3331. In order to determine the transition probability p_{34} we must determine the corresponding 1-month survival probability. Let p denote that 1-month survival probability. Then p^2 would be the probability the patient survives 2 months, p^3 would be the probability the patient survives 3 months, and so forth. Therefore, the probability the patient survives for a year is p^{12}, which we know to be 0.3331. That is

$$p^{12} = 0.3331$$

Using a little high school algebra, the probability the patient survives 1 month is then

$$p = 0.3331^{1/12} = 0.9125$$

The second row in Table 12.1 repeats this calculation for several follow-up periods. Note the agreement between the implied 1-month survival probabilities. The average value for these 1-month survival probabilities is 0.9260/month.

What have we computed so far? The value 0.9260 approximates the average probability that a patient will survive each month while they have a distant recurrence of breast cancer. In other words, one minus 0.9260/month, or 0.0740/month, is the probability of death during a 1-month period for the patient in the **Distant recurrence** health state. This means,

$$p_{34} = 0.0740/\text{month}$$

Therefore, we have determined the mortality rates for two of the health states: **Successful treatment** and **Distant recurrence**. It turns out that we already determined the mortality rate for the **Local recurrence** health state.

Recall the observation made earlier that the increased risk faced with an uncontrolled local recurrence is not because of the local recurrence itself. A recurrence usually is not life threatening as long as it remains at the original site in the patient's breast. Of course, a local recurrence is not a pleasant experience. Therefore, the quality of life is less for the **Local recurrence** health state than it is for the **Successful treatment** health state. However, both health states have roughly the same mortality rates. This means that

$$p_{24} = p_{54} = 0.0067/\text{month}$$

The remaining mortality rate that must be determined is for the initial **Breast cancer recurrence** health state. Recall that this health state represents the experience of a patient who will undergo treatment because breast cancer has recurred. The transition probability p_{14} represents the corresponding mortality rate. In general, recall that a transition probability measures the likelihood of a transition during the time unit used to define the model, which is 1 month in this example. Therefore, the transition probability p_{14} measures the likelihood of death during the 1 month period following the detection of the cancer recurrence. Presumably, the patient will undergo treatment starting at the beginning of that month.

Breast cancer treatments are painful and can be disfiguring; however, usually, they are not dangerous. Therefore, we will ignore the risk of death from the procedure itself. However, two other issues affect the patient's chance of dying during the initial month. The first issue is the extent of the breast cancer recurrence that has been detected. As we have already discussed, the cancer itself does not threaten the patient's life if the recurrence is local. However, with a metastasis, the patient does face an increased mortality rate from the cancer, since it has spread to what may be a vital organ.

The second issue affecting the chance of death for the patient in the initial **Breast cancer recurrence** health state is the success of the salvage treatment. If the treatment is successful, the patient then faces the mortality rate for a typical 75-year-old woman during the first month because that is what we mean when we say the treatment is successful.

If the treatment is not successful, the mortality rate for the first month depends on the extent of the cancer recurrence. With a local recurrence, the patient still faces the mortality rate for a typical 75-year-old woman during the first month.

That local recurrence will eventually spread and become a distant recurrence, which will increase the mortality rate. However, that mortality rate increase will occur during a later month. On the other hand, unsuccessful treatment of a distant recurrence means the patient faces elevated risk during that first month.

Therefore, during the first month, the patient will face the mortality rate for a 75-year-old woman (0.0067/month) if either (1) the recurrence is local or (2) the recurrence is distant, but the treatment is successful. Otherwise, the patient will face the mortality rate associated with a distant recurrence, which we found to be 0.0740/month when we determined the value for p_{34}.

Combining these observations into a single expression for p_{14} benefits from the use of a more compact notation. Denote the probabilities for a local and distant recurrence as follows:

$$P[\text{Local recurrence}] = p_{\text{Local}}$$

and

$$P[\text{Distant recurrence}] = p_{\text{Distant}}$$

Similarly, the following notation will denote the probability of success given the type of recurrence:

$$P[\text{Successful treatment of local recurrence}] = \sigma_{\text{Local}}$$

and

$$P[\text{Successful treatment of distant recurrence}] = \sigma_{\text{Distant}}$$

As noted earlier, the patient's mortality will be 0.0067/month during the first month if either (1) the recurrence is local or (2) the recurrence is distant but the treatment is successful. Using the notation we just defined

$$P[\text{Local recurrence}] = p_{\text{Local}}$$

Similarly,

$$P[\text{Distant recurrence and successful treatment}] = p_{\text{Distant}} \times \sigma_{\text{Distant}}$$

Therefore,

$$P[\text{Mortality rate} = 0.0067/\text{month}] = p_{\text{Local}} + p_{\text{Distant}} \times \sigma_{\text{Distant}}$$

Similarly, the patient's mortality will be 0.0740/month during the first month if they have a distant recurrence and unsuccessful treatment. That is

$$P[\text{Mortality rate} = 0.0740/\text{month}] = p_{\text{Distant}} \times (1 - \sigma_{\text{Distant}})$$

Combining these two results leads to the following expression for the patient's mortality rate in the **Breast cancer recurrence** health state:

$$p_{14} = (p_{\text{Local}} + p_{\text{Distant}} \times \sigma_{\text{Distant}}) \times 0.0067/\text{month} + p_{\text{Distant}} \times (1 - \sigma_{\text{Distant}}) \times 0.0740/\text{month}$$

The probabilities used in this expression can be determined from the study that provided the survival curve for distant recurrences, shown in Figure 12.13. That same study also provided survival data for local recurrences. In addition to the 622 patients with distant recurrences, there were 958 patients with local recurrences. Since these patients were found in a population of unselected breast cancer cases, the patient counts of 958 and 622 represent the relative proportion of recurrences that are local or distant, respectively. That is

$$\text{Proportion of recurrences that are local} = \frac{958}{958 + 622} = 0.6063$$

$$\text{Proportion of recurrences that are distant} = \frac{622}{958 + 622} = 0.3937$$

Therefore,

$$p_{\text{Local}} = 0.6063 \text{ and } p_{\text{Distant}} = 0.3937$$

In order to determine the probability that treatment will be successful, recall how the two-part survival model was developed in the previous chapter for a patient with a distant recurrence of breast cancer. The number of expected deaths were subtracted from the deaths observed in the 622 patients during follow-up. This calculation implied that 550 patients, or 87.57%, died from cancer. Dying from cancer means treatment was not successful, implying

$$P[\text{Successful treatment of distant recurrence}] = \sigma_{\text{Distant}} = 1 - 0.8757 = 0.1243$$

A similar analysis of the 958 patients with local disease implies that

$$P[\text{Successful treatment of local recurrence}] = \sigma_{\text{Local}} = 1 - 0.5459 = 0.4541$$

We now have the values needed to compute the mortality rate for the patient during the first time interval.

$$p_{14} = \left(p_{\text{Local}} + p_{\text{Distant}} \times \sigma_{\text{Distant}}\right) \times 0.0067/\text{month} + p_{\text{Distant}} \times \left(1 - \sigma_{\text{Distant}}\right) \times 0.0740/\text{month}$$

$$= \left(0.6063 + 0.3937 \times 0.1243\right) \times 0.0067/\text{month} + 0.3937 \times \left(1 - 0.1243\right) \times 0.0740/\text{month}$$

$$= 0.0299/\text{month}$$

This completes the determination of the mortality rates for the Markov model.

12.3.3 Determining probability for transitions between stages of recurrence

Next, we will determine the probability of a transition between the **Local recurrence** health state and the **Distant recurrence** health state (p_{23}). This transition represents the inevitable spread of a local recurrence when treatment has not been successful. As has already been emphasized, the possibility of this transition is how a local recurrence reduces the patient's survival.

Figure 12.13 showed the survival model for a group of patients with breast cancer recurrence that had spread to distant locations by the time of diagnosis. Figure 12.14 shows the corresponding survival model for patients from the same study with a local recurrence of breast cancer. In other words, the newly diagnosed recurrences in this second group of patients were near the sites of the original tumors in the patients.

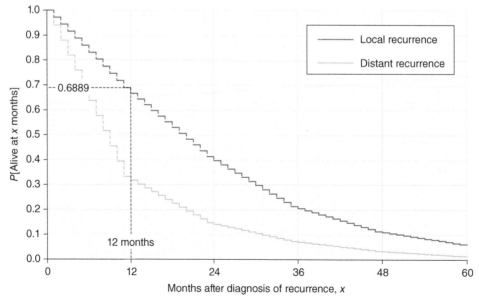

Figure 12.14 Kaplan–Meier survival model for patients diagnosed with a local recurrence of breast cancer. The corresponding survival curve for local recurrence also is shown. Adapted from Stokes *et al.* (2008).

Table 12.2 Monthly mortality rates for local recurrence of breast cancer.

	Months since first detection of distant recurrence					
	12	*24*	*36*	*48*	*60*	*Average*
Observed survival probability	0.6889	0.4138	0.2190	0.1320	0.0796	0.3067
Implied 1-month survival probability	0.9694	0.9639	0.9587	0.9587	0.9587	0.9619

Notice in Figure 12.14 that the 1-year survival probability increases from 0.3331 for a distant recurrence to 0.6889 for a local recurrence. Using the same logic as before, a 1-year survival probability of 0.6889 implies a 1-month survival probability of $0.6889^{1/12}$, or 0.9694. Table 12.2 repeats these calculations for several follow-up periods. As before, the implied monthly survival probabilities are consistent. The average value for the 1-month survival probabilities shown in Table 12.2 is 0.9619/month implying an average 1-month mortality rate of one minus 0.9619/month, or 0.0381/month.

Earlier, when we analyzed the mortality rate for the **Distant recurrence** health state in the Markov model, we noted that the life expectancy is one over the mortality rate. Therefore, the survival curve in Figure 12.14 implies that the life expectancy for a patient in the **Local recurrence** health state is

$$\text{Life expectancy starting in } \textbf{Local recurrence} \text{ health state} = \frac{1}{0.0381 \, / \, \text{month}} = 26.2 \text{ months}$$

However, consider the portion of the Markov model shown in Figure 12.15. This figure focuses on the health states related to the transition probability p_{23}. Note that if our patient remained in the **Local recurrence** health state until death, they would live for the remainder of their life with a monthly mortality rate of 0.0067/month. Put in other words, if the transition probability p_{23} is zero, the patient's life expectancy would be one over 0.0067/month, or 149.3 months. At the other extreme, if p_{23} is one, the patient would immediately move to the **Distant recurrence** health state. In this case the patient would face a monthly mortality rate of 0.0740/month, implying a life expectancy of only 13.0 months.

Together, these two extremes show how the transition probability p_{23} determines the life expectancy for the patient when they are in the **Local recurrence** health state. Small values for p_{23} mean a long time is spent in the **Local recurrence** health state, where the life expectancy is 149 months. Large values for p_{23} mean a long time is spent in the **Distant recurrence** health state, where the life expectancy is 13 months. The proper value for p_{23} balances the time spent in these two health states so that our patient's life expectancy matches the 26 months observed in a population of similar patients.

Determining the value for p_{23} that achieves this balance is not difficult, but it requires several steps.

Think about the patient's remaining life once they reach the **Local recurrence** health state. The patient will spend part of their life in the **Local recurrence** health state. The patient could next move to the **Distant recurrence** health state. This means the patient's life expectancy also could include the average time they spend in the **Distant recurrence**

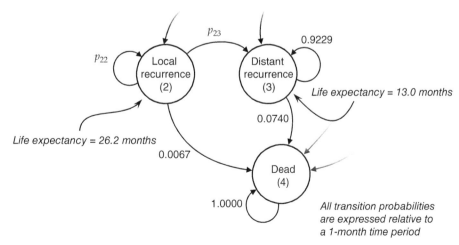

Figure 12.15 Portion of Markov model used to determine the transition probability p_{23}. The life expectancies for an outcome starting in the **Local recurrence** health state and the **Distant recurrence** health state are shown.

health state. However, the patient also can leave the **Local recurrence** health state by dying. Therefore, there is only a possibility that the patient's life expectancy also includes time spent in the **Distant recurrence** health state.

We can summarize these observations with the following expression for the patient's life expectancy starting in the **Local recurrence** health state:

Life expectancy starting in **Local recurrence** = Average time in **Local recurrence**

   +P[Distant recurrence follows Local recurrence]× Average time in Distant recurrence

The steps that follow will translate this expression into an equivalent expression containing the transition probability we would like to know (p_{23}) as well as several terms we already know. Solving this new expression for p_{23} will let us compute the value for this transition probability.

As a first step, recall that we just determined

Life expectancy starting in **Local recurrence** = 26.2 months

We also determined the average time a patient will spend in the **Distant recurrence** health state because a departure from this health state is the end of the patient's life. This means the average time a patient will spend in the **Distant recurrence** health state equals the patient's remaining life expectancy once they reach the **Distant recurrence** health state. Earlier we determined that the life expectancy in the **Distant recurrence** health state is 13.0 months. Therefore,

Average time in **Distant recurrence** = 13.0 months

Next, we must determine P[**Distant recurrence** follows **Local recurrence**]. This is a conditional probability. Recall the definition of conditional probability from Chapter 3. Suppose that A and B are two events. The probability for event A conditioned on event B is the probability event A occurs given that event B has occurred and is defined as

$$P[A \mid B] = \frac{P[A \text{ and } B]}{P[B]}$$

In our case, event A is the patient is in the **Distant recurrence** health state and event B is the patient has left the **Local recurrence** health state. The intersection of events A and B is the occurrence of a transition from the **Local recurrence** health state to the **Distant recurrence** health state Therefore, we can express the probability of reaching the **Distant recurrence** health state from the **Local recurrence** health state as follows:

$$P[\text{Distant recurrence follows Local recurrence}] = \frac{P[\text{Transition from Local recurrence to Distant recurrence}]}{P[\text{Leave Local recurrence}]}$$

By definition, the probability of a transition from the **Local recurrence** health state to the **Distant recurrence** is the transition probability p_{23}. Also, notice in Figure 12.15 that there are two transitions that leave the **Local recurrence** health state: (1) the local recurrence becomes a distant recurrence or (2) the patient dies. This means the probability of leaving the **Local recurrence** health state, during any given time interval, is the sum of the transition probabilities for the two arcs leaving the **Local recurrence** health state. That is,

$$P[\text{Leave } \textbf{Local recurrence}] = p_{24} + p_{23}$$

We already know that p_{24} is 0.0067/month. So, we can write

$$P[\text{Leave } \textbf{Local recurrence}] = 0.0067/\text{month} + p_{23}$$

We can summarize these observations as

$$P[\text{Distant recurrence follows Local recurrence}] = \frac{P[\text{Transition from Local recurrence to Distant recurrence}]}{P[\text{Leave Local recurrence}]}$$

$$= \frac{p_{23}}{0.0067/\text{month} + p_{23}}$$

Finally, we must determine the average stay for the patient in the **Local recurrence** health state. We determine this average stay using the same approach we used to determine the patient's average stay in the **Distant recurrence** health state. In the case of the **Distant recurrence** health state, the average stay equals the life expectancy since life ends when the patient leaves this health state. The probability of leaving the **Distant recurrence** health state is the mortality rate. Therefore, the average stay in the **Distant recurrence** health state is one over the mortality rate.

A similar logic applies to the **Local recurrence** health state except that there are two ways the patient can leave this health state. As we just noted, the probability of leaving the **Local recurrence** health is the sum of the corresponding two transition probabilities. That is

$$P[\text{Leave } \textbf{Local recurrence}] = 0.0067/\text{month} + p_{23}$$

As with the **Distant recurrence** health state, the average stay in the **Local recurrence** health state is one over the probability of leaving the **Local recurrence** health state. Therefore,

$$\text{Average time in } \textbf{Local recurrence} = \frac{1}{P[\text{Leave } \textbf{Local recurrence}]} = \frac{1}{0.0067/\text{month} + p_{23}}$$

This derivation has been a long journey but recall that we started with the expression

Life expectancy starting in **Local recurrence** = Average time in **Local recurrence**
$+ P[\text{Distant recurrence follows Local recurrence}] \times$ Average time in Distant recurrence

We then determine the following values for each of the four terms in this expression:

Life expectancy starting in **Local recurrence** $= 26.2\,\text{months}$

Average time in **Local recurrence** $= \dfrac{1}{0.0067/\text{month} + p_{23}}$

$$P[\textbf{Distant recurrence} \text{ follows } \textbf{Local recurrence}] = \frac{p_{23}}{0.0067/\text{month} + p_{23}}$$

Average time in **Distant recurrence** $= 13.0\,\text{months}$

Using these values in the original expression yields:

$$26.2\,\text{months} = \frac{1}{0.0067/\text{month} + p_{23}} + \frac{p_{23}}{0.0067/\text{month} + p_{23}} \times 13.0\,\text{months}$$

Solving this expression for the transition probability we would like to know yields

$$p_{23} = \frac{1 - 26.2\,\text{months} \times 0.0067/\text{month}}{26.2\,\text{months} - 13.0\,\text{months}} = 0.0647/\text{months}$$

Deriving this transition probability may have required multiple steps. However, as will be discussed later in the final section, this derivation demonstrated one approach to how Markov models are analyzed.

12.3.4   Determining transition probabilities for treatment response

The remaining transition probabilities represent the response of the patient to treatment during the first time interval. Figure 12.16 shows the corresponding portion of the Markov model.

Determining these transition probabilities will use notation and probabilities that were introduced earlier in this section. Recall that

p_{Local} $= P[\text{Local recurrence}]$ $= 0.6063$
p_{Distant} $= P[\text{Distant recurrence}]$ $= 0.3937$
σ_{Local} $= P[\text{Successful treatment of local recurrence}]$ $= 0.4541$
σ_{Distant} $= P[\text{Successful treatment of distant recurrence}]$ $= 0.1243$

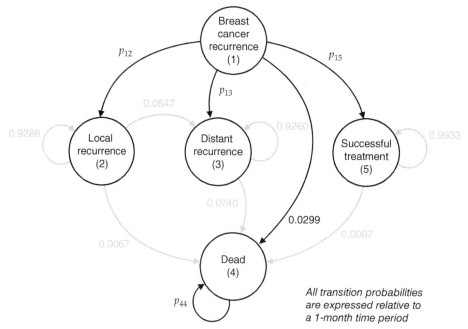

Figure 12.16 Portion of Markov model representing the treatment response.

We already used these probabilities to determine the mortality rate for the patient in the **Breast cancer recurrence** health state (p_{14}). That discussion derived the following expression to account for the different ways the patient might die during the first time interval represented by the Markov model

$$p_{14} = \left(p_{\text{Local}} + p_{\text{Distant}} \times \sigma_{\text{Distant}} \right) \times 0.0067 / \text{month} + p_{\text{Distant}} \times \left(1 - \sigma_{\text{Distant}} \right) \times 0.0740 / \text{month}$$

$$= 0.0299 / \text{month}$$

The following discussion will derive similar expressions that determine the transition probabilities for the other possible outcomes of treatment.

Perhaps the probability of the transition to the **Successful treatment** health state (p_{15}) is the simplest of these transition probabilities. Of course, in order for this transition to occur, the patient must survive. As we just saw, the probability that the patient survives the first time interval is

$$P\left[\text{Survive first time interval} \right] = 1 - p_{14} = 1 - 0.0299 = 0.9701$$

Assuming the patient survives, the treatment must successfully treat either a local recurrence or a distant recurrence, depending on the stage of the patient's disease.

Therefore, there are two cases that must be considered. First, the patient can have a local recurrence. The probability of a local recurrence is denoted by p_{Local} and the probability of a successful treatment with a local recurrence is denoted by σ_{Local}. Second, the patient can have a distant recurrence. The probability of a distant recurrence is denoted by p_{Distant} and the probability of a successful treatment with a local recurrence is denoted by σ_{Distant}. Therefore, the probability of a transition from the initial **Breast cancer recurrence** health state and the **Successful treatment** health state is

$$p_{15} = \underbrace{\left(1 - p_{14} \right)}_{\substack{\text{Survival} \\ \text{probability}}} \times \left(\underbrace{p_{\text{Local}} \times \sigma_{\text{Local}}}_{\substack{\text{Probability local} \\ \text{recurrence is cured}}} + \underbrace{p_{\text{Distant}} \times \sigma_{\text{Distant}}}_{\substack{\text{Probability distant} \\ \text{recurrence is cured}}} \right)$$

Inserting the values for the probabilities into this expression

$$p_{15} = \left(1 - 0.0299 \right)\left(0.6063 \times 0.4541 + 0.3937 \times 0.1243 \right) = 0.3146 / \text{month}$$

The similar expressions for the possible transitions to the **Local recurrence** and **Distant recurrence** health states are slightly more complicated. The important property of a local recurrence is that it can become a distant recurrence.

That transition can occur during the first time interval. This means the transition probabilities from the initial **Breast cancer recurrence** health state to the **Local recurrence** and **Distant recurrence** health states must account for this possibility.

However, we quantified the probability that a local recurrence will become distant recurrence when we determined the transition probability p_{23}. Deriving that transition probability was the focus of the previous subsection. What we found was

$$P[\text{Transition from Local recurrence to Distant recurrence}] = 0.0647/\text{month}$$

Therefore, consider the probability of a transition from the **Breast cancer recurrence** health state to the **Local recurrence** health state (p_{12}). As before, in order for the patient to make this transition, the following must be true:
1. The patient must survive ($1 - p_{14} = 0.9701$).
2. The recurrence must be local rather than distant ($p_{\text{Local}} = 0.6063$).
3. Treatment of that local recurrence must fail ($1 - \sigma_{\text{Local}} = 0.5459$).
4. The local recurrence cannot become a distant recurrence ($1 - p_{23} = 0.9353/\text{month}$).
Combining the probabilities for these four events

$$p_{12} = \left(1 - p_{14}\right) \times p_{\text{Local}} \times \left(1 - \sigma_{\text{Local}}\right) \times \left(1 - p_{23}\right)$$

Inserting the values for the probabilities into this expression

$$p_{12} = 0.9701 \times 0.6063 \times 0.5459 \times 0.9353/\text{month} = 0.3003/\text{month}$$

The corresponding expression for the probability of a transition from the **Breast cancer recurrence** health state to the **Distant recurrence** health state (p_{13}) is

$$p_{13} = \left(1 - p_{14}\right) \times \left(p_{\text{Local}} \times \left(1 - \sigma_{\text{Local}}\right) \times p_{23} + p_{\text{Distant}} \times \left(1 - \sigma_{\text{Distant}}\right)\right)$$

or

$$p_{13} = 0.9701 \times \left(0.6063 \times 0.5459 \times 0.0647/\text{month} + 0.3937 \times 0.8757/\text{month}\right)$$
$$p_{13} = 0.3552/\text{month}$$

We can check the transition probabilities derived in this subsection by recalling that the transition probabilities for the arcs from the **Breast cancer recurrence** health state must add up to one. That is

$$p_{12} + p_{13} + p_{14} + p_{15} = 1$$

Indeed

$$0.3003/\text{month} + 0.3552/\text{month} + 0.0299/\text{month} + 0.3146/\text{month} = 1.0000/\text{month}$$

Figure 12.17 summarizes this section by showing the Markov model we have discussed with the corresponding values for the transition probabilities.

12.4   Markov model analysis – an overview

This final section provides a high-level overview of two different approaches to analyzing Markov models. One approach uses the mathematical properties of a Markov model to directly determine the statistical properties of the outcomes faced by the patient. We will call this the *direct approach* to analyzing a Markov model. The second approach uses a computer program to randomly generate a large number of examples of the outcomes implied by the Markov model. The computer program is designed so that the probability an outcome will be generated equals the probability a patient would experience that outcome in the medical condition represented by the model. Therefore, the statistical properties of the outcomes faced by a patient can be determined from the statistical properties of those randomly generated outcomes. For example, the average length of an outcome in real life will equal the average length of the generated outcomes. This second approach is called *Monte Carlo simulation*.

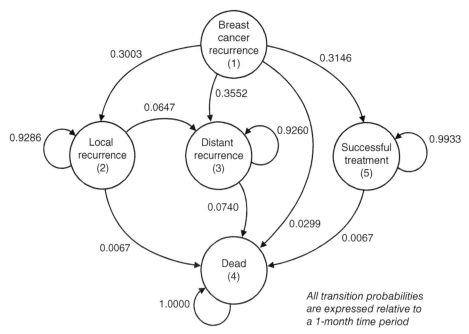

Figure 12.17 Markov model of breast cancer showing values for the transition probabilities expressed as the probability of a transition per month.

12.4.1 Direct approach to Markov model analysis

As was emphasized in the introduction to this chapter, Markov models extend the survival models described in Chapter 11. The extensions provided by Markov models account for the dynamics as well as the uncertainty in how a patient's outcome will unfold following a decision. As such, the goals of Markov model analysis are much like the goals of survival model analysis. For example, survival models can be analyzed to compare the life expectancies that will follow a treatment decision. Similarly, Markov models imply the life expectancies for the represented medical condition.

Definition: direct approach to Markov model analysis

The direct approach to Markov model analysis uses the mathematical properties of the model to determine the statistical properties of the outcomes represented by the Markov model.

Clearly, the life expectancy implied by a Markov model depends on the transition probabilities used in the model. The previous section showed how to reverse this link between life expectancy and transition probabilities to determine values for the latter. The life expectancy implied by the transition probabilities in a Markov model should match the average length of life observed in a group of similar patients experiencing the medical condition represented by the model. The previous section showed how to use observational data, together with a life expectancy calculation, to infer the corresponding transition probabilities. The life expectancy calculation that was used illustrates a direct approach to analyzing a Markov model.

The basis for that life expectancy calculation is a simple observation. The patient's life expectancy, starting in a health state, includes the average time the patient remains in that health state plus the weighted sum of the average times the patient spends in the other health states they might experience. The weighting in that sum depends on the probabilities of reaching those subsequent health states. In turn, the transition probabilities determine the probability that a health state will be reached.

For example, Figure 12.17 contains the Markov model used in the previous section to show how to determine transition probabilities. This model described the survival of a patient experiencing either a local recurrence or a distant recurrence of breast cancer.

The Markov model in Figure 12.17 is acyclic, meaning the patient never returns to a health state once it has been left. The life expectancy calculation described earlier depends on that acyclic property. Life expectancy is the average value for the weighted sum of the times the patient spends in each of the health states encounter before reaching death.

The probability that each health state is reached provides the weighting in that sum. Because the Markov model in Figure 12.17 is acyclic, a health state's contribution to that sum is fully captured by the average length of stay for a single visit to the health state. There will be no additional time spent in a health state once it is left because the patient will never return to that health state. Therefore, the acyclic property plays a central role in this example of how direct analysis can be applied to a Markov model.

In addition to determining the patient's life expectancy, the probabilities for different lengths of life – what we called the lifetime probabilities in Chapter 11 – also can be determined. For example, Figure 12.18 shows the lifetime probabilities for the outcomes represented by the Markov model in Figure 12.17. The steps used to calculate the curves in Figure 12.18 are complicated and will not be covered here. However, those complicated calculations extend the same reasoning used in the life expectancy calculations.

The transition probabilities for the Markov model shown in Figure 12.17 were derived in the previous section under the assumption that the probability of a local recurrence is 0.6 and a distant recurrence is 0.4. This assumption was based on data for over 1500 patients with either local or distant recurrences.

Treatment of a recurrence requires knowing the extent of the recurrence. Therefore, Figure 12.19 shows the lifetime probabilities when the transition probabilities in the Markov model have been adjusted to represent scenarios where the extent of the recurrence is known. Comparing the lifetime probabilities for local recurrence and distant recurrence in Figure 12.19, notice that with a distant recurrence, the probabilities are greater for lengths of life less than 15 months. That is as it should be. The risk to the patient's survival is greater with a distant recurrence. Therefore, the lifetime probabilities should reflect that shorter lifetimes are more likely with a distant recurrence than with a local recurrence.

Of course, the validity of any analysis depends on the validity of the assumptions used in the Markov model. Recall that the Markov model shown in Figure 12.17 is called stationary because the transition probabilities are assumed to not change as the patient ages. For example, the patient's mortality rate after successful treatment is set equal to 0.0067/month. This value is used as the transition probability between the **Local recurrence** and **Dead** health states for the remainder of the patient's life.

The discussion of actuarial survival models in Chapter 11 described how mortality rates actually increase with age. As an example, Figure 12.20 shows the age-specific morality rates for women over the age of 75 ($R_{75}(t)$). The monthly mortality rates in this figure are derived from the annual mortality rates shown back in Figure 11.14.

In other words, the mortality rates shown in Figure 12.20 are what the 75-year-old woman in our example actually would face after successful treatment of a recurrence. So far, our analysis has ignored how mortality rates change with time and instead used an intermediate constant value of 0.0067/month. How much does this approximation affect the life probabilities that have been computed?

Figure 12.21 shows a *nonstationary* Markov model that does represent how mortality rates change. Note that in the original version of the Markov model (see Figure 12.17), the mortality rate for the **Successful treatment** health state (p_{54}) was set so that the patient's life expectancy would be that of a 75-year-old woman (0.0067/month). We used

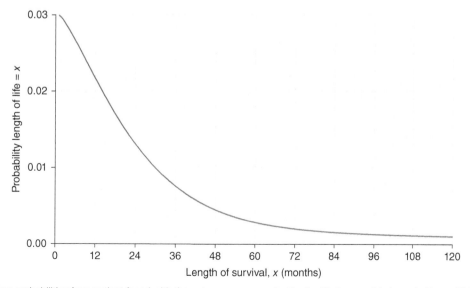

Figure 12.18 Lifetime probabilities for a patient faced with the outcomes represented by the Markov model shown in Figure 12.17.

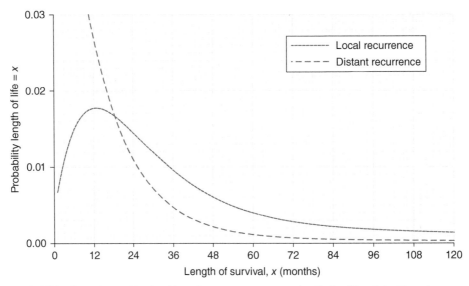

Figure 12.19 Lifetime probabilities for patients with a local breast cancer recurrence and patients with a distant breast cancer recurrence, determined from the Markov model in Figure 12.17.

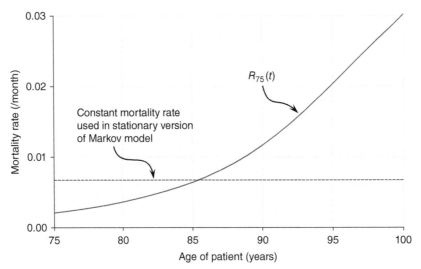

Figure 12.20 Age-specific mortality rates ($R_{75}(t)$) for women based on the life tables published by the Social Security Administration.

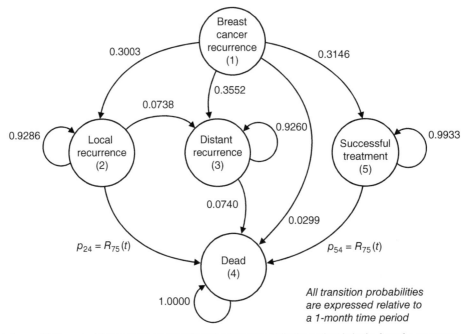

Figure 12.21 Nonstationary Markov model showing how mortality rates increase while the patient is in the **Local recurrence** and **Successful treatment** health states. The corresponding transition probabilities equal the actuarial mortality rates for a 75-year-old woman, which is denoted by $R_{75}(t)$. See Figure 12.21 for a graph of the values for $R_{75}(t)$.

the same mortality rate (0.0067/month) for the **Local recurrence** health state (p_{24}) because the chance of death with the local occurrence would not increase until the cancer progressed to the **Distant recurrence** health state.

In Figure 12.21, the probabilities for both the transition between the **Local recurrence** and **Dead** health states and between the **Successful treatment** and **Dead** health states are set equal to the age-specific mortality rates ($R_{75}(t)$) shown in Figure 12.20. Using direct analysis to determine the lifetime probabilities for the resulting nonstationary, Markov model is more difficult than it was for the stationary version of the same model. Nevertheless, Figure 12.22 shows the result of that more difficult analysis. Figure 12.21 also shows the lifetime probabilities determined using the original stationary model.

At first glance, the differences between the lifetime probabilities for distant recurrences are difficult to see in Figure 12.22 because the two curves are almost identical. That is to be expected. Successful treatment is the only way the patient will experience the actuarial mortality rates if the recurrence is distant. The transition probabilities used in this Markov model assume that the chances treatment will be successful with a distant recurrence is only 12%. Otherwise, the mortality rates for the patient will be that of someone who is likely to die from breast cancer. As we saw in the previous chapter, survival probabilities when death comes from a known cause, such as breast cancer, usually match the constant mortality rate of an exponential survival model.

On the other hand, the corresponding differences in Figure 12.22 increase when the recurrence is local. To see why this is true, notice in Figure 12.20 that the constant mortality rate used in the stationary Markov model is greater than the age-specific mortality rates for a 75-year-old woman until the patient's age reaches about 85 years. In other words, the stationary Markov model, with its constant mortality rate, assumes a higher likelihood of death in the near term. The resulting distortion is greater when the recurrence is local because the Markov model assumes the chance of successful treatment is higher for a local recurrence (45%). Also, with a local recurrence, the patient will spend time in the **Local recurrence** health state if the treatment is not successful. Therefore, the same overestimation of the patient's mortality rate occurs in the **Local recurrence** health state.

How significant are the differences in Figure 12.22? Recall how the concept of certainty equivalents was used to characterize the differences between survival curves in Chapter 11 (see Subsection 11.6.4). The certainty equivalent for a gamble is the guaranteed outcome the patient believes is equivalent to the gamble. A comparison between the guaranteed outcome and the gamble reflects the patient's risk attitudes. Therefore, a certainty equivalent provides a number that measures the patient's preferences for a gamble based on the patient's risk attitudes.

The lifetime probabilities shown in Figure 12.22 represent a gamble between the possible lengths of life the patient might live. Chapter 9 showed how to compute the certainty equivalent for a gamble, based on the assumption of constant risk attitudes (see Subsection 9.3.3). Figure 12.23 shows the resulting certainty equivalents for the lifetime probabilities in Figure 12.22 for different levels of risk aversion. The risk parameter (γ), described in Chapter 9, quantifies the patient's risk aversion in this figure.

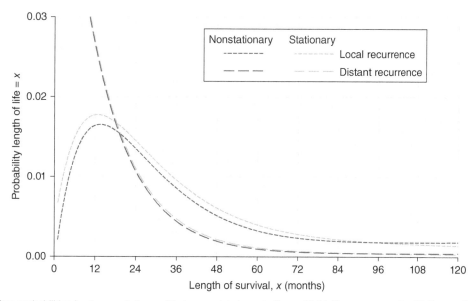

Figure 12.22 Lifetime probabilities for the nonstationary Markov model shown in Figure 12.21. The corresponding lifetime probabilities for the stationary Markov model (see Figure 12.17) are shown in grey.

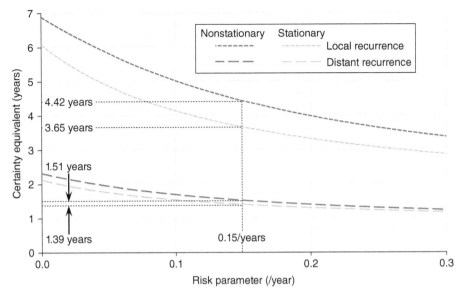

Figure 12.23 Comparison of the certainty equivalents for experiencing the lifetime probabilities for the nonstationary Markov model shown in Figure 12.21 and the corresponding lifetime probabilities for the stationary Markov model shown in Figure 12.17.

In summary, direct analysis of a Markov model usually depends on assuming the transition probabilities do not change – what we called the stationarity property. Figure 12.23 shows that with a distant recurrence, the direct analysis of a stationary Markov model can differentiate between alternatives even when the differences are small. Using the nominal value of 0.15/year as a measure of risk aversion, with patients experiencing a distant recurrence of breast cancer, treatment differences as small as less than 2 months (1.51 years minus 1.39 years) can be found by analyzing a stationary Markov model.

On the other hand, with a patient experiencing a local recurrence of breast cancer, the distortions caused by using a stationary model are much larger. Again using a risk parameter value of 0.15/year, the size of the distortion caused by using a stationary model increases to almost 9 months (4.42 years minus 3.65 years). That is because the longer lifetimes possible with this medical condition mean that mortality rate changes will be larger since the patient is likely to live a longer life. For these medical conditions, a nonstationary Markov model is necessary. Analyzing nonstationary Markov models is difficult using the direct methods outlined so far in this section. This brings us to consideration of an alternative approach called Monte Carlo simulation.

12.4.2 Using Monte Carlo simulation to analyze Markov models

Monte Carlo simulation is the alternative to directly analyzing the mathematical properties of the Markov model. Monte Carlo simulation was first used by the same John von Neumann who co-discovered the utility model discussed in earlier chapters.

Definition: Monte Carlo simulation of a Markov model

Monte Carlo simulation of a Markov model uses a computer program to generate a large number of possible outcomes for the medical condition represented by the Markov model. The probability that an outcome is generated equals the probability that the patient will experience that outcome as a result of the medical condition. Statistical properties of the generated outcomes determine the corresponding statistical properties of the outcomes faced by the patient.

The principle underlying Monte Carlo simulation follows from the fundamental relationship between probability and prevalence. Suppose we would like to know the probability that a patient with a symptom has a disease. As was discussed in Chapter 3, an observed prevalence can inform the subjective concept we call a probability. For example, the usual method for determining the disease probability for a patient with a symptom starts with the disease prevalence in a large population of similar patients who have that same symptom. Presumably, the probability of the disease determines the number of patients with the disease in that large population. Therefore, the prevalence suggests the probability.

Starting with this relationship between prevalence and probability, Monte Carlo simulation randomly generates a large set of possible outcomes based on the structure of the Markov model. By "outcome" we mean a path that starts with the initial health state for the problem and proceeds through a series of health states until the final trapping state is reached. Suppose the goal of the analysis is to determine the probability that the medical condition represented by the Markov model means the patient will live at least 10 more years. That probability would be determined by the prevalence of generated outcomes that last at least 10 years before the trapping state is reached.

Therefore, the key requirement in Monte Carlo simulation is that the probability of generating an outcome must equal the probability that the patient will experience that same outcome. The simple three-state Markov model shown in Figure 12.24 will be used to illustrate how this requirement is met.

This model assumes the patient starts in a **Disease-free** health state. The patient ultimately proceeds to either the **Disease** health state or directly to the **Dead** health state. A transition to the **Disease** health state (0.2/year) is twice as likely as a transition to the **Dead** health state (0.1/year). The mortality rate in the **Disease** health state (0.4/year) is 4 times what the mortality rate is in the **Disease-free** health state (0.1/year).

In order to keep things simple, we will assume that all transitions occur at the *beginning* of a time interval, which will last 1 year in this example. Therefore, the patient's health state during a year is the health state occupied by the patient, after the transition has occurred.

Given this assumption, what is the probability the patient will experience the following sequence of health states representing a life lasting 3 years?

Year 1: **Disease-free** health state
Year 2: **Disease-free** health state
Year 3: **Disease** health state
Year 4: **Dead** health state

The patient starts in the **Disease-free** health state. Therefore, the probability for the first health state in this outcome is 1.0. Based on the transition probabilities shown in Figure 12.24, the probability for the transition that happened at the beginning of the second year is 0.7/year. This first transition kept the patient in the **Disease-free** health state. The probability for the second transition that moves the patient to the **Disease** health state at the beginning of the third year is 0.2/year. The probability for the final transition to the **Dead** health state at the beginning of the fourth year is 0.4/year. This means the probability the patient will experience this outcome is

$$P[\text{Disease-free, Disease-free, Disease, Dead}] = 1.000 \times 0.7000 \times 0.2000 \times 0.4000 = 0.0560$$

Therefore, the probability that Monte Carlo simulation generates this particular outcome must equal 0.0560.

Monte Carlo simulation meets this requirement by the following iterative process. At the beginning of each iteration, a transition from the current health state is randomly selected and the resulting health state is added to the outcome as

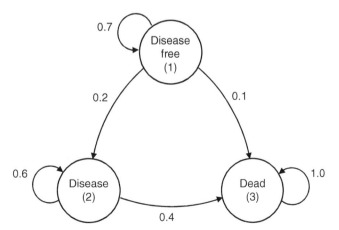

Figure 12.24 Three-state Markov model of survival with hypothetical disease used to illustrate Monte Carlo simulation. The transition probabilities are expressed relative to a 1-year time period.

the new current health state. For example, suppose the current health state is **Disease-free**. The process randomly selects between adding (1) the **Disease-free** health state, (2) the **Disease** health state, or (1) the **Dead** health state as the new current health state for the year.

These random selections are made by first generating a random number between zero and one. By "random" we mean that any possible value between zero and one is equally likely. Since we are starting in the **Disease-free** health state, if the random number is less than 0.7, another **Disease-free** health state is added as the new current health state in the outcome. If the random number is between 0.7 and 0.7 + 0.2, the **Disease** health state is added as the new current health state. If the random number is greater than 0.7 + 0.2, or 0.9, the selected transition adds the **Dead** health state as the current health state.

Notice that a randomly selected number has a 70% chance of being less than 0.7. Starting in the **Disease-free** health state, according to the Markov model, the probability the patient remains in the **Disease-free** health state is 0.7. Therefore, the probability that the **Disease-free** health state is added to the generated outcome equals the probability that the patient would experience the corresponding transition. Similarly, the randomly selected number has a 20% chance of being more than 0.7 and less than 0.7 + 0.2. Therefore, the probability that the **Disease** health state is added as the next current health state equals the probability of the corresponding change in the patient's life. Finally, the chance the randomly selected number is greater than 0.9 is 10%. Therefore, the probability that the **Dead** health state is added equals the probability of the patient will die. This sequential selection process is repeated, using additional random numbers, until the trapping health state is reached.

This example shows that the probability for an outcome generated by Monte Carlo simulation equals the probability the patient would experience the corresponding sequence of health states in real life. In effect, the collection of outcomes and their relative proportions generated by the random process simulates what would be found in a large population of patients facing the same uncertainty as the patient represented by the Markov model. In this sense, a prevalence observed in the generated population would determine the corresponding probability for the patient.

The outcomes generated by Monte Carlo simulation can answer a variety of questions about the medical condition represented by the Markov model. For example, calculating the life expectancy for the generated outcomes determines the life expectancy for the patient. Similarly, the lifetime probabilities described in the discussion of the direct analysis approach, earlier in this section, also can be determined by Monte Carlo simulation. The resulting lifetime probabilities can be combined with the patient's utility for the length of life to incorporate risk attitudes into the analysis of a Markov model.

Quality of life adjustments is one type of analysis that is far more easily addressed with Monte Carlo simulation. As mentioned in the introduction, the possible health states encountered as a medical condition evolves can affect the quality of the patient's life. The onset of disabilities and the appearance of symptoms can be an important consideration when evaluating the possible outcomes of a decision. The structure of a Markov model characterizes when health states are encountered and for how long the patient will experience those symptoms. The properties of those events can be determined by analyzing the set of outcomes generated by Monte Carlo simulation. This supports a version of the quality of life adjustments described in Chapter 10.

The Markov model used to demonstrate Monte Carlo simulation has only three health states and the transition probabilities are all constant. However, the random selection process used by Monte Carlo simulation works just as well with many more health states and transition probabilities that change with time. Therefore, the restrictions imposed by direct analysis of Markov models are not an issue with Monte Carlo simulation. For this reason, Markov models and Monte Carlo simulation has become an important tool for the analysis of complex health care decisions. Chapter 15 will provide examples of the use of this important methodology.

Finally, the direct analysis approach, discussed earlier in this section, still has a role in the use of Markov models. The relationship between transition probabilities and the observable properties of outcomes, such as life expectancy, often is used to determine the values for transition probabilities. Therefore, the direct analysis of the mathematical properties used in Markov models is important even when the actual analysis is conducted using Monte Carlo Simulation.

Summary

1. This chapter has presented a mathematical model that represents both the uncertainty as well as the dynamics of how the outcomes of a medical decision unfold over time. These are called Markov models, named after the early twentieth-century Russian mathematician who first described their use.

2. A Markov model consists of a collection of health states, linked by transitions, representing how the patient's experience and risks change over time.

3. A health state is a collection of symptoms and levels of disability a patient will experience during the unfolding of an outcome. The health states used in a Markov model are collectively exhaustive and mutually disjoint. This means that at any point in the unfolding of an outcome, the patient's condition must be represented by exactly one of the health states in the Markov model.

4. Suppose that a Markov model includes health states A and B. The transition probability from health state A to health state B is the probability that the patient is in B at the end of a time interval if the patient had been in health state A at the beginning of the time interval.

5. The survival probability for health state A is the probability that the patient is in A at the end of a time interval if the patient was in health state A at the beginning of the time interval.

6. A health state is a trapping state if there are no possible transitions to other health states in the Markov model.

7. Let n equal the total number of health states in a Markov model. Then:

For any health state j : $p_{j1} + p_{j2} + \ldots + p_{jj} + \ldots + p_{jn} = 1$

8. Markov independence means that the transition probabilities from any health state are independent of how the health state is reached.

9. A Markov model has stationarity if the values for the transition probabilities are constant.

10. Methods for representing nonstationary transition probabilities:
    - Use an average value to represent the range of values for a transition probability that changes over time.
    - Add health states that represent the different values for a transition probability that changes over time.
    - Use a nonstationary Markov model.

11. In a Markov model, a mortality rate is the transition probability for an arc connecting a health state to a trapping state representing death.

12. A Markov model is acyclic if, for every health state, there is no possible sequence of transitions that return to health state once it has been left.

13. The direct approach to Markov model analysis uses the mathematical properties of the model to determine the statistical properties of the outcomes represented by the Markov model.

14. Monte Carlo simulation of a Markov model uses a computer program to generate a large number of possible outcomes for the medical condition represented by the Markov model. The probability that an outcome is generated equals the probability that the patient will experience that outcome as a result of the medical condition. Statistical properties of the generated outcomes determine the corresponding statistical properties of the outcomes faced by the patient.

Epilogue

This chapter concludes a series of chapters that described the basic tools and concepts used to analyze medical decisions. The discussion started with probability as a quantification of the uncertainty faced in most medical decisions. Chapters 6 and 7 presented decision trees as diagrams that capture the structure of a decision problem. Chapters 8, 9, and 10 showed how the patient's preferences for the possible outcomes of a decision can be quantified. Chapters 11 and 12 presented modeling techniques that represent the uncertainty about the length of the patient's life following a decision. We also saw how to represent the timing of events in the progression of the patient's life.

The remaining chapters apply these tools and concepts to a range of specific problems, starting with the selection and interpretation of diagnostic tests.

Bibliography

Stokes, M.E., Thompson, D., Montoya, E.L. *et al.* (2008) Ten-year survival and cost following breast cancer recurrence: estimates from SEER-Medicare data. *Value in Health*, **11**(2), 213–20.

CHAPTER 13

Selection and interpretation of diagnostic tests

Do that test only if the result could change what you do for the patient.

Anonymous

This precept challenges clinicians to be thoughtful about ordering tests. How to meet this challenge is the subject of this chapter. It will provide a logical, patient-centered approach to deciding when to do a test, when to do nothing, and when to start treatment.

13.1 Introduction

The clinical principle behind the threshold model is easy to grasp: "Do a test only if the results could change your mind about the next step."

Applying this principle to clinical practice takes three steps:

1. Establish a probability scale. Divide it into two parts: a "Treat" range and a "Do Not Treat" range. The dividing point is the treatment threshold probability, the point of indifference between "treat" and "do not treat."
2. Determine the patient's probability of the target condition.
3. Ask, "if I do a test, could the patient's probability cross the treatment threshold?" Answer that question by using Bayes' theorem to calculate the post-test probability.

Expected value decision making uses numbers to inform choices. Probabilities and utilities are numerical proxies for the clinical characteristics and preferences of patients. Although the logic of the three steps is clear, its translation into action requires numbers and a mathematical framework for using them. This chapter describes such a framework.

The chapter is organized into four main sections. Section 13.1 establishes four clinical principles for clinical decision making under uncertainty. Section 13.2 starts the process of expressing these four principles as mathematical concepts by defining a treatment threshold. This threshold is the lowest probability that justifies the use of a treatment. Similarly, treatment is justified when the probability of the disease exceeds that threshold. Section 13.3 extends the use of threshold probabilities from "Treat or No Treat" decisions to "No Treat, Test, or Treat" decisions. Section 13.4 provides an extended clinical example: threshold probabilities applied to the management of suspected pulmonary embolism (PE). The chapter ends with several shorter sections that address related topics.

Medical Decision Making, Third Edition. Harold C. Sox, Michael C. Higgins, Douglas K. Owens, and Gillian Sanders Schmidler.
© 2024 John Wiley & Sons Ltd. Published 2024 by John Wiley & Sons Ltd.

13.2   Four principles of decision making

The following principles lead directly to a method for deciding when a diagnostic test could alter the patient's treatment.

Principle 1

Seek more information if, and only if, it could change your plan.

Clinicians often start treatment before they know the patient's true disease state. Sometimes the clinical circumstances require prompt action before the diagnosis is certain: starting antibiotics for suspected bacterial pneumonia is nearly always a good practice. The treatment is safe and usually effective, and delay could cause harm.

Based on the history of the illness and a physical examination, the clinician forms an opinion about the diagnosis and chooses between three options: start treatment, withhold treatment, or get more information. Getting more information could simply be close follow-up, watching closely for diagnostic clues as the illness evolves. Often, it means obtaining a diagnostic test. According to Principle 1, the information sought should have the potential to change the plan.

For example, a clinician may order a test to confirm their clinical reasoning before starting treatment. A positive test result would be reassuring but not necessary, but if a negative test result would not change the plan, the test should not play a decisive role. Alternatively, a test result that refutes one's suspicions could lead to a change of plan that avoids unnecessary costs and the risks of treatment. The motivation for getting more information is the *possibility* that it might change the plan. The topic of this chapter is learning how to decide if a test result *could* make a difference.

The next principle of clinical decision making under uncertainty is:

Principle 2

When you suspect a disease but are uncertain, establish the patient's probability of the disease and then choose what has worked best for similar patients.

Often, a diagnosis is uncertain, but the circumstances require action. Based on the clinical circumstances, the clinician decides on the most probable cause and the patient's probability of that condition. The outcome of an intervention in patients with a similar probability of the probable cause is the best guide to further action.

The third principle is

Principle 3

Starting treatment when the diagnosis is uncertain means treating some who may suffer harm – and no benefit – because they do not have the target condition.

Figure 13.1 depicts a probability scale and a visual representation of each decile of probability (see next page). Each point on the scale corresponds to a population in which some patients have a disease (closed circles) and some do not have the disease (open circles). Those who are not diseased can suffer the harms of treatment but get no benefit.

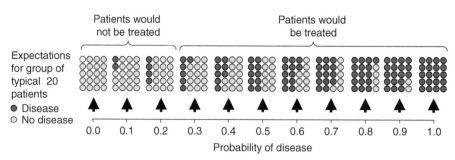

Figure 13.1 Probability scale with visual depiction of each decile of probability. Dark circles denote patients with a disease. Open circles denote patient who do not have the disease.

Of course, in a clinical situation, there is only one patient, but because the patient's true disease state is unknown, it may be helpful to imagine that patient as two people coexisting in one body. One person has the target condition and can benefit from treatment. The other person does not have the target condition and therefore can experience only its harms. The relative proportions of these two people in this imaginary "hybrid" patient depend on the patient's probability of the target condition.

How certain must the clinician be before deciding to act? The clinician must find the best tradeoff between benefit and harm at the patient's probability of the target condition. We will see that the best tradeoff depends on the magnitude of the benefits and harms and on the probability of the target condition. *Finding the best compromise between the potential benefits and harms of an action is the core challenge in medical decision making in the face of uncertainty.* Two examples will illustrate this point.

13.2.1 Two examples of decision making under uncertainty

Example 1: a life-and-death situation

You recall a patient that you saw during your medical training. The patient had a sudden onset of stabbing pain in the right anterior chest a few days after total knee replacement. Despite a normal physical examination, your pre-test probability of pulmonary embolism (PE) was 0.75 (pre-test odds 3:1). So, you were very concerned but unsure. A D-dimer test was negative, which surprised you. You looked up the likelihood ratio-negative (LR-) for the D-dimer test (0.11), and calculated the odds of PE in your patient after a negative D-dimer (now approximately 1 to 3 odds: 1 patient with PE for every 3 with no PE). Your dilemma was whether to send the patient home without starting treatment, start anticoagulation (the correct treatment for PE) straightaway, or obtain a CT pulmonary arteriogram. You analyzed the problem by considering the harms if you made the wrong choice. Suppose you sent the patient home with no treatment. There is 1 chance in 4 that the patient had a PE. A second PE could be fatal. Not treating was not an option, you decided. But if you started anticoagulation, 3 patients out of 4 would not have a PE but would get a treatment that could cause serious bleeding. Failing to treat a patient with PE was unthinkable. So, you opted for the CT pulmonary arteriogram. Thankfully, it did not show a PE.

Comment: You ordered the CT pulmonary angiogram because you thought that the probability of serious harm was unacceptably high if you either started treatment or withheld treatment at a p(PE) of 0.25. Many people represented by the open circles in Figure 13.1 would get a risky treatment that could not benefit them. However, not treating would mean that the people represented by the closed circles would not receive treatment for a potentially fatal disease. Whether to treat is a difficult decision.

Doing the CT pulmonary arteriogram minimizes the chance of harm in a perilous situation. If the test is positive, the p(PE) is high, and treatment is indicated. The high p(PE) means that only a few patients do not have a PE yet get the risky treatment. If the test is negative, the p(PE) is low, and treatment is not indicated. A low p(PE) means that only a very few have a PE and would be harmed for lack of treatment.

Example 2: management of a minor illness

A pediatrician is examining an adolescent with a sore throat. The patient has low-grade fever, a confluent tonsillar exudate, and very tender anterior cervical lymph nodes. The pediatrician estimates the probability of streptococcal pharyngitis to be 0.20. After asking about a penicillin allergy, the pediatrician writes a prescription for amoxicillin.

Comment: Why is the pediatrician willing to give amoxicillin when the patient probably does not have a strep infection? The pediatrician believes that the consequences of taking amoxicillin are minor. Therefore, patients who do not have a strep infection are unlikely to suffer harm from the treatment they do not need.

These two examples and Figure 13.1 give rise to a fourth principle:

> **Principle 4**
>
> The need for greater diagnostic certainty depends on the benefits of treatment relative to its harms at the patient's probability of the target condition.

13.2.2   The four principles as a framework

We can build a framework for decision making from the four principles discussed in this section. You can use them as a set of guideposts about what to do when faced with a difficult decision. The result will be a decision based on informed intuition, which is how clinicians make many difficult decisions.

The four principles also serve as the foundation for a model that goes beyond informed intuition to incorporate tools and facts that are the product of research. One tool is a clinical prediction model for estimating the probability of a disease of concern. Another fact is the sensitivity and specificity of a diagnostic test. Other facts include the natural history of the disease and the effectiveness and adverse effects of treatment. The patient provides other facts: their risk tolerance and their utilities for the outcomes they may experience.

This chapter describes such a model: the threshold model for decision making. With this model, the clinician and patient can use the products of scientific observations to identify the action (treat, get more information, or observe) that is best for the patient. Moreover, that action can reflect how the patient feels about the potential outcomes of that decision. The first and most difficult step is to establish the treatment threshold probability for a clinical condition.

13.3   The threshold probability for treatment

13.3.1   The rationale for a treatment threshold probability

The preceding two illustrations of Principle 4 – one a life-and-death situation and the other a minor illness – had one point in common: the preferred action depended on the harms and benefits of treatment at the patient's probability of the disease. This section addresses the problem of representing those relationships in a clinically useful form.

The interplay of harms, benefits, and probability is a key element in clinical reasoning. Imagine a treatment that benefits 70% of patients with the target condition and causes harm to 5% of them. Only patients with the target condition can benefit from treatment. However, the harms of treatment can affect the healthy as well as the sick. Therefore, up to 5% of the healthy could suffer harm but cannot benefit because they do not have the target condition.

Figure 13.1 is a graphic reminder that at every probability of the disease, the proportion of patients who have the target condition – and can benefit from treatment – differs relative to the proportion who do not have the target condition and can only experience treatment harms. As the patient's probability of the disease increases, the probability of benefit from correct treatment increases and the probability of harm to those without the condition decreases. Conversely, as the probability of the target condition falls, the patient is more and more likely to suffer harm but receive no benefit from treatment (Figure 13.2).

Figure 13.2 illustrates circumstances in which the decision-maker must choose between treating and not treating. The figure shows that the expected benefit of treating is low when the probability of Disease X is low. The reason: very

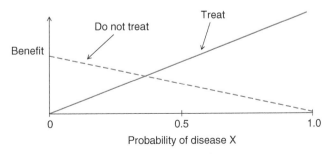

Figure 13.2 The effect of probability on the expected benefit of treating or not treating.

few patients would have Disease X when the probability of X is low. Conversely, the expected benefit of not treating is high, because nearly all patients would not have Disease X and would benefit from avoiding exposure to treatment.

When the probability of X is very high, the expected benefit of treatment is high because nearly all patients would have disease X. At that probability, the expected benefit of not treating is low because very few patients would have disease X and benefit from avoiding exposure to treatment.

Decision making at these two extremes is easy. Away from the extremes, a patient may or may not have Disease X, and both benefit and harm can happen. To decide about treating, the clinician must try to estimate the relative amount of benefit and harm, which, as seen in Figure 13.1, varies with the probability of X.

Assessing the proportion of benefit and harm of treatment is hard cognitive work except at one probability: the probability of X where the two lines in Figure 13.2 intersect. At that point the benefits of treating and not treating are the same. That point is called the *treatment threshold probability*. At *any* probability above it, treating is better for the patient. At *any* probability below it, not treating is better. The treatment threshold probability simplifies the problem of deciding whether to treat when the diagnosis is uncertain.

> **Definition: treatment threshold probability**
>
> The *treatment threshold probability* is the probability of the disease at which one should be indifferent between treating and withholding treatment.

13.3.2 Deriving an expression for the treatment threshold probability

Determining the treatment threshold requires us to be explicit about the meaning of "harm" and "benefit" as consequences of a decision. Just as probability provides the conceptual framework for quantifying uncertainty, utility is the conceptual framework for quantifying what outcomes mean to the patient (see Chapter 8).

Consider the following situation. A patient has symptoms and signs of a pulmonary embolus. The clinician has taken the history, done the physical examination, and received the results of the recommended diagnostic tests. After estimating the patient's probability of PE, the clinician must now choose whether to start or withhold treatment. We can represent that decision problem with the simple decision tree shown in Figure 13.3. Note the labels adjacent to the nodes. Decision node **A1** represents the choice between treating and not treating. Chance nodes **A2** and **A3** represent the probability that the patient has a PE.

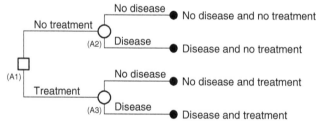

Figure 13.3 Tree for treatment decision given uncertainty about the diagnosis.

The treatment threshold probability is the probability of PE such that the expected utility of the Treat and No Treat alternatives is the same. The discussion of expected utility decision making in Chapter 6 showed how to calculate the expected utilities for Treat and No Treat, which will be the same at the treatment threshold probability.

Implementing this approach to determining the treatment threshold probability requires some notation. Let

$D+$ denotes the disease is present
$D+$ denotes the disease is absent
$A+$ denotes treatment is started
$A-$ denotes no treatment

Then

$p(D+)$ = Probability that the disease is present
$1-p(D+)$ = Probability that the disease is absent

and

$U(D+A+)$ = Outcome utility when the disease is present and treatment is started
$U(D-A+)$ = Outcome utility when the disease is absent and treatment is started
$U(D+A-)$ = Outcome utility when the disease is present and treatment is withheld
$U(D-A+)$ = Outcome utility when the disease is absent and treatment is withheld

The expected utility calculations for the two alternatives depicted in Figure 13.3 can then be expressed as follows:

Expected utility for withholding treatment $= p(D+) \times U(D+A-) + (1-p(D+)) \times U(D-A-)$
Expected utility for starting treatment $\quad = p(D+) \times U(D+A+) + (1-p(D+)) \times U(D-A+)$

The treatment threshold probability is the probability of a disease such that the expected utility of Treat and No treat are the same. Therefore, we can determine the threshold probability by solving for the value for $p(D+)$ in the following equation, in which Utility of No Treat = Utility of Treat:

$$p(D+) \times U(D+A-) + (1-p(D+)) \times U(D-A-) = p(D+) \times U(D+A+) + (1-p(D+)) \times U(D-A+)$$

The value for $p(D+)$ that solves this equation is

$$p(D+) = \frac{\big(U(D-A-)-U(D-A+)\big)}{\big(U(D-A-)-U(D-A+)\big)+\big(U(D+A+)-U(D+A-)\big)}$$

This equation becomes easier to understand if we use the following notation. Let

$B = U(D+A+) - U(D+A-)$, where B stands for Benefit

$H = U(D-A-) - U(D-A+)$, where H stands for Harm

Here, the difference between $U(D+A+)$ and $U(D+A-)$ is the net benefit of treatment in the patient who has the target disease. Likewise, the difference between $U(D-A-)$ and $U(D-A+)$ is the harm done by treatment if the patient does not have the disease. Note that both B and H are *net effects* or the *absolute risk differences* of treatment. For example, $U(D+A+) - U(D+A-)$ takes account of improvements that occur in the absence of treatment.

> **Definition: the harm and benefit of treatment**
>
> The *harm* of treatment measures the loss in utility when treatment is given when the disease is absent.
>
> $H = U(D-A-) - U(D-A+)$
>
> The *benefit* of treatment measures the increase in utility when the treatment is given when the disease is present.
>
> $B = U(D+A+) - U(D+A-)$

Letting p^* denote the treatment threshold probability, we can then write:

$$p^* = \frac{H}{H+B}$$

This expression for the threshold probability has face validity. If the benefit of treatment is large relative to the potential harm, then p^* is close to zero, and we would treat even if the probability of the disease was low. On the other hand, if the benefits of treatment are small relative to the potential harm, p^* would be close to 1.0, and we would not start treatment unless we were sure of the diagnosis.

Figure 13.4 depicts how the treatment threshold probability depends on the harm and benefit of the treatment (see next page). The horizontal axis is the probability of the disease. The vertical axis is the outcome utilities. The dashed line labelled "No treatment" shows how the expected utility for withholding treatment varies with the probability of the disease.

Expected utility for No Treat $= p(D+) \times U(D+A-) + (1-p(D+)) \times U(D-A-)$

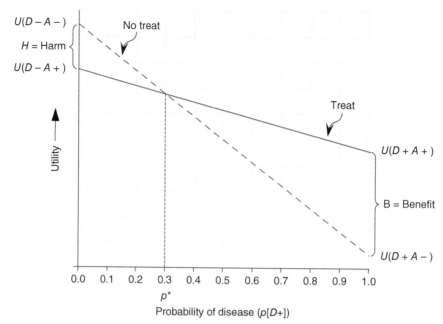

Figure 13.4 Graphic depiction of the relationship between the utility of treating or not treating and the probability of the target condition.

The solid line labelled "Treat" shows how the expected utility for starting treatment varies with the probability of the disease.

Expected utility for Treat $= p(D+) \times U(D+A+) + (1-p(D+)) \times U(D-A+)$

The probability of the disease at which the two lines cross is the treatment threshold probability p^*. The expected utility of Harms and Benefits is the same for Treatment and No Treatment at p^*.

Figure 13.4 shows graphically how the interplay of probability, harms, and benefits drives optimal treatment decisions through their effect on p^*. It echoes lessons imparted at the beginning of this section and in Figure 13.2, which is a simplified representation of Figure 13.4.

The treatment causes net harm when the expected utility of No Treat exceeds the utility of Treat. Net harms are largest when $p[D+] = 0$ and decrease as $p[D+]$ approaches p^*. The treatment causes net benefit when the utility of Treat exceeds the utility of No Treat. Net benefit is largest when $p[D+] = 1.0$ and decrease as $p[D+]$ approaches p^*. Figure 13.4 shows that $p[D+]$ drives the relationship between net benefit and net harm of treatment.

Varying the harms and benefits will shift the location of the threshold probability. When the benefit line is stationary, increasing the size of the harm $[(U(D-A-)- U(D-A+)]$ relative to the benefit moves the threshold toward a higher probability of the disease. Conversely, decreasing the size of the harm relative to the benefit moves the threshold toward a lower probability of the disease.

Result: determining the treatment threshold probability

For a given treatment, let H and B denote the harm and benefit, respectively. The treatment threshold probability p^* is determined by the following ratio:

$$p^* = \frac{H}{H+B}$$

This relationship between harms and benefits is one of the great insights that you will encounter in this book. That the decision to treat should reflect the balance of benefits and harms of treatment is a basic principle of clinical practice. This expression frames this principle in terms of harms and benefits that can be quantified using the concepts described earlier in this chapter. It personalizes the decision for two reasons. First, the treatment threshold probability (p^*) can depend on the patient's utilities for the outcome states they may experience downstream from the decision. Second, whether the patient's probability of the disease is above or below the threshold probability drives the treatment decision.

These observations have some important implications:

- When benefits are high and harms are low, we should be willing to treat even when the probability of the target condition is well below the outcome of a coin flip. Recall the earlier case of treating an adolescent with a sore throat with amoxicillin, a safe drug.
- When benefits are low and harms are high, we should be cautious about starting treatment unless we are quite sure that the patient has the target condition. Getting more information, e.g., doing a biopsy of a lung mass may be the best action, as in confirming a suspected cancer diagnosis.
- When the benefits equal the harms, the treatment threshold probability is 0.50. The benefits of most treatments exceed their harms, which means the treatment threshold probability will often be less than 0.50.

Finally, as an example of what we have discussed in this section, consider the decision about when to give an antibiotic for suspected pneumococcal pneumonia. Antibiotics are generally safe for those who are not allergic to them and usually cure pneumococcal pneumonia. With minimal harms and a large benefit, the treatment threshold probability should be low. The conclusion: if you have a good reason to suspect pneumococcal pneumonia, you should start an antibiotic.

13.3.3 Heuristics for setting a treatment threshold probability

If asked, clinicians do have subjective treatment threshold probabilities. The author has given medical grand rounds on the diagnosis and treatment of suspected PE to audiences of experienced clinicians. Anticoagulation, the standard treatment for PE, is life-saving but sometimes leads to fatal bleeding. Early in these talks, he asked members of the audience to write down the lowest probability of suspected PE at which they would give anticoagulation, in effect disclosing their treatment threshold probability. Similar numbers of clinicians raised their hands for each decile of probability from 10–20 to 80–90. Perhaps the wide range of threshold probabilities would have been narrower if the clinicians had taken the following formal approach to formulating a treatment threshold probability for PE:

Think about the dangers of making a mistake: either treating when the patient does not have a PE or withholding treatment when the patient does have a PE. Which mistake is worse, and why? How much worse? This line of thinking may help you answer the following question:

"At what probability of PE would I be indifferent between treating and withholding treatment?"

Test the strength of your convictions: "Would I really be willing to withhold treatment if the probability of the disease was just below my threshold probability? Would I be willing to treat if the probability of the disease were just above the threshold probability?"

Looking beyond a purely subjective estimate, clinicians could use this relationship to guide their thinking:

$$p^* = \frac{H}{H + B}$$

Note that the right side of this expression is a ratio. The denominator is the sum of the harms and benefits. But for many treatments, the harms are much less than the benefits. Therefore, often we can approximate our expression for the threshold probability as follows:

$$p^* \approx \frac{H}{B}$$

This simple expression suggests that we can think about the threshold probability as reflecting the relative importance of errors of commission and errors of omission. What we call the harm of a test result measures the loss to a patient when subjected unnecessarily to the treatment. Subjecting a patient to this harm would be an error of commission. What we call the benefit of a test result measures the gain to a patient from receiving the treatment when they have the targeted disease. Withholding this benefit would be an error of omission.

Consider the following heuristic for determining a treatment threshold probability:

$$p^* \approx \frac{\text{Errors of comission}}{\text{Errors of omission}} \approx \frac{\text{Overtreatment}}{\text{Undertreatment}}$$

If you think undertreatment is 10 times worse than overtreatment, your treatment threshold probability is 0.10.

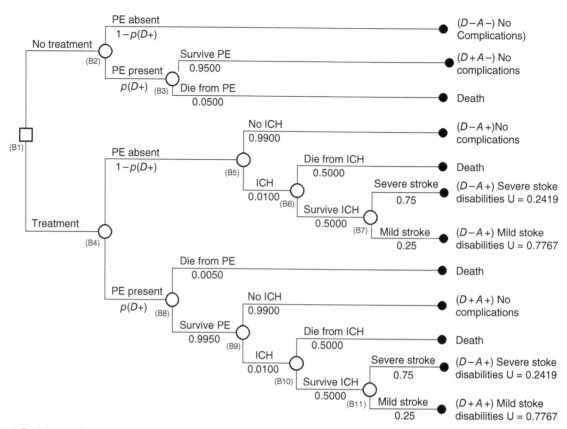

Figure 13.5 Decision tree for estimating the treatment threshold probability for pulmonary embolism. The initial decision node **B1** represents the decision whether to withhold or start treatment. The open circular chance nodes **B2** and **B4** represent the uncertainty about whether the patient has had a PE. Note that node **B2** leads to two states: *D−A−* and *D+A−* and Node **B4** leads to *D−A+* and *D+A+*.

13.3.4 Determining the treatment threshold probability for pulmonary embolism – a formal approach

To illustrate the treatment threshold probability model, we will use suspected PE, a common high-stakes diagnostic problem with a well-developed body of evidence. The estimated annual US death toll from PE is 100 000. The most common findings leading to suspicion of PE are chest pain (typically sharp and increased by a deep breath), shortness of breath, unilateral leg pain, tenderness, warmth, and swelling. A history of cancer, blood clots, and recent immobility are common settings for PE.

The first step in a formal decision analysis is to construct a decision tree, as shown in Figure 13.5.

D−A−: The patient who does not have a PE and does not receive treatment faces the outcome of *Survival without complications*, the most desirable outcome state. The utility for this outcome is $U(D−A−)$.

D+A−: The chance node **B3** represents the uncertainty faced by the patient who has a PE but does not receive treatment. The expected value for this chance node is the outcome utility $U(D+A−)$ that we will use in our treatment threshold probability calculation. The expected utility at node **B3** is $p[\text{survive PE}] \times 1.0 + p[\text{die of PE}] \times 0$. The probability of death from untreated PE is uncertain since treatment of PE has become mandatory. The death rate for untreated PE was 30% 60 years ago, but the general care of very sick patients has improved and patients are now more likely to survive. This analysis assumes a 5% mortality rate for untreated PE. A sensitivity analysis (Figure 13.17) appears in Section 13.7.

D−A+: A similar calculation will determine the expected utility for chance node **B5**, which represents what happens if the patient does not have a PE but is treated for PE. However, the outcomes of treatment are the same as when PE is present: survive and leave the hospital or experience an intracranial hemorrhage (ICH) due to anticoagulation (chance node **B6**). If they survive the ICH (node **B6**), they still face uncertainty about the severity of the stroke caused by the bleed (node **B7**). The expected utility for chance node **B5** is the outcome utility for the term $U(D−A+)$.

D+A+: Determining the outcome utility for treated PE, $U(D+A+)$ involves the branches originating at chance node **B8** in the decision tree. If PE is present, the patient may die of PE (chance node **B8**). The patient who survives the PE may leave the hospital or may experience an ICH, which will cause either death or a stroke. The outcome utility $U(D+A+)$ is the expected utility for chance node **B8**.

The branch probabilities for the decision tree shown in Figure 13.5 and Table 13.1 are taken from two sources: randomized trials of drugs to treat PE and DVT and observational data sets. The patients from these two sources may differ. Participants in randomized trials of drugs are often selected to have few co-morbid conditions that would cause them to leave the study before experiencing a study endpoint. This analysis assumes that the PE-related death rate is 0.5%, a figure taken from a community-based observational data set of unselected patients with PE.

The remaining task is to determine the utilities for the possible outcomes in the decision tree. These are taken from Chapter 10 and are listed in Table 13.2.

Table 13.1 Probabilities for treatment decision for suspected pulmonary embolism.

Outcome	Probability
Death with treatment for PE	0.005
Death with no treatment for PE	0.05
With treatment	
Intracranial hemorrhage	0.01
Survival after intracranial hemorrhage	0.50
Mild stroke after surviving intracranial hemorrhage	0.25
Severe stroke after surviving intracranial hemorrhage	0.75
Survival without PE or treatment	1.0000

Table 13.2 Outcomes and utilities for treatment decision for suspected pulmonary embolism.

Outcome	Outcome utility
Death	0.0000
Survival with severe stroke	0.2419
Survival with mild stroke	0.7767
Survival with no complications	1.0000

The worst outcome is *death* and the best outcome is *survival without complications*. The utilities for these two outcomes are 0.0 and 1.0, respectively. With survival and no complications, the patient in our example would have the life expectancy of a typical 55-year-old woman, an additional 35 years.

If the patient suffers a stroke due to ICH, she will face a reduced life expectancy and a reduction in the quality of her life. The final section of Chapter 10 used the example of the four outcomes in Table 13.2 to show how to assess a patient's outcome utilities, taking account of the patient's risk attitudes and preferences for the quality of their life. The outcome utilities determined in that example are shown in Table 13.2.

We now have what we need to calculate the expected utilities for the four outcome states. Table 13.3 is based on the decision tree (Figure 13.5). In Table 13.3, probabilities are shown in normal font and utilities in boldface. Refer to Figure 13.5 for help in understanding the calculations.

Table 13.3 Path probabilities and utilities for decision tree for suspected pulmonary embolism.

Outcome	Calculation	Expected utility
$U(D-A-)=$	$+1.0000 \times \mathbf{1.0000}=$	1.0000
$U(D+A-)=$	$+0.9500 \times \mathbf{1.0000} + 0.0500 \times \mathbf{0.0000}=$	0.9500
$U(D-A+)=$	$+0.9900 \times \mathbf{1.0000} + 0.0100 \times 0.5000 \times \mathbf{0.0000} + 0.0100 \times 0.5000 \times 0.7500 \times \mathbf{0.2419}$	
	$\quad +0.0100 \times 0.5000 \times 0.2500 \times \mathbf{0.7767} =$	0.9919
$U(D+A+)=$	$+0.0050 \times \mathbf{0.0000} + 0.9950 \times 0.9900 \times \mathbf{1.0000}$	
	$\quad +0.9950 \times 0.0100 \times 0.5000 \times \mathbf{0.0000} + 0.9950 \times 0.0100 \times 0.5000 \times 0.7500 \times \mathbf{0.2419}$	
	$\quad +0.9950 \times 0.0100 \times 0.5000 \times 0.2500 \times \mathbf{0.7767} =$	0.9870

The harm and benefit are:

$$H = U(D-A-) - U(D-A+) = 1.0000 - 0.9919 = 0.0081$$
$$B = U(D+A+) - U(D+A-) = 0.9870 - 0.9500 = 0.0370$$

Accordingly, the treatment threshold probability is

$$p^* = \frac{H}{H+B} = \frac{0.0081}{0.0081+0.0370} = 0.180$$

This treatment threshold probability for PE may seem quite low. The rationale for treating PE when its probability could be as low as 18% is straightforward: PE is a deadly disease, and while treatment has infrequent but serious harms, it is very effective.

For the examples in this chapter, we will use $p^* = 0.18$. It is *a* treatment threshold probability for PE, not *the* treatment threshold probability. Section 13.7 reinforces this point by showing how p^* changes depending on the value of several parameters in the decision tree in Figure 13.5.

Readers should take the specifics of the examples as illustrative of how to use a treatment threshold probability to guide clinical practice, not as a guide to the care of patients with PE. For the latter, clinicians should use evidence-based practice guidelines for managing PE.

13.4 Threshold probabilities for testing

This chapter is about making the best of situations in which the benefits of treatment are accompanied by harms. In clinical decision making under uncertainty, the approach to balancing the benefits of treatment against its harms is to choose the action that maximizes the patient's expected utility at the patient's $p[D]$. The focus of this chapter has been the treatment threshold probability (p^*), which governs the Treat-No Treat decision. Getting more information is the clinician's third option. The topic now shifts to choosing between taking no action, ordering a test, or starting treatment.

13.4.1 The criteria for doing a test
Criterion 1. Test when the pre-test probability is *below* the treatment threshold and the post-test probability after a positive test would be above the treatment threshold

Criterion 2. Test when the pre-test probability is *above* the treatment threshold and the post-test probability after a negative test would be *below* the treatment threshold:

> The rationale for these criteria is **Principle 1**: *seek more information if, and only if, a test result could change your plan.*

Criterion 1 and Criterion 2 restate the teaching precept that you should do a test if and only if a test result could change your management of the patient. This precept is easy to remember, but potentially difficult to use in practice because it does not address the particulars of the patient's situation. Ideally, the approach would include factors like the effect of treatment, the patient's probability of the target condition, the sensitivity and specificity of the test, and how the patient feels about potential downstream health states. The next topic is a method that uses these factors to inform the decision to do a test.

13.4.2 A method for deciding when to perform a diagnostic test
The potential for treatment-related harm is a recurring theme in this chapter. The decision maker's goal is to optimize the balance of harms and benefits at the patient's probability of the target condition (Principle 4). The basic strategy for optimizing care is to choose the option that maximizes the patient's expected utility. In this section, we learn how to make utility-maximizing decisions about when to get more information. The simple tree shown in Figure 13.6 represents the choice between do not treat, do a test, and treat.

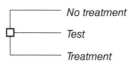

Figure 13.6 Decision tree for choosing between no treatment, test, and treat.

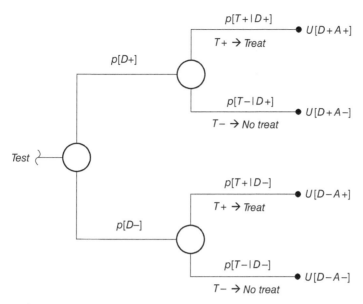

Figure 13.7 Outcomes of the Test option.

To decide between these three alternatives, we must calculate the expected utility of each option and act upon the one with the highest expected utility at each probability of the target condition. Here is an opportunity to take a short-cut. Instead of calculating the expected utility at each probability, we divide the probability scale into three zones, one for No Treat, one for Test, and one for Treat. As with the treatment threshold probability (Section 13.2), the action with the highest expected utility will be the same within each zone: No Treat, Test, or Treat. On the probability scale, the transition from the No Treat zone to the Test zone is a threshold probability, as is the transition from Test to Treat. If we identify these two thresholds, we simplify the task of choosing between No Treat, Test, and Treat.

Figure 13.7 depicts the outcomes of the Test option. The probabilities at the chance nodes that depict the outcome of the test are written in conditional probability notation. For example, if the patient is diseased and the test is positive, the probability of the test being positive is the conditional probability, $p[T+|D+]$ ("probability of a positive test given that the disease is present"), also known as the sensitivity (abbreviated as SE). To simplify the notation in the rest of this chapter, we will use the abbreviations SE for sensitivity and SP for specificity.

Recall the following definitions from Chapters 4 and 5:

Target condition present	Target condition absent
$p[T+|D+]$ = sensitivity (SE)	$p[T-|D-]$ = specificity (SP)
$p[T-|D+]$ = 1−sensitivity (1−SE)	$p[T+|D-]$ = 1−specificity (1−SP)

Using this notation, we may calculate the expected utility of the test option portrayed in Figure 13.7. A+ denotes Treat, and A− denotes No Treat, and we assume that the result of the test will determine the treatment.

$$EU[\text{Test}] = p[D+] \times SE \times U[D+A+] + p[D+] \times [1-SE] \times U[D+A-]$$
$$+ (1-p[D+]) \times [1-SP] \times U[D-A+] + (1-p[D+]) \times SP \times U[D-A-]$$

The equations for the expected utility of the No treat (A−) and Treat (A+) options are obtained by averaging out at the chance nodes in the trees for these options (Figures 13.8 and 13.9, see next page). Similar equations were used earlier in this chapter to derive the expression for the treatment threshold probability.

$$EU[\text{No Treat}] = EU[A-] = p[D+] \times U[D+A-] + (1-p[D+]) \times U[D-A-]$$
$$EU[\text{treat}] \quad = EU[A+] = p[D+] \times U[D+A+] + (1-p[D+]) \times U[D-A+]$$

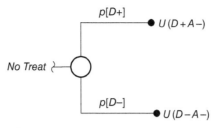

Figure 13.8 Expected outcomes for the No treat option.

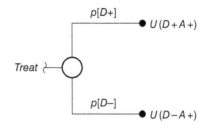

Figure 13.9 Expected outcomes for the Treat option.

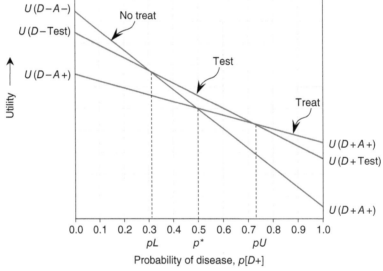

Figure 13.10 Graphical representation of equations for EU[Test], EU[No Treat], and EU[Treat].

Figure 13.10 represents the equations for EU[Test], EU[A-], and EU[A+] graphically by plotting the expected utility of the decision alternatives (vertical axes) against $p[D+]$, the probability of the target condition (horizontal axis). Each of the lines intersects the vertical axes at a point determined by the utility of one of the disease-treatment states and, in the case of the testing option, also by the SE and SP of the test. The points of intersection with the vertical axes determine the slope of the lines and, therefore, where they intersect. The points of intersection determine the testing threshold probabilities.

To maximize the patient's utility, the clinician should choose the alternative that has the highest expected utility at each $p[D+]$. Figure 13.10 shows that, given the slopes of the Test, Treat, And No Treat lines and the $p[D+]$ where they intersect, the preferred option depends on the probability of the target condition ($p[D+]$).

Low probability of the disease: Below a certain probability (the No Treat-Test threshold, pL), observation without treatment (No Treat) has the highest expected utility. Below pL, the post-test probability after a positive test result would still be below the treatment threshold probability (p*). Management would not change. Note that pL indicates the lower testing threshold.

High probability of the disease: Above a certain probability (the Test-Treat threshold, pU), treatment has the highest expected utility. Above pU, the post-test probability after a negative test result would still be above the treatment threshold probability (p*). Management would not change. Note that pU indicates the upper testing threshold.

Intermediate probability of the disease: Between pL and pU, testing has the highest expected utility; the post-test probability could cross the treatment threshold and alter the decision to treat or not treat. Above p*, this outcome would require a negative test result; below p*, it would require a positive test result.

To recapitulate, you should recommend, and the patient should prefer, the alternative with the highest expected utility at the patient's probability of the target condition ($p[D+]$). The uppermost lines in Figure 13.10 represent the expected utilities of the No Treat, Test, and Treat options at the probabilities of the disease for which they are the options with the highest expected utility.

Definitions

pL: the No Treat-Test threshold probability
pU: the Test-Treat threshold probability

In these abbreviations, p stands for probability and *L* and *U* stand for the lower (No Treat-Test) and upper (Test-Treat) treatment threshold probabilities.

13.4.3   Equations for calculating testing thresholds

We next derive expressions for calculating pL and pU. They are important because they define the zones of probability at which No Treat, Test, or Treat has the highest expected utility and should be the preferred option at the patient's $p[D]$.

Definition

No Treat-Test threshold (pL): The minimum probability at which the Test option has the highest expected utility. At pL, No Treat and Test have the same expected utility.

If the patient's initial pre-test probability of the disease falls below the No Treat-test threshold probability (pL), the post-test probability after a positive test result ($p[D+\,|\,T+]$) would still fall below the treatment threshold ($p*$), and the test result would not affect the decision to withhold treatment. If pL is the pre-test probability, the post-test probability after a positive test is the treatment threshold probability. Note a key distinction: $p*$ is a *treatment* threshold probability, while pL is a *testing* threshold probability.

Definition

Test-Treat threshold (pU): The maximum probability at which the Test option has the highest expected utility. At pU, Treat and Test have the same expected utility.

Referring again to Figure 13.10, when the probability of the target condition is above the Test-Treat threshold probability (pU), Treat has the highest expected utility. Above pU, the post-test probability after a negative test result would be above the treatment threshold probability ($p*$), and the test result would not affect the decision to treat. If pU is the pre-test probability, the post-test probability after a negative test is the treatment threshold, $p*$.

Identifying the preferred action (do nothing, test or treat) simply requires knowing pL and pU and the pre-test probability. The next step is to derive expressions for pL and pU as follows:

Recall the equations for solving the trees for the No Treat, Test, and Treat decisions:

No Treat: $EU[A-] = p[D+] \times U[D+A-] + (1-p[D+]) \times U[D-A-]$

Test: $EU[\text{Test}] = p[D+] \times SE \times U[D+A+] + p[D+] \times [1-SE] \times U[D+A-]$
$$+ (1-p[D+]) \times (1-SP) \times U[D-A+] + (1-p[D+]) \times SP \times U[D-A-]$$

Treat: $EU[A+] = p[D+] \times U[D+A+] + (1-p[D+]) \times U[D-A+]$

At the No Treat-Test threshold probability (pL) for $p[D+]$, the expected utility of the "No Treat" option is, by definition, equal to the expected utility of the "Test" option. To determine pL, we set the right sides of the No Treat and Test equations equal to each other and rearrange terms to obtain the following equation that can be solved for pL.

$$pL \times \{SE \times U[D+A+] + (1-SE) \times U[D+A-] - U[D+A-]\}$$
$$= [1-pL] \times \{U[D-A-] - (1-SP) \times U[D-A+] - SP \times U[D-A-]\}$$

This expression may be simplified by rearranging terms and substituting the following relationships:

$H = U[D-A-] - U[D-A+]$, the harms of treating patients without the target condition
$B = U[D+A+] - U[D+A-]$ the benefits of treating patients with the target condition

The result is this equation: $pL \times (SE \times B) = (1-pL) \times ([1-SP] \times H)$
Solving this expression for pL

$$pL = \frac{(1-SP) \times H}{(1-SP) \times H + SE \times B}$$

Similarly, set the Test Equation equal to the Treat Equation and solve for pU

$$pU = \frac{(SP) \times H}{(SP) \times H + (1-SE) \times B}$$

These equations for pL and pU do not contain p^*, the treatment threshold probability, but they can be reformulated in terms of p^* which is related to H and B, the harms and benefits of treatment (from Section 13.3). From the following relationship, pL and pU may be obtained in terms of p^*.

$$p^* = \frac{H}{H+B}$$

This equation for p^* can be solved for B, expressing B in terms of H and p^*, and, similarly, solved for H. Substituting the expressions for B and H in the preceding equations for pL and pU, we obtain the following relationships between p^* and pL and pU.

$$pL = \frac{(1-SP) \times p^*}{(1-SP) \times p^* + SE \times (1-p^*)}$$
$$pU = \frac{(SP) \times p^*}{(SP) \times p^* + (1-SE) \times (1-p^*)}$$

Do these equations have face validity? Imagine an exceptionally good test whose SP and SE are both 1.0. For this test, pL would be zero, and pU would be 1.0. Therefore, with a perfectly accurate test, testing would be preferred for all pre-test probabilities.

To summarize, the derivation of the equation for pL is conceptually straightforward: set the expected utility of No Test equal to the expected utility of Test and solve for pL. Likewise for pU: set the expected utilities of Test and Treat equal to one another and solve for pU. The equations for pL and pU require only the sensitivity and specificity of the test and the treatment threshold probability (p^*). Of course, as we saw in the preceding section, setting p^* is hard work.

However, when someone takes the next step – to represent the completed model in a computer – the effect of changing one or more of these parameters on pL and pU takes but a moment.

13.5   Clinical application of the threshold model of decision making

13.5.1   Test selection for suspected pulmonary embolism: an example

We are now prepared to apply the threshold model to an important clinical problem: deciding when to test for suspected PE. In Section 13.3.4, we showed the process for determining a treatment threshold probability (p^*) for PE. In our example, $p^* = 0.18$. We then derived equations for determining the two testing thresholds (pL, the No Treat-Test threshold, and pU, the Test-Treat threshold) that divide the probability scale into three zones: No Treat, Test, and Treat. These equations require p^* and the SE and SP of tests for PE.

In clinical practice, when PE is suspected, a typical first test is D-dimer, an inexpensive rapid test for blood clotting. If indicated by the D-dimer results, the second test is CT pulmonary angiography (CTPA), an expensive imaging test for detecting a PE. Table 13.4 shows their test performance characteristics. The sources for the SE and SP of the tests are in the references list at the end of the chapter.

Table 13.4 Performance measures of tests for PE.

Test	Sensitivity (SE)	Specificity (SP)
D-dimer	0.95	0.44
CT pulmonary angiogram	0.83	0.96

D-dimer: The following equations determine pL and pU for D-dimer in suspected PE. In these equations, p^* is 0.18.

$$pL = \frac{(1-SP) \times p^*}{(1-SP) \times p^* + (1-p^*) \times SE} = \frac{0.56 \times 0.18}{0.56 \times 0.18 + (1-0.18) \times 0.95} = 0.115$$

$$pU = \frac{(SP) \times p^*}{(SP) \times p^* + (1-p^*) \times (1-SE)} = \frac{(0.44) \times 0.18}{(0.44) \times 0.18 + (1-0.18) \times (1-0.95)} = 0.66$$

CT pulmonary angiography: CTPA would seldom be the first test in suspected PE: it is expensive, it uses radiocontrast dye which can harm the kidneys, and it exposes the patient to considerable ionizing radiation. A high-quality multisite study measured the SE (0.83) and SP (0.96) of CTPA in 2006.

$$pL = \left((1-SP) \times p^*\right) / \left((1-SP) \times p^* + (1-p^*) \times SE\right) = \frac{0.04 \times 0.18}{0.04 \times 0.18 + (1-0.18) \times 0.83} = 0.011$$

$$pU = \frac{(SP) \times p^*}{(SP) \times p^* + (1-p^*) \times (1-SE)} = \frac{(0.96) \times 0.18}{(0.96) \times 0.18 + (1-0.18) \times (1-0.0.83)} = 0.55$$

13.5.2   Incorporating a clinical prediction model into a probabilistic framework for test selection for suspected pulmonary embolism

This section describes a sequence of assessments, starting with the use of a clinical prediction model (the Wells criteria) and followed by a blood test for blood clotting (D-dimer) and, if required, an imaging procedure (CTPA). Figure 13.11 describes this sequence.

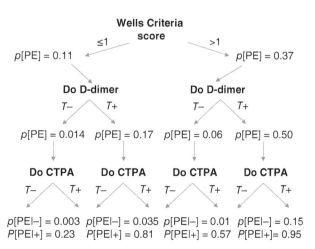

Figure 13.11 Sequence of assessments for suspected pulmonary embolism.

The pre-test probability of PE: the Wells Criteria
When PE is suspected, the first step is to establish the patient's $p[PE]$ and then determine the zone it lies within (No Treat, Test, Treat). The Wells Criteria is a well-tested clinical prediction model for estimating $p[PE]$.

Wells and colleagues identified 7 predictors of PE. Each has a weight of 1. With a score of 1 or zero, the $p[PE]$ is 0.11. With a score of 2 or more, the $p[PE]$ is 0.37. These two probabilities (0.11 and 0.37) are the output of applying the Wells Criteria. For the source, see the bibliography for this chapter.

When to use the D-dimer test after estimating the pre-test probability of PE with the Wells Criteria
If p^* for PE is 0.18, pL for the D-dimer is 0.115, and pU is 0.66 (Table 13.5). With a low Wells Criteria score (1 or zero), the corresponding $p[PE]$ is 0.11, which is just below the test zone for D-dimer. Many clinicians would say "that's close enough to the Test range to be within the range of statistical uncertainty" and would do a D-dimer.

Table 13.5 Test performance and testing threshold probabilities for D-dimer and CTPA.

	Sensitivity	Specificity	pL	pU
D-dimer	0.95	0.44	0.115	0.66
CTPA	0.83	0.96	0.011	0.55

With a Wells Criteria score of 1 or zero and a negative D-dimer, $p[PE]$ becomes 0.014, which is below p^* for treating PE (0.18). Withholding treatment for PE in patients with a low Wells Criteria score and a negative D-dimer test is a common clinical practice based on the low rate of PE during several months of follow-up of such patients. Figure 13.12 depicts the situation.

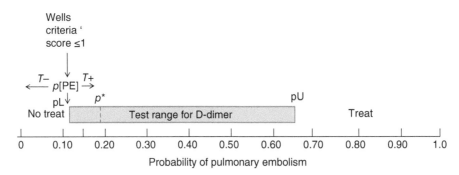

Figure 13.12 Using the Wells Criteria to decide about doing a D-dimer. The blue bar denotes the Test range for D-dimer. To its left is the No Treat zone. To its right is the Treat zone. Per the Wells Criteria, the $p[PE]$ is 0.11, just below pL, which is 0.115. As discussed in the text, doing a D-dimer when the $p[PE]$ is this close to the Test zone is a reasonable decision. After a negative D-dimer, $p[PE] = 0.014$, which is in the No Treat zone for D-dimer.

Table 13.6 Probability of PE based on the Wells Criteria and D-dimer results.

Wells criteria score	p[PE]	p[PE] after positive D-dimer	p[PE] after negative D-dimer
1 or zero	0.11	0.17	0.014
≥2	0.37	0.50	0.063

Use of D-dimer and CTPA in sequence after estimating the pre-test probability of PE with the Wells Criteria
The logical approach to diagnostic testing is to start with inexpensive, safe diagnostic tools and use more expensive and potentially harmful tools if needed to make a treatment decision. The diagnosis of suspected PE illustrates this sequential approach: apply the Wells Criteria, do a D-dimer if a result could change management, and do a CTPA only when it could resolve uncertainty about whether treatment would maximize the patient's expected utility.

The Wells Criteria score is ≤1 As described in the preceding section, a low Wells Criteria score is an indication for doing a D-dimer. Figure 13.12 depicts the post-test $p[PE]$ for a positive D-dimer ($T+$) and a negative D-dimer ($T-$). Table 13.6 lists the corresponding post-test probabilities after a D-dimer.

Low Wells Criteria score and D-dimer negative: After these findings, the post-test probability of PE is 0.014. What is the next step? Do nothing or do a CTPA? The $p[PE]$ of 0.014 is just above pL for the CTPA (pL = 0.011). Therefore, doing a CTPA would be a utility-maximizing decision. After a positive CTPA (*T+*), the $p[PE]$ would be 0.23, which is above p^* for pulmonary embolism ($p^* = 0.18$). After a negative CTPA, $p[PE]$ would be 0.003. Figure 13.13 shows this sequence of events, and Table 13.7 shows the post-test probabilities of PE for the CTPA result.

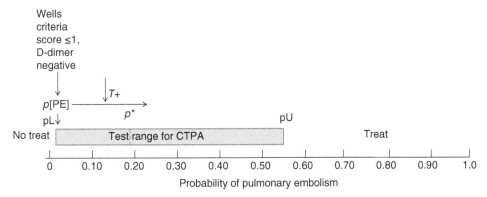

Figure 13.13 Deciding about doing a CTPA. With a low Wells Criteria score and a negative D-dimer, the $p[PE]$ is 0.014, just above pL for the CTPA (0.011). A positive CTPA would raise $p[PE]$ to 0.23, which is above p^*. Starting treatment would maximize the patient's expected utility. *T+* represents a positive test for D-dimer.

Table 13.7 The probability of PE with the Wells Criteria score 1 or zero ($p[PE]$ = 0.11) and corresponding D-dimer and CTPA results.

D-dimer result after low Wells Criteria score	p[PE] after D-dimer result	p[PE] if CTPA positive	p[PE] if CTPA negative
Positive	$p = 0.17$	0.81	0.035
Negative	$p = 0.014$	0.23	0.003

Discussion: Current clinical practice would be to observe the patient without treating them after a low Wells Criteria score and a negative D-dimer. Why, when the $p[PE]$ is 0.014, might doing a CTPA have the highest expected utility of the alternative actions? What are the consequences of Do nothing, Test, or Treat in this situation?

As a reminder, when reading about the three alternatives: with a probability of 0.014, the diagnosis remains uncertain, which means that any action (Do nothing, Test, or Treat) has potential harms or benefits.

Alternative 1: Start treatment. Treating when the probability of PE is 0.014 would mean giving anticoagulation to everyone in a population in which only 1.4 persons per 100 would have the target condition and could benefit. The other 98.6 per 100 would not have the target condition, could not benefit, and might be harmed by treatment. Given concerns about ICH because of anticoagulation, treating would seem imprudent.

Alternative 2: Do a CTPA and start treatment if it is positive. The probability of a positive CTPA would be 0.05. If the CTPA were positive, the post-test $p[PE]$ would be 0.23. Compared with Alternative 1, 23 persons per 100 treated would have the target condition and could benefit from treatment. Conversely, 77 per 100 with a positive CTPA would not have PE, yet would be treated. Therefore, the probability of harm without benefit in treating after a positive CTPA would be lower than treating with a $p[PE]$ of 0.014 (Alternative 1). Treatment would seem safer. Another consideration: with a negative CTPA, the post-test probability would be 0.003, well below p^* and a clear indication for no treatment. With a pre-test $p[PE]$ of 0.014, the probability of a negative CTPA would be 0.95.

Alternative 3: Observe the patient after a negative D-dimer. This would eliminate any risk of hemorrhage but would fail to treat 1.4 patients per 100 with PE, leaving them at an unknown risk of death from untreated PE.

This discussion illustrates some of the considerations in decision making. Other factors are statistical uncertainty in point estimates of probabilities derived from measurements of SE and SP and the output of clinical prediction rules. CTPA SE and SP may differ according to the results of other tests and patient factors (as discussed in Chapter 5). Long-term cancer risk from radiation exposure, not represented in the decision model in Section 13.3.4, would be a concern in younger patients who would face many years of living with a small increase in the risk of cancer.

Low Wells Criteria Score and D-dimer positive: With a low Wells Criteria score ($p[PE]$ = 0.11), the post-test probability of PE after a positive D-dimer is 0.17, which is within the Test range for the CTPA. If the CTPA was positive, the $p[PE]$ would be 0.81, well above pU and a clear indication to treat. If the CTPA was negative, the $p[PE]$ would be 0.035, well below p^* and an indication to withhold treatment. Doing a CTPA after a positive D-dimer would give a clear answer regardless of the result of the CTPA.

Wells Criteria score of ≥2 The pre-test $p[PE]$ is 0.37, within the Test range for the D-dimer test (0.115–0.66). Therefore, a D-dimer is indicated. $p[PE]$ after a positive D-dimer $(T+)$ would be 0.50 (Table 13.8). After a negative D-dimer $(T-)$, $p[PE]$ would be 0.06. Both probabilities are within the Test range for CTPA (0.011–0.55). Since $p[PE]$ is within the Test zone for CTPA regardless of the D-dimer result, the D-dimer result does not help decide whether to do a CTPA. Thus, it would be logical to proceed directly to a CTPA if the Wells Criteria score was 2 or greater. Figure 13.14 shows the situation graphically.

Table 13.8 Post-test $p[PE]$ with the Wells Criteria score ≥2 ($p[PE]$ = 0.37) and D-dimer and CTPA results.

D-dimer result after high Wells Criteria score (≥2)	$p[PE]$ after D-dimer	$p[PE]$ if CTPA is positive after D-dimer result	$p[PE]$ if CTPA is negative after D-dimer result
Positive	$p = 0.50$	0.95	0.15
Negative	$p = 0.06$	0.57	0.01

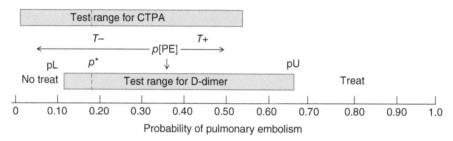

Figure 13.14 Testing for D-dimer with a high Wells Criteria score. The $p[PE]$ when the Wells Criteria is ≥2 is 0.37, within the Test zone for D-dimer. The post-test $p[PE]$ after a negative D-dimer is 0.06 and 0.50 after a positive D-dimer, both within the Test zone for CTPA (0.011–0.55).

The example of decision making for suspected PE shows the power of the treatment threshold model. It provides a transparent, evidence-based approach to the sequence of a testing decision followed by a treatment decision. It shows how to maximize your patient's expected utility by following the guidance of the testing and treatment threshold probabilities. When test results become known, using the guidance of the treatment threshold probability about whether to treat will maximize your patient's expected utility. Said differently, when uncertain about what to do, choose the option that will maximize the patient's expected utility.

13.6 Accounting for the non-diagnostic effects of undergoing a test

From this book's perspective, the role of a diagnostic test is to change the probability of the target condition. Tests do have adverse effects, and they could outweigh the benefit of testing. In principle, given a large-enough utility loss from undergoing a test, the patient would be better off deciding between Treat and No Treat without undergoing the test.

Tests often cause the patient some discomfort, and some can cause very unpleasant adverse effects. Claustrophobia-prone patients can become very anxious undergoing an MRI. Doing a test can delay the start of treatment when the test result is needed to decide whether to treat. Tests cost money. Are these effects of testing bad enough to forgo an otherwise indicated test? In the framework of this chapter, will the adverse effects shrink the testing zone to the point where the patient's probability is no longer within the Test zone defined by pL and pU?

The adverse effects of testing mean that using a test to reach a treatment decision usually decreases the patient's utility for the resulting outcome. In principle, even sitting in the waiting room prior to a test reduces one's utility. The exception: when the patient asks for a test to reassure themselves.

Consider two scenarios. In the first scenario, the patient has the targeted medical condition $(D+)$ and the treatment is started $(A+)$ without doing the tests. (Notation: in this section $A+$ has the same meaning as A+ elsewhere in this chapter). The patient's outcome utility for this scenario is $U(D+A+\text{No test})$. The second scenario is exactly like the first except that the test result is used to make the treatment decision. The patient's outcome utility is $U(D+A+\text{Test})$.

Stating that testing usually decreases the patient's utility implies the following:

$$U(D+A+\text{No test}) > U(D+A+\text{Test})$$

Therefore, let Δ denote the amount that testing reduces the patient's utility for this outcome. That is

$$\Delta = U\left(D + A + \text{No test}\right) - U\left(D + A + \text{Test}\right)$$

Note that since testing usually reduces the patient's utility for an outcome, Δ is usually a positive number.

So far, we have only discussed the utility loss from testing when the patient has the disease and receives treatment. We denote this state by the pair $D+A+$. What about the other possible combinations of the disease state ($D+$ and $D-$) and treatment ($A+$ and $A-$)?

In general, the amount that testing reduces the patient's utility will depend on the patient's actual disease state and treatment decision. To simplify the presentation, we assume that the utility reduction is roughly the same for all outcomes. That is, if Δ is such that

$$U\left(D + A + \text{No test}\right) = U\left(D + A + \text{Test}\right) + \Delta$$

then we assume the following approximations:

$$U\left(D + A - \text{No test}\right) \approx U\left(D + A - \text{Test}\right) + \Delta$$
$$U\left(D - A + \text{No test}\right) \approx U\left(D - A + \text{Test}\right) + \Delta$$
$$U\left(D - A - \text{No test}\right) \approx U\left(D - A - \text{Test}\right) + \Delta$$

These approximations will help us see how nondiagnostic effects of testing can affect the testing thresholds PL and PU.

Assuming that the utility loss from testing is roughly the same for the four possible outcome states, the expected utility for testing is as follows:

$$
\begin{aligned}
\text{Expected utility for testing} = \ & p[D+] \times \text{SE} \times U(D + A+) \\
& + \ p[D+] \times (1 - \text{SE}) \times U(D + A-) \\
& + \ p[D-] \times (1 - \text{SP}) \times U(D - A+) \\
& + \ p[D-] \times \text{SP} \times U(D - A-) - \Delta
\end{aligned}
$$

Figure 13.15 uses this equation to show how the patient's utility with testing varies with the probability of the disease. Notice in Figure 13.15 that the lower testing threshold increases, and the upper testing threshold decreases, as Δ increases. In other words, an increase in the adverse effects of testing leads to a narrower zone of the disease probabilities within which testing has the highest expected utility (Figure 13.15).

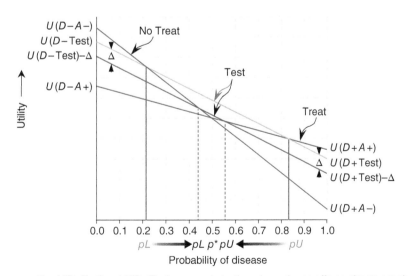

Figure 13.15 The gray line connecting $U(D-$ Test) and $U(D+$ Test) represents testing when adverse effects of tests are absent. The solid blue line connecting $U(D-$ Test)$-\Delta$ with $U(D+$ Test)$-\Delta$ represents the utility of testing when adverse effects (signified by Δ) of testing are present. The left solid vertical gray line indicates the probability of disease at the intersection of the No Treat line and the $U(D-$ test) line. The right solid vertical gray line indicates the probability of disease at the intersection of the Treat and the $U(D-$ test) lines. The left vertical dashed line represent the probability of disease at the intersection of the No Treat line and the $U(D-$ Test)$-\Delta$ line. The right dashed vertical gray line indicates the probability of disease at the intersection of the Treat line and the $U(D+$ Test)$-\Delta$ line. The dashed vertical lines are much closer to each other than the solid gray vertical lines, indicating that taking the harms of treatment into account narrows the range of disease probabilities at which Testing is indicated.

A constant utility loss from testing changes the expressions used to calculate the testing thresholds. Under the constant utility loss assumption, the following equations show how the nondiagnostic effects of a test affect the testing thresholds. In these equations, H is the harm from treatment, and B is the benefit from treatment, as defined in Section 13.3.2.

$$pL = \frac{p^* \times (1-SP) + \dfrac{\Delta}{H+B}}{p^* \times (1-SP) + (1-p^*) \times SE}$$

$$pU = \frac{p^* \times SP - \dfrac{\Delta}{H+B}}{p^* \times SP + (1-p^*) \times (1-SE)}$$

13.7 Sensitivity analysis

Sensitivity analysis tests the stability of the output of a decision model as the model's parameters vary (see **Chapter** 7 for a full discussion). Consider a decision analysis that compares the expected utility of two actions. One-way sensitivity analysis measures the effect of varying one model parameter on the expected utility of the two actions. The analyst starts by substituting the lowest plausible value for the parameter, recalculates the expected utility of the two actions, and repeats the process over the full range of plausible values for the parameter. If the expected utility of one of the actions is always higher than the other action, the parameter is not critical to the decision.

With the threshold model, the main drivers of decision making are:
- SE and SP of the test
- The treatment threshold probability, $p^* = H/(H + B)$
  - $B = U[D+A+] - U[D+A-]$
  - $H = U[D-A-] - U[D-A+]$
- The pre-test probability
- The patient's utility for a health state that they may experience.

In this section, one illustrative sensitivity analysis addresses an unknown quantity, the mortality rate when a patient with a PE ($D+$) does not receive anticoagulation ($A-$). This quantity is needed to estimate $U(D+A-)$ and thus the benefit of treating PE, which is $U(D+A+) - U(D+A-)$. As noted earlier, the only published studies date from the 1950s, when the reported mortality rate was approximately 30%. The current mortality rate of untreated PE is unknown but probably much lower. The author set the mortality of untreated PE at 5% in the decision tree to calculate p^* (Figure 13.4). The sensitivity analysis models p^* for several hypothesized mortality rates for untreated PE, ranging from 3.2% to 32%.

Figure 13.16 shows that p^* increases sharply as the mortality of untreated PE, falls below 5%. This result is consistent with the following reasoning: as the mortality without treatment approaches the mortality with treatment, the value of treatment declines, and one should require more diagnostic certainty before treating with potentially lethal drugs.

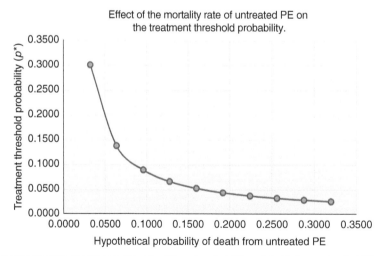

Effect of the mortality rate of untreated PE on the treatment threshold probability.

Figure 13.16 Treatment threshold probability for PE calculated for different probabilities of death from untreated PE.

A second sensitivity analysis (Table 13.9) uses the decision model depicted in Figure 13.5 to calculate p^* for different probabilities of intracranial hemorrhage while taking anticoagulation to treat a PE. A lower probability of hemorrhage, which implies safer treatment, lowers p^*, widening the range of probabilities at which treatment has the highest expected utility.

Table 13.9 Effect of the probability of intracranial hemorrhage on the treatment threshold probability.

Probability of intracranial hemorrhage	Treatment threshold probability
0.002	0.036
0.004	0.072
0.006	0.108
0.008	0.146
0.01	0.181
0.015	0.271
0.02	0.451

A third sensitivity analysis (Table 13.10) describes the effect of varying the utility for severe stroke after an intracranial hemorrhage. The baseline utility is very low, 0.2419 on a scale of 0–1.0, implying a low value placed on very poor quality of life. In the sensitivity analysis, as the utility for severe stroke is increased up to 1.0 (perfect health), p^* goes down, enlarging slightly the range of $p[PE]$ at which treatment should be preferred. This effect suggests that with fewer concerns about the state of health after a severe stroke due to bleeding, a person would want more opportunity for treatment with anticoagulation, which implies treatment at a lower probability of PE.

Table 13.10 Effect of utility for severe intracranial hemorrhage on the treatment threshold probability.

Utility of severe stroke after intracranial hemorrhage	Treatment threshold probability, p^*
0	0.201
0.2	0.184
0.4	0.167
0.6	0.151
0.8	0.134
1.0	0.118

A final sensitivity analysis (Table 13.11) explores the relationship between the incidence of treatment-related intracranial hemorrhage (ICH) and the testing threshold probabilities pL and pU. Here, a rising incidence of ICH is associated with a convex-upward rising curve for the width of the Test zone. The result seems to imply that a clinician should be more willing to test for PE when the patient has an increased risk of a catastrophic cerebral hemorrhage.

Table 13.11 Effect of utility for severe intracranial hemorrhage on the width of the Test zone.

p[ICH]	No treat-test threshold probability (pL) for D-dimer	Test-Treat threshold probability (pU) for D-dimer	Width of Test zone (pU–pL)
0	0	1.0	
0.002	0.022	0.248	0.226
0.004	0.044	0.407	0.363
0.006	0.067	0.517	0.450
0.008	0.108	0.601	0.493
0.010	0.115	0.760	0.545
0.015	0.180	0.832	0.586
0.020	0.250	0.912	0.582

ICH = intracranial hemorrhage.

13.8 Decision curve analysis

Decision Curve Analysis (DCA) addresses the same problem as the expected utility treatment threshold model of decision making described in this chapter: "given this patient's findings, do I treat, get more information, or do neither?" With the expected utility threshold model, the patient's probability of the target condition determines which of these options should be preferred. With the DCA approach, the clinician's subjective threshold probability for treating the target condition determines the preferred option.

The expected utility treatment threshold model may require assessing the patient's utilities for the outcomes they may experience, depending on their effect on the treatment threshold probability (p^*) in a sensitivity analysis (see Table 13.10 in the preceding section). Clinicians probe the patient's concerns about possible treatment, but they seldom, if ever, assess a patient's utilities by the methods described in this book. Vickers and Elkin, the developers of DCA, describe a method that uses the clinician's subjective treatment threshold probability, which might serve as a proxy for the patient's utilities, to decide whether to treat, get more information, or do neither.

The product of DCA is a plot of net benefit (y-axis) vs. the clinician's p^* (x-axis) for the individual patient, as shown in Figure 13.15 (Notation: p^* has the same meaning here as elsewhere in this chapter: the probability at which the decision maker is indifferent between treating and not treating). The clinician chooses to do nothing, get more information, or treat everyone, depending on which option has the largest net benefit at the clinician's estimate of p^* (Figure 13.17).

DCA defines net benefit as follows:

Net benefit = (proportion of positive test results that are true-positives in the total population) – (proportion of positive test results that are false-positives in the total population) × ($p^*/(1-p^*)$).

DCA weighs the potential harms of a false-positive test result by ($p^*/(1-p^*)$), where p* is equivalent to the Harms of treatment divided by Harms + Benefits of treatment. The larger the ratio of harms to benefits, the larger the weight and, by the definition of Net Benefit, the lower the Net Benefit.

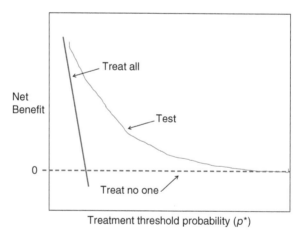

Figure 13.17 A hypothetical decision curve. The horizontal line represents treating no one. The slanting straight line represents treating everyone. The curve represents getting more information, such as a diagnostic test or using a clinical prediction model.

13.8.1 Making the plot of net benefit vs. p^*

The task of making the plot of net benefit (y-axis) vs. the clinician's p^* (x-axis) will fall to a researcher who has access to a data set of many patients suspected of having a disease. The record for each patient in the data set contains the clinical predictors of $p[D]$ for the prediction model or the results of the diagnostic test being assessed. The end point is a plot of net benefit (vertical axis) vs. the clinician's treatment threshold probability (p^*, horizontal axis) for (1) treat no one; (2) use the clinical prediction model or diagnostic test, or (3) treat everyone. A clinician could use this plot to decide between these options at the clinician's treatment threshold probability (Figure 13.17).

The process of making the plot assumes that every person in the data set is treated. The DCA definition of a TP and FP test result refers to whether the patient was treated correctly. The definition of "treated correctly" is a probability *above* the clinician's p^* as determined by the clinical prediction model or test result. "Treated incorrectly" is defined as a probability *below* the clinician's p^*. The role of the clinical prediction model or diagnostic test result is to estimate the patient's posterior probability.

- *True-positive result*: The patient's posterior $p[D]$ exceeds p^*. Therefore, the patient would have been treated correctly.
- *False-positive result*: The patient's posterior $p[D]$ is below p^*. Therefore, the patient would have been treated incorrectly.

To summarize, the product of DCA is a plot of net benefit (y-axis) vs. the clinician's p^* for the individual patient (x-axis). The goal of the analysis is a value of net benefit across all patients in the data set for each value of p^* within a clinically plausible range. For each value of p^*, the process generates a count of true-positive and false-positive results and uses that to calculate the proportion of results that are true-positive or false-positive across all patients in the data set.

To generate a plot of the Net Benefit of getting more information vs. p^* proceed as follows:

1. Set p^* equal to the lowest plausible value, say 0.05.
2. For each patient in the data set, determine if the probability of the target condition, from the prediction model or post-test probability, is above or below $p^* = 0.05$ and classify the result as a true-positive or a false-positive, respectively.
3. Using as the denominator all patients in the data set, calculate the proportion with a true-positive result and the proportion with a false-positive result.
4. Use the DCA Net Benefit formula to calculate net benefit as a point on the y-axis corresponding to $p^* = 0.05$ on the x-axis.
5. Using the data set, repeat steps 2–4 for every value of p^* from 0.05 to a higher but plausible number, perhaps 0.50.
6. Plot the Net Benefit of getting more information (y-axis) vs. p^* (x-axis).

The Decision Curve Analysis approach compares the net benefits of (1) getting more information, as described earlier; (2) assuming that no one has the target condition and therefore does not receive treatment for any value of p^*; (3) assuming that everyone has the target condition and is treated for all values of p^*.

Net benefit of treating no one: Assume that no patients receive treatment regardless of their probability of the target condition. The DCA defines a true-positive (the patient's probability is >p^* and treatment is given), and a false-positive (the patient's probability is <p^* and treatment is given). If no one is treated, no one has a true-positive or false-positive result. Therefore, the Net Benefit of testing will be zero at all values of p^*, which is represented on the plot of Net Benefit vs. p^* by a horizontal line intersecting the y-axis at Net Benefit = 0.

Net benefit of treating everyone: Assume that all patients would be treated ("treat all"), regardless of their probability of the target condition. Using the DCA definitions of true-positive and false-positive, p^* is the cut-point to define whether a positive test is a TP or an FP result. As p^* increases, the proportion of all positive test results that are above p^* decreases, which means that the proportion of positive results that are true-positive results decreases and, correspondingly, the proportion that are false-positive results increases. Remembering the formula for Net Benefit, as p^* increases, the first term (true positives) decreases while the second term (false positives) increases. The overall result is a decrease in Net Benefit as p^* increases.

13.8.2 Use of DCA in practice

1. The clinician must become adept at choosing a p^* that fits the clinical context and the patient's preferences. How do clinicians choose an appropriate p^*? Ideally, they know the harms and benefits of the proposed treatment and adjust them to fit the individual patient. They can use the heuristics for setting a treatment threshold probability as described in Section 13.3.4.
2. The forgoing advice is aspirational. In this writing, little is known about whether clinicians try to characterize their treatment threshold probability as a number, let alone how well those numbers match up with a gold-standard treatment threshold probability.

Summary

DCA has attracted considerable interest. It is the first new approach to using decision analysis in clinical care in many decades. Its value is to bypass the decision modeling – and the utility assessment – required to estimate p^*.

Both expected utility treatment threshold models and DCA share one characteristic: neither, to the author's knowledge, have been incorporated into day-to-day patient care at scale. The opportunities for research are endless.

Summary

1. The topic of this chapter is deciding if a test result *could* make a difference. If the result could make a difference, the clinician *should* order the test.

2. The clinical principle behind the threshold model is: "Do a test only if the results could change your mind about the next step."

3. Starting treatment when the diagnosis is uncertain means treating some who do not have the target condition and may suffer harm – and no benefit – from treatment.

4. As the probability of the target condition changes, so does the relative likelihood of benefit or harm from treatment which, in turn, drives the need for greater diagnostic certainty.

5. The *treatment threshold probability* is the probability of the target condition at which one should be indifferent between giving and withholding treatment.

6. The treatment threshold probability p^* is determined by the following ratio:

$$p^* = \frac{H}{H+B}$$

where H is the net harm from treatment and B is the net benefit from treatment.

7. Two testing thresholds divide the probability scale into three zones: No Treat, Test, and Treat. The testing thresholds are determined by the treatment threshold probability and the sensitivity and specificity of the test.

8. The harms of a test narrow the range of probabilities within which testing should be preferred.

9. A logical approach to diagnostic testing is to start with inexpensive, safe diagnostic tools and use more expensive and potentially harmful tools if needed to make a treatment decision.

Bibliography

Cohen, A.T., Gitt, A.K., Bauersachs, R. *et al*. (2017) The management of acute venous thromboembolism in clinical practice: results from the European PREFER in VTE Registry. *Thrombosis and Haemostasis*, **117**, 1326–37.

Outcomes and adverse effects of treatment in a large cohort of patients with VTE followed for one year.

Doubilet, P. (1983) A mathematical approach to interpretation and selection of diagnostic tests. *Medical Decision Making*, **3**, 177–96.

This article describes how the decision threshold concept for test ordering can be extended to tests with multiple discrete results or continuous results.

Gibson, N.S., Sohne, M., Marieke, J.H.A. *et al*. (2008) Further validation and simplification of the Wells clinical decision rule in pulmonary embolism. *Thrombosis and Haemostasis*, **99**, 229–34.

The accuracy of the Wells' Criteria clinical prediction model in its simplest form.

Pauker, S.G. and Kassirer, J.P. (1975) Therapeutic decision making: a cost-benefit analysis. *New England Journal of Medicine*, **302**, 1109–17.

A threshold approach to therapeutic decision making.

Pauker, S.G. and Kassirer, J.P. (1980) The threshold approach to clinical decision making. *New England Journal of Medicine*, **302**, 1109–17.

An extension of the threshold approach to test ordering decisions. This chapter is based on this article.

Stein, P.D., Hull, R.D., Patel, K.C. *et al*. (2004) D-Dimer for the exclusion of acute venous thrombosis and pulmonary embolism: a systematic review. *Annals of Internal Medicine*, **140**, 589–602.

A systematic review of the sensitivity and specificity of D-dimer.

Stein, P.D., Fowler, S.E., Goodman, L.R. *et al*. (2006) Multidetector computed tomography for acute pulmonary embolism. *New England Journal of Medicine*, **354**, 2317–27.

A large, multi-site, carefully performed study of the sensitivity and specificity of computed tomography for pulmonary embolism.

Vickers, A.J. and Elkin, E. (2006) Decision curve analysis: a novel method for evaluating prediction models. *Medical Decision Making*, **26**, 585–74.

This article describes a now widely used method for relating the net benefit of using a prediction model or a test to a clinician's subjective treatment threshold probability.

CHAPTER 14

Medical decision analysis in practice: advanced methods

The reader may be wondering how the principles in this book have been applied in the real world. The framework for this chapter is three example analyses. The first of these has informed policy for screening for HIV, the second has informed clinical evaluation and management in lung cancer, and the third has demonstrated the cost-effectiveness of a promising new therapy. One of the most important examples in current practice is the systematic use of decision analysis to inform the cancer-screening recommendations of the US Preventive Services Task Force (USPSTF) (see Barry *et al.*, 2023; Owens *et al.*, 2016; Petitti *et al.*, 2018). The USPSTF recommendations for screening for lung cancer, colorectal cancer, breast cancer, and cervical cancer all are based in part on sophisticated models developed by the Cancer Intervention and Surveillance Modeling Network (see for example, Knudsen *et al.*, 2021). In each of these cases, decision analysis has informed guidelines for practice that clinicians implement without being aware that decision analysis has shaped the actions they take in their daily work. A remaining goal, as yet out of reach, is to inform decisions custom-tailored to the clinical characteristics and preferences of an individual. The last section of this chapter touches upon this topic.

The purpose of this chapter is to show the reader how the concepts covered in the book are used in real-world analyses that shape daily practice. These real-world analyses are much more complex than the examples used in previous chapters, but the underlying concepts are the same. The models we discuss here have been published in leading medical journals, and each required over a year of full-time effort to develop.

14.1 An overview of advanced modeling techniques

Many of the real-world problems that people analyze are quite complex. In this book, we showed how to use decision trees to represent a decision problem. Analysts typically use a decision tree to represent problems in which all the events occur either immediately or within a short time frame (as shown in Chapter 6). If events may occur at different points in time, decision trees may become very large and difficult to understand. In general, for clinical problems in which events occur over long time horizons (e.g., cancer), events occur repeatedly, or one group interacts with another, the decision tree representation usually is not sufficient. We will discuss briefly several advanced modeling methods that can represent such events faithfully (also see Chapter 12 on Markov models). The publications at the end of the chapter provide more detailed explanations of these methods.

Medical Decision Making, Third Edition. Harold C. Sox, Michael C. Higgins, Douglas K. Owens, and Gillian Sanders Schmidler.
© 2024 John Wiley & Sons Ltd. Published 2024 by John Wiley & Sons Ltd.

14.1.1 When are advanced modeling approaches needed?

The decision about when to use more advanced methods depends on the decision problem. Modeling approaches other than decision trees are usually needed when the clinical problem:

- Requires representing the natural history of a chronic disease (e.g., cancer);
- Has events that occur over long time horizons (e.g., heart disease);
- Has events that can occur multiple times (e.g., opportunistic infections in people living with HIV);
- Requires representing the transmission of an infectious disease (e.g., HIV, tuberculosis, and influenza);
- Involves interactions among groups (e.g., patients and clinicians in a model that addressed how to treat patients more efficiently);
- Involves resource constraints (e.g., a limited number of hospital beds in a model that addressed how to triage patients in an influenza pandemic).

Each of these situations would be difficult to represent in a decision tree. For complex problems with long time horizons, the decision tree would become too large. For problems that require modeling interactions between groups over time, the decision tree is not suitable because it cannot depict such interactions.

14.1.2 Types of modeling approaches

A variety of modeling frameworks are suitable for representing complex medical decision problems. All of the approaches described here use computer-based mathematical simulations. The analysts can implement these models in software developed specifically for the modeling approach, in more general programming software, and for some of the approaches, in spreadsheet software.

The most common type of model used currently for medical decision problems is the state-transition model (see Siebert *et al.*, 2012). This general term describes several modeling approaches that we will define and explain briefly. Interested readers should read the publications at the end of the chapter for more detail and guidance on how to develop these models.

State-transition models characterize the health states of a disease (e.g., HIV) or of an epidemic (e.g., the at-risk population) as a sequence of transitions from one state of nature (or health state) to another. For example, a health state-transition model of the natural history of HIV infection in a given individual might define health states in terms of CD4 lymphocyte counts or HIV-RNA levels. Analysts can use state-transition models to estimate the changes in length and quality of life and costs for a cohort of persons who undergo a particular intervention, either preventive or therapeutic. These models allow for a running tally of all clinical events, the length of time spent in each health state, and the costs and quality of life associated with each health state. These, in turn, make it possible to compute overall health and economic outcomes such as average life expectancy, quality-adjusted life expectancy, cost, and cost-effectiveness.

There are several types of state-transition models. **Markov models**, introduced in Chapter 12, are a special class of state-transition models. They are relatively easy to specify and are used widely. The Markov assumption specifies that the probability of transition to another state depends only on the current health state. Because past history is often important in clinical problems, the Markov health states must be specified with care to avoid violations of the Markov assumption. For example, the probability of recurrence of breast cancer may depend on how many years have elapsed since treatment. To represent this clinical history in a Markov model therefore often requires expanding the number of health states. A breast cancer model might need to include a state for each year after initial treatment (e.g., year 1, year 2, . . ., year 20). Markov models are very useful, but if the relevant clinical history is very complex, the models may require so many health states that they become difficult to develop, debug, and understand.

In such situations, another approach is to use a generalized health state-transition model, often called an "individual-level state-transition model," or **microsimulation model**. These models provide a means of flexibly modeling events over time when a Markov model would have too many states to be tractable. In a microsimulation model, the model comprises specific individuals that have particular attributes (such as age and gender) and can have a complex history (such as a history of a disease, associated treatment, and complications). As time progresses in the model, the history of each person can develop as events occur (e.g., a stroke) with specified probabilities. The approach allows for complex health states, but the model must track the trajectory of each of many individuals (usually thousands or more). So, this approach is often more computationally intensive than are Markov models. For example, see the paper by Bendavid *et al.* (2008) in the list of references at the end of the chapter.

For problems in which the population-wide effects of an infectious disease are important, **dynamic transmission models** are a useful approach (see the paper by Pitman *et al.*, 2012). These models divide the population into compartments (e.g., the infected population and the uninfected-susceptible population), and the transitions between the compartments occur as specified by systems of equations. These equations account for the fact that the number of people in one compartment influences the rate of transition to other compartments. For example, up to a point, as the number of people in the infected population increases, transmission becomes more likely. Then at some point, transmission slows because there are fewer uninfected people to become infected. See the article by Long *et al.* (2010) for an example.

Other types of models

We also note two additional modeling approaches that do not fall into the category of state-transition models. **Discrete-event simulation models** can be used for a variety of applications (see the article by Karnon *et al.*, 2012). In these models, *entities* (e.g., a patient) have *attributes* (e.g., demographic information and clinical history), are subject to *events* (e.g., a stroke), can interact with other entities (e.g., patients and physicians), and use *resources* (e.g., money or a hospital bed). These models allow for complex interactions over time. Discrete-event simulation models are particularly useful when interactions between agents are important, or when there are resource constraints. For example, a discrete-event simulation may be useful for modeling the interactions of patients with parts of the health care system (say, the number of available clinic visits or beds in a hospital) in an analysis of health care system capacity. **Network models** can be useful when detailed disease transmission patterns are especially important. For example, an analysis of how influenza spreads in a population might use a network model that captures detailed relationships between people, such as family members, coworkers, and classmates.

14.1.3   Choosing among modeling approaches

The choice of a modeling approach depends on the purposes of the analysis, the problem under consideration, and the expertise of the analyst. For some problems, several different approaches may be applicable. In the example we will turn to next, we used a Markov model to evaluate the cost-effectiveness of screening for HIV. This problem can also be analyzed with microsimulation models, dynamic transmission models, or discrete event simulation models.

The choice between a Markov model and a microsimulation model depends in large part on the number of health states required to represent the problem. If the natural history of the disease, or the clinical history, is very complex, many health states would be required in a Markov model. Therefore, a microsimulation model may be preferable. In the example of HIV screening in the next section, the screening and treatment Markov model had several hundred health states. Although the model was still manageable, a microsimulation approach would have also been a good option. Analysts often find that the complexity of the model and health condition is not fully apparent until the project is far along. Consultation with an experienced decision modeler is advisable before starting a project.

If a major focus of the analysis is to determine the population-wide effects of an intervention for an infectious disease, a dynamic transmission model is often preferred, although microsimulation models are also an option. A network model is especially useful for a detailed analysis of disease transmission patterns.

The goal in choosing a modeling framework is to use an approach that can capture the necessary complexity to represent a problem faithfully, while preserving its essential features in a form that an expert colleague and clinicians can understand well enough to offer useful criticism. The word "transparency" is often used to describe this characteristic of a model. Transparency is important for both the modeling team and the end user of the analysis. Highly complex models are more difficult to develop and debug. They are also more difficult for readers to understand, and to the extent that critical readers cannot understand the model, they will be more skeptical of the results. Unfortunately, despite the desire for simplicity, most challenging medical problems require relatively sophisticated models.

In the next section, we turn to an extended example of a Markov-model-based analysis of the health and economic outcomes of HIV screening.

14.2   Use of medical decision-making concepts to analyze a policy problem: the cost-effectiveness of screening for HIV

In the second and third parts of this chapter, we illustrate analyses of real-world problems using the concepts covered in the book. The first example is an analysis of a policy question: Is routine screening for HIV cost-effective? We will discuss several aspects of the analysis, and interested readers may want to read the journal article by Sanders *et al.* (2005).

Table 14.1 Steps in performing an analysis.

1. Define the problem, objectives, and perspective
2. Identify alternatives
3. Choose the modeling framework
4. Structure the problem, define chance events, and represent the time sequence
5. Determine the probability of chance events
6. Value the outcomes
7. Estimate costs
8. Discount costs and health outcomes appropriately
9. Calculate the expected value (utility) and costs of each alternative
10. Calculate cost-effectiveness and eliminate dominated alternatives
11. Analyze uncertainties
12. Address ethical issues
13. Discuss results

Adapted data from: Office of Technology Assessment, *The Implications of Cost-Effectiveness Analysis of Medical Technology*, US Congress, 1980.

14.2.1 The policy question

The problem we will assess is whether routine, voluntary HIV screening is cost-effective. This question was important at the time of the analysis because national guidelines for screening recommended risk-based screening in many different clinical situations. The guidelines recommended that clinicians screen people who had behaviors that put them at increased risk for HIV infection (such as having multiple sexual partners or injection drug use). Although this approach seemed as if it should be efficient because only people at increased risk would be screened, it had not been successful in reaching people at risk. Many high-risk patients were not screened and were therefore diagnosed with HIV very late in the course of the disease when they could not receive the maximum benefit from antiretroviral therapy and may have infected others. An alternative strategy would be to screen all patients, regardless of risk. But such a strategy could have high total costs, and it was not known whether routine screening of all patients would be cost-effective relative to practice at the time.

14.2.2 Steps of the analysis

The main steps in such an analysis are listed in Table 14.1. The first step is to define the problem, objectives, and perspective. Then the analyst should identify the alternatives, choose a modeling framework, and structure the problem. Structuring the problem includes defining chance events and the sequence of decisions and chance events. Depending on the condition under study, it may also include defining and modeling the natural history of the disease. The next step is to define the probabilities of chance events, which requires reviewing the available evidence on the natural history of the disease, the accuracy of diagnostic tests, and the benefits and harms of interventions or treatments. If the analysis is a cost-effectiveness or cost–benefit analysis, the analyst will need to estimate costs, and discount costs and benefits appropriately (see Chapter 15). Then the analyst can calculate the expected value (utility) and costs of the alternatives, calculate cost-effectiveness, analyze uncertainties, address ethical issue, and discuss the results.

We will illustrate some of these steps in the next sections.

14.2.3 Define the problem, objectives, and perspective

The problem is whether routine HIV screening is cost-effective. The objective of the analysis is to estimate the health benefits, costs, and cost-effectiveness of HIV screening. We will evaluate this problem from the societal perspective, which considers all benefits and all costs, regardless of who benefits or who pays.

14.2.4 Identify alternatives and choose the modeling framework

The alternatives we will compare are routine voluntary screening of all patients presenting for medical care and a strategy in which only patients who presented with symptoms or signs that suggested HIV would be tested. To choose the modeling framework, we first consider the natural history of HIV. Without treatment, HIV infection causes progressive destruction of the immune system and susceptibility to infections that healthy people do not get. These infections, called opportunistic infections, occur over time as the immune system becomes weaker. As of 2023, HIV requires lifelong treatment. Therefore, to understand the long-term benefits and costs of a screening program, we need a modeling framework that enables us to model medical events and costs that occur over the entire lifetime of the cohort that will be screened (or not screened). Because of the long time horizon, a decision tree is not practical, as it requires hundreds or thousands of chance nodes to represent the uncertain events that could occur over many years. The options include Markov models, microsimulation models, and dynamic transmission models.

For this analysis, we chose a Markov model because we believed it would be more transparent and more easily debugged. In the end, because of the complicated history associated with antiretroviral treatment, the model contained a large number of health states. So, a microsimulation model would also have been a good alternative approach for representing the complex treatment history. Another analysis was published at the same time based on a microsimulation model (see the article by Paltiel *et al.*, (2005) referenced at the end of the chapter). Our analysis did account for HIV transmission to partners but did not model population-wide effects of HIV transmission. A dynamic transmission model would be an alternative for a more complete analysis of transmission, but we wanted to model treatment regimens in substantial detail. A detailed treatment model would be more challenging in a dynamic transmission model because of the large number of compartments the model would require.

14.2.5 Structure the problem, define chance events, represent the time sequence

An analysis of screening must represent both the events related to screening and the events related to treatment that follows screening. We must model treatment because the benefit of screening comes from treatment, presumably earlier treatment than would be prescribed in the absence of screening. An analysis of the cost-effectiveness of screening therefore includes the costs of screening and the costs, benefits, and harms of treatment over the lifetime of the patient.

Modeling the time course of disease

To understand how treatment affects the length and quality of life with HIV, we must model the events that occur during HIV disease. As HIV disease progresses, a certain kind of white blood cell, called a CD4 lymphocyte, declines in number, which reflects progressive immune system destruction. HIV replicates rapidly and clinicians can measure ribonucleic acid (RNA) from the virus in the blood, which is called the viral load. If HIV antiretroviral therapy is successful, viral replication is stopped and the viral load drops, and the virus becomes undetectable in the blood. With successful antiretroviral therapy, CD4 counts generally increase or remain stable, but if viral replication begins again and remains unchecked, CD4 counts drop. Opportunistic infections and death occur when the CD4 count gets low. Although we will not explore these details further, the actual model that we used to analyze screening and treatment contained health states that represented screening status, CD4 count, viral load, and antiretroviral treatment regimens. As noted, this complexity resulted in a Markov model with several hundred health states. The technical appendix for the published paper by Sanders *et al.* (2005) contains further details about the model. See Chapter 12 for more on Markov models.

To illustrate the concept of modeling the course of HIV disease, Figure 14.1 shows a simplified schematic of a Markov model of disease and treatment health states. In the figure, we have grouped stages of HIV disease into asymptomatic (high CD4 counts), symptomatic (medium CD4 counts), and AIDS (low CD4 counts). In this type of figure, circles represent health states and arrows represent the allowed transitions among health states. An arrow that loops back to the same health state indicates that a person could stay in the same health state during the next cycle. The schematic shows the transitions associated with the natural history of untreated HIV, and the transitions to health states associated with antiretroviral treatment.

Modeling screening

Our model of HIV screening must reflect both the outcomes of testing and the effect of treatment on the course of HIV disease. In the discussion that follows, we are representing screening from a population perspective, rather than that of an individual. A possible structure is shown in Figure 14.2. The model reflects the outcomes of testing in a decision tree, followed by Markov models that reflect early treatment in the Screening strategy and later treatment in the No Screening strategy.

This structure, with modifications to make it more realistic, could represent a 1-time screening program in which all patients are screened at the initiation of the program. However, a more realistic scenario is that screening would occur over time rather than all at once. In addition, another important question is whether screening should be repeated. Guidelines at the time of our analysis called for periodic screening of high-risk individuals; the model in Figure 14.2 could not address repeat screening.

To address repeat screening, say every year or every 5 years, we could use the structure shown in Figure 14.3. In this figure, the Markov model is represented in a tree format rather than as circles and arrows as in Figure 14.1. Figures 14.1 and 14.3 show two alternative methods for representing the Markov model schematically, but the underlying model itself is the same. Health states shown as circles in Figure 14.1 (Uninfected, Asymptomatic HIV Infection, Symptomatic

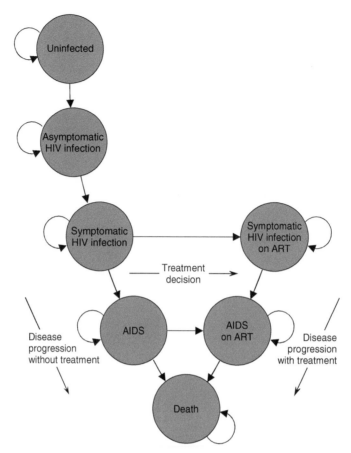

Figure 14.1 Schematic diagram of a Markov model of HIV disease. The circles indicate health states and the arrows indicate allowed transitions between health states. Arrows that point downward indicate transitions due to disease progression. Arrows that point from left to right indicate transitions that occur because of the initiation of treatment. ART = antiretroviral therapy.

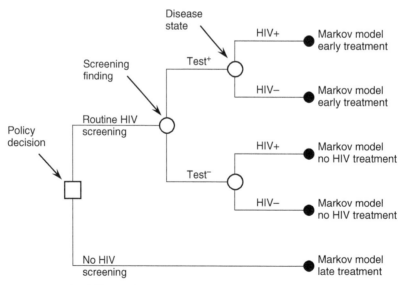

Figure 14.2 Decision tree representation of an HIV screening model. The square indicates a decision and circles indicate chance events. At the end of each branch in the decision tree, a Markov model is attached, similar to the Markov model in Figure 14.1.

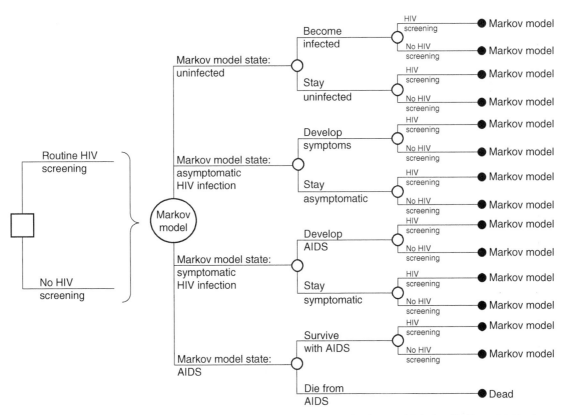

Figure 14.3 Tree representation of a Markov model of HIV screening. In the diagram, the Markov model depicted in Figure 14.1 is shown as a tree structure. After the decision to screen or not, the Markov model has the health states Uninfected, Asymptomatic HIV Infection, Symptomatic HIV Infection, and AIDS. The branches of the tree after these states indicate the allowed transitions to other health states in the Markov model. The last chance node in each branch indicates that screening could occur during that cycle of the Markov model. At the end of each branch, Markov model indicates that the next cycle of the Markov model then begins. Adapted from Sanders *et al.* (2005).

HIV Infection, and AIDS) are shown in Figure 14.3 as branches in a tree, with "Markov" in the circle to indicate that it is a Markov node. In this format, we denote the possible transitions from a health state as branches in the tree, rather than as arrows. For example, the branches from the uninfected health state are labeled Become Infected and Stay Uninfected. These correspond to the arrows from the uninfected health state in Figure 14.1.

In Figure 14.3, we represent whether or not someone is screened as a chance node at the end of each branch in the Markov model, rather than as a decision node in the decision tree. Although whether someone is screened is actually a decision, the standard Markov model can represent chance events only, not decisions. To work around this constraint, we use the chance node to represent screening. We can model periodic screening by setting the probability of screening to 1 in the years that screening occurs and 0 in the other years, or we can model ongoing screening by having a probability of screening each year.

People identified as having HIV, either through screening or case finding, can begin antiretroviral treatment if they are eligible. Figure 14.1 shows treatment-associated health states. We model the benefit of treatment as a reduction in the probability of transitioning to more advanced states of HIV disease or to death.

Our next step is to determine the probability of chance events in the model.

14.2.6   Determine the probability of chance events

When the analyst believes the structure of the model adequately represents the clinical problem, the next step is to specify the probability of chance events (see the paper by Briggs *et al.*, 2012). To do so, the analyst will review the relevant medical literature. This process is labor intensive, but as we note later, the analyst can use the model to help identify important parameters. The model we used for evaluating the cost-effectiveness of HIV screening had over 80 parameters, many of which were chance events.

Although the analyst may not be able to perform a comprehensive review of the literature for all model parameters, they should do so for all parameters likely to be important, such as the probability of transitioning to more advanced

HIV disease for patients who are on treatment, which depends on the effectiveness of antiretroviral therapy. To estimate the relevant probabilities for parameters, we reviewed the available literature on the effectiveness of antiretroviral therapy. This task alone required substantial effort. Other important parameters included the sensitivity and specificity of the tests used to screen, the probability of death by stage of HIV infection, the probability of HIV transmission to sexual partners, and the probability of treatment failure.

Given that a complex model may have many parameters and a comprehensive review of the literature is time intensive, how can an analyst approach this task efficiently? For important parameters, we recommend that the analyst search for high-quality systematic reviews, and then update those reviews selectively as necessary. The analyst may also search for clinical prediction models that help estimate probabilities for specific clinical settings or risk factors. We also recommend using the decision model early in the process to help determine which parameters are crucial to the analysis. To do this, the analyst can perform a preliminary review of the literature and consult experts to get rough estimates of the model parameters. The analyst can then use sensitivity analysis to determine which parameters are most important. The sensitivity analyses can direct the effort of the subsequent literature review. The analyst can use this process iteratively to use resources efficiently in the literature review. The analyst should also aim to estimate a probability distribution for important parameters, rather than a single-point estimate of the probability because such distributions are necessary to perform probabilistic sensitivity analysis (see Briggs *et al.*, 2012).

When the analysts are convinced that they have the best estimates possible for the important model parameters, they can move to the next step, valuing the outcomes.

14.2.7 Value the outcomes

The analysts can now turn to valuing the outcomes. They could use any of the metrics we have discussed in previous chapters, including life expectancy or quality-adjusted life years (QALYs). We chose to use QALYs as our primary metric because HIV and antiretroviral therapy affect both length and quality of life. If we used life expectancy only, we would not capture the effect of screening and treatment, for better or worse, on quality of life. Estimation of how screening changes quality of life is challenging, however, so we also used life expectancy as an outcome.

Quality of life is important in the HIV screening analysis because untreated HIV reduces quality of life, screening may reduce or increase quality of life, and treatment, at least for patients with advanced disease, increases quality of life. The effect of screening itself on quality of life is complex. You could imagine that a person with asymptomatic HIV infection might feel that their quality of life had been diminished by discovering through screening that they had HIV. Alternatively, a person with symptoms of HIV might find quality of life to be improved by effective therapy. Published studies suggest that both of these scenarios do occur.

To estimate QALYs, we had to specify the quality of life associated with each health state in the Markov model. Using the health states in Figure 14.1 as an example, we note that we must estimate the quality of life for people who are uninfected, and for people both on and off treatment with asymptomatic HIV, symptomatic HIV, and AIDS. To do this, we reviewed the literature to find quality-of-life estimates for these health states. Many studies have measured the quality of life with HIV based on standard gambles, time tradeoffs, and with other quality-of-life assessment instruments such as the health utilities index and the EQ-5D. See the study by Joyce *et al.* (2009) for an example of analysts using all of these quality-of-life assessment instruments.

More generally, analysts will need to review the literature to find quality-of-life assessments for the health states in their models. They can also conduct sensitivity analyses to determine how important quality-of-life estimates are for their analysis. For some topics, the quality of life of health states has a large impact on model-based outcomes, but for other analyses, they have minimal influence on outcomes.

14.2.8 Estimate costs and discount outcomes

To estimate the costs associated with an intervention, the analyst must determine the cost of the intervention itself and the costs of any subsequent care that occurred because a person decided to undergo the intervention (see Chapter 15). We include these subsequent costs because they result from the use of the intervention; these downstream costs would not have occurred had the intervention not been performed. In the analyses, we compare these costs to those in the No Screening strategy to estimate the incremental cost associated with screening.

For our HIV screening example, this principle means that we must estimate the cost of screening and of all care that follows screening. The screening costs include the cost of the initial and confirmatory tests and the cost of associated counseling. The analyst should also include the costs of follow-up tests or treatment that result from a false-positive test result, and, if there are any, the costs from a false-negative test result. The treatment costs include the costs of tests, office visits, procedures, drugs, and hospitalizations.

For an analysis that uses a Markov model or other state-transition model, the analyst must assign costs for each health state. We used the literature to estimate the cost of the health states depicted in Figure 14.1. The cost of care increases as HIV disease progresses. Therefore, the annual cost for a patient with asymptomatic HIV infection is less than the annual cost for a patient with more advanced disease.

As explained in Chapter 15, the analyst should discount costs. By using appropriate formulas, the analyst can specify the Markov model so that the model discounts future costs appropriately. The further a cost occurs in the future, the more it will be discounted. If the analysis has a long time horizon, the effect of discounting may be substantial. For example, HIV treatment costs that occur 15–20 years in the future will have less influence on cost-effectiveness than do treatment costs that occur in the first 5 years.

14.2.9 Calculate the expected utility, costs, and cost-effectiveness

Once the analysts have specified the probability of chance events, estimated costs, and valued the outcomes, they can analyze the model to calculate expected utility, costs, and cost-effectiveness. In a Markov model, this analysis occurs differently than in the decision trees that we evaluated in earlier chapters. While a decision tree is evaluated by averaging and rolling back the tree from right to left (see Chapter 7), a Markov model is evaluated as a mathematical simulation that begins at a specified time and goes forward in time until predetermined stopping criteria are met.

For our HIV screening example, we can think of the model as performing two mathematical simulations: one for the Screening strategy and one for the No Screening strategy. Consider the Screening strategy first. The software for the model begins the analysis at time 0 and, as time moves forward, the model keeps track of how long an individual spends in each health state. For example, a person might spend a year in the uninfected state before becoming infected, and then progress through each of the health states associated with HIV disease. The person would be diagnosed as having HIV (depending on when screening occurs), and then be treated. At each new cycle of the Markov model, people either stay in the same health state or transition to other health states according to the specified transition probabilities. Based on these transition probabilities, the model determines the duration of time a person is in each health state. The model also accounts for the quality of life and costs in the health states. To calculate life expectancy, QALYs, and total costs, the model sums these amounts (with appropriate discounting of costs and QALYs) over all the health states. The model also performs the same simulation for the No Screening strategy.

The results of the analysis for HIV screening are given in Table 14.2. The table shows the lifetime costs and benefits of each strategy, based on a prevalence of undiagnosed HIV infection of 1%. We note that No Screening is the least expensive strategy, and the least effective. The 1-time screening strategy costs $194 additional dollars over the lifetime of the person screened and increases life expectancy by 5.48 days and quality-adjusted life expectancy by 4.70 days relative to the No Screening strategy. We emphasize that a cost-effectiveness analysis estimates the incremental benefit and incremental costs of one strategy relative to another. Compared with 1-time screening, every 5 years result in slightly higher costs ($206 per person screened) and slightly larger increases in life expectancy (1.52 days) and QALYs (1.31 days).

Table 14.2 Health outcomes, costs, and cost-effectiveness of HIV screening.

Strategy	Lifetime cost ($)	Incremental cost relative to no screening ($)	Life expectancy (years)	Incremental life expectancy (days)	Incremental cost-effectiveness ($/LY)	Quality-adjusted life expectancy (years)	Incremental quality-adjusted life expectancy (days)	Incremental cost-effectiveness ($/QALY)
No screening	52 623		21.015			18.576		
One-time screening	52 816	194	21.030	5.48	12 919	18.589	4.70	15 078
Screening every 5 years	53 022	206*	21.034	1.52*	49 509*	18.592	1.31*	57 138*

*Relative to 1-time screening.

LY = life year, QALY = quality-adjusted life year. Based on a prevalence of 1% of undiagnosed HIV infection, and includes the benefit from the reduction in transmission (we did not discuss transmission in our example, but it was included in the published analysis). Health and economic outcomes were discounted at 3%, including benefits and costs of transmission to partners. Based on data from Sanders *et al.* (2005).

The increases in life expectancy and QALYs are approximately 5 days per person screened. You may wonder if such a benefit is important. To understand this result, we first note that the analysis assumes that the prevalence of undiagnosed HIV infection is 1%. This prevalence means that of 100 people who are screened, 99 do not have HIV infection and receive no benefit from screening, while 1 person does have HIV and will receive a benefit of approximately 1.5 additional years of life (see the published study by Sanders *et al.* (2005) for more detail). The fairly large benefit to the one person is averaged across all 100 people screened, which results in *per person* benefit of about five quality-adjusted days. Of course, a specific individual either receives no benefit or a relatively large benefit, but our results represent the average per-person benefit for each person screened. Although the per-person benefit is modest, the total benefit from the screening program may be very substantial. For example, a program that screened 1 million people would result in almost 13 000 additional QALYs in the screened population.

We can also calculate the incremental cost-effectiveness ratio of screening compared to case finding from the results in Table 14.2. One-time screening costs $15 078 per QALY gained. This result means that if we implement a screening program, we would expect to spend about $15 000 dollars for each additional QALY gained from screening. In the United States, that would be considered good value. Screening every 5 years relative to 1-time screening costs $57 138 per QALY gained. In our example, repeated screening is a less efficient use of resources than 1-time screening.

14.2.10 Evaluate uncertainty

In Chapter 7, we discussed how to do sensitivity analyses and why they are important. We now discuss sensitivity analysis in the context of the HIV screening example.

The most important sensitivity analysis of the HIV screening analysis assessed how the cost-effectiveness of screening changed with the prevalence of undiagnosed HIV infection. This analysis is important because it answers a key clinical question. The Centers for Disease Control and Prevention (CDC) HIV screening guideline recommended routine screening only if the prevalence of HIV was above 1%. If screening at a prevalence lower than 1% were cost-effective, routine screening might be warranted in more clinical settings.

The results of the sensitivity analysis indicated that screening was cost-effective even at a much lower prevalence than 1%. At a prevalence of 0.5%, 1-time screening cost about $19 000 per QALY gained. Even at a prevalence of 0.05%, 20 times lower than the CDC guideline threshold for routine screening, the cost-effectiveness of screening was approximately $50 000 per QALY gained, which most observers would agree is a good value in the United States.

The critical insight from the sensitivity analysis was that routine screening was cost-effective even at a much lower HIV prevalence than was recommended in guidelines at the time. We discuss the implications of this finding in the next section.

14.2.11 Address ethical issues, discuss results

The analyst should always consider whether the results raise important ethical issues. Ethical questions may include whether a policy is fair to all individuals, whether a policy might benefit one group at the expense of the other, whether the analysis fairly captures benefits and harms, and whether a policy based on the analysis may have unintended consequences. Independent of the analysis we have discussed, other ethical considerations shaped several aspects of HIV screening policy in the United States, including recommendations that screening should be voluntary, that people should be informed before being tested for HIV, and that people diagnosed with HIV should be protected from stigmatization.

The final step in an analysis is to discuss the importance and implications of the results and the limitations of the analysis. The content of this discussion depends on the nature of the problem, the context for the analysis, the intended audience, and the goals of the analysis. The purpose of the discussion is to help the reader understand the insight that the analysis provides and to appreciate limitations of the data or analytic approach.

For our HIV screening example, the finding that screening is cost-effective at a low prevalence of HIV had important implications. The analysis we have described, and an independent analysis by Paltiel *et al.* (2005) had similar results. In part based on these studies, the CDC recommended routine screening in all health care settings in which the prevalence of HIV was above 0.1%, a threshold that was 10 times lower than the previously recommended prevalence of 1% for routine screening. Because there were few, if any, health care settings with a documented prevalence of less than 0.1%, the new guideline was essentially a recommendation to switch from risk-based screening to routine voluntary screening in health care settings. This new recommendation represented a major change in screening policy.

We will now turn to an example in which we evaluated a testing strategy for a complicated diagnostic problem.

14.3   Use of medical decision-making concepts to analyze a clinical diagnostic problem: strategies to diagnose tumors in the lung

We now turn to an example that evaluates a challenging diagnostic and treatment problem in the evaluation of possible lung cancer (this example is based on the article by Gould *et al.*, 2003; the reader can refer to this article and its appendix for details of the analysis, assumptions, inputs, and results). The question is how best to evaluate and manage an abnormality on a chest x-ray known as a solitary pulmonary nodule. A solitary pulmonary nodule is a circumscribed lesion on a chest x-ray and may be caused by lung cancer or by other disease processes, such as infectious or inflammatory diseases. The clinician has many possible diagnostic tests to choose from. This problem has high stakes for the patient, as early diagnosis of lung cancer may be life-saving. Alternatively, an erroneous diagnosis of cancer could result in unnecessary surgery or other treatments.

14.3.1   Define the problem, objectives, and perspective

The problem we will address is the cost-effectiveness of alternative management strategies for patients with a solitary pulmonary nodule on chest x-ray. The management strategies include both the diagnostic evaluation and the treatment. Because there are several possible diagnostic tests, we will by necessity evaluate many different strategies.

14.3.2   Identify alternatives and choose the modeling framework

The diagnostic tests we will consider are computed tomography (CT), which localizes the nodule within the lung, and positron emission tomography (PET). PET scans measure the metabolic rate of tissues; because malignant tumors have increased metabolic rates, PET scans can also distinguish cancer from benign lesions. The strategies to manage pulmonary nodules include surgical resection, transthoracic needle biopsy, and watchful waiting. Surgical resection is the definitive treatment if the nodule is malignant and the cancer has not spread to other locations. However, the surgery has risks, and clinicians would not want to recommend lung surgery to a patient who did not have lung cancer. Transthoracic needle biopsy is a technique for sampling the tissue from the nodule to see if it is cancer. The watchful waiting strategy involves repeating the imaging test (CT or PET) periodically to see if the nodule is getting bigger. If the nodule stays the same size, it is unlikely to be cancer.

We will use a hybrid modeling strategy: a decision tree to represent the multiple possible initial strategies to be compared, followed by a Markov model that represents the natural history of lung cancer and the effect of treatment. We could have also chosen a microsimulation modeling framework.

14.3.3   Structure the problem, define chance events, and represent the time sequence

We start by defining the initial management decision, as shown in Figure 14.4. As shown by the decision node labeled with an A, the options the clinician could choose are imaging with CT or PET, observation (watchful waiting), immediate surgery, or transthoracic biopsy. The decision tree in Figure 14.4 shows the events that could occur after each of these choices. If the clinician chooses to perform a CT scan, the scan could be negative (i.e., indicate that the nodule is benign) or positive, which indicates that the nodule is possibly malignant. A CT scan cannot prove that a nodule is malignant. So, we will use the phrase "possibly malignant" to denote a positive CT. The clinician must then decide what to do about the results of the CT scan; the decision node labeled B shows the options. The clinician could choose watchful waiting, surgery, biopsy, or further imaging with PET scan. With further imaging using PET scan, then the clinician must decide what to do, as shown by decision node D, about the results of the PET scan. Figure 14.5 shows the subtrees for biopsy and surgery, which indicate the events that can occur if the clinician chooses those options.

Note that the time sequence of the decisions is represented by their place within the decision tree. Going from left to right in Figure 14.4, decision A occurs first, and decisions B, C, and D occur subsequently or not at all, depending on the clinician's choice for decision A. We can see from the tree that decision D occurs only if the clinician chooses to obtain both CT and PET.

The decision tree captures the complexity of the choices facing the clinician. We can evaluate 40 clinically plausible strategies, based on different choices in decisions A, B, C, and D.

14.3.4   Determine the probability of the chance events

As in our previous example, to determine the probability of chance events, the analyst should search the literature carefully, seeking out the best available evidence, which is usually found in systematic reviews, and clinical prediction rules for estimating the probabilities in the model. For this analysis, we had to determine the prior probability that a solitary pulmonary nodule is malignant given the patient's history and the features of the nodule on the chest x-ray.

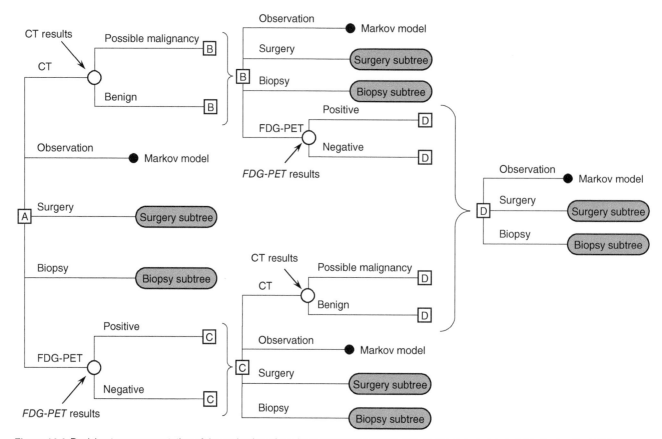

Figure 14.4 Decision tree representation of the evaluation of a solitary pulmonary nodule. The decision node labeled A indicates the initial alternatives the clinician can choose. The decision node labeled B indicates the management choices after an initial CT scan. The decision node labeled C indicates the management choices after an initial PET scan. The decision node labeled D indicates management choices after both PET and CT. See Figure 14.5 for the structure of the Biopsy Subtree and the Surgery Subtree. CT = computed tomography; FDG-PET = 18-flourodeoxyglucose positron emission scanning. Adapted from Gould *et al.* (2003).

Other important information is the sensitivity and specificity of the diagnostic tests, and the probability of the outcomes of surgery and biopsy, including complications. We combined the results of studies of the sensitivity and specificity of CT and PET so that we could maximize the validity of estimates of test performance. We also developed a model of the natural history of lung cancer, which included estimates of the rate of growth of malignant tumors, the probability of death from cancer at different stages, and the probability of recurrence of cancer for various stages of cancer and treatments. The estimates of these and all other input parameters are available in the appendix of the article by Gould *et al.* (2003).

14.3.5 Value the outcomes

Because lung cancer affects both length and quality of life, we chose to measure the outcomes for the management of lung nodules in QALYs. To do so, we estimated the mortality with lung cancer, the effectiveness of treatment, and the quality of life with lung cancer, with lung cancer treatment (e.g., with partial or complete removal of the lung containing the nodule), and with complications of treatment. We also estimated decrements in quality of life caused by diagnostic biopsy and surgery. Invasive procedures will reduce quality of life for a while, even if no complications occur. Modeling these changes is straightforward.

14.3.6 Estimate costs and discount outcomes

To evaluate the cost-effectiveness of management strategies for pulmonary nodules, we estimated the costs of the tests and treatment alternatives. These include the cost of CT, PET, biopsy, surgery, costs of complications, the cost of cancer treatment, including the cost of follow-up care, and long-term costs associated with cancer and other conditions that cause pulmonary nodules. We also estimated the costs of health care unrelated to cancer that patients would receive over their lifetime. We included these costs because a treatment that changes length of life will change the cost of non-cancer care over a lifetime.

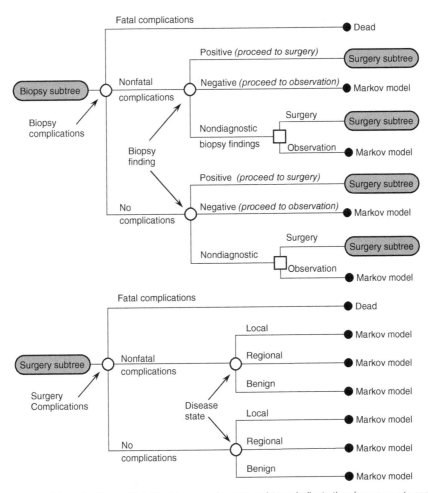

Figure 14.5 Biopsy and surgery subtrees for Figure 14.4. The biopsy and surgery subtrees indicate the chance events and outcomes that occur after a decision to perform a biopsy or surgery. Adapted from Gould *et al.* (2003).

14.3.7   Calculate expected utility, costs, and cost-effectiveness

The analysis resulted in estimates of the costs, life expectancy, QALYs, and cost-effectiveness of each of the 40 clinical strategies, at different pre-test probabilities. Here, we will focus on the main clinical insights from the analysis. First, a CT scan was the initial best choice unless the pre-test probability of cancer was greater than 0.9. When the pre-test probability of cancer was greater than 0.9, surgery was the preferred option. Second, the choice of subsequent management strategy after a CT scan depends strongly on the pre-test probability of cancer. That is, the strategies that were most effective and cost-effective varied depending on the pre-test probability of disease. This finding reinforces the lessons of previous chapters about the importance of pre-test probability in the interpretation of diagnostic tests. Third, PET, a very expensive test, could still be cost-effective, if clinicians used it selectively.

Figure 14.6 shows the next preferred test after CT based on the pre-test probability of disease. The top panel in the table shows the next test after a positive (possibly malignant) CT result, and the bottom panel shows the next test after a negative (benign) CT result. At low pre-test probabilities (0.05–0.1), after a positive CT, the post-test probability is sufficiently high (0.10–0.20) that biopsy is preferred (top panel). At pre-test probabilities between 0.10 and 0.55, PET is preferred as the next test after a positive CT. At higher pre-test probabilities, surgery is preferred without further testing. In contrast, if at low pre-test probabilities (0.05–0.10), CT is negative, then the post-test probability of cancer is less than 0.01, and watchful waiting is preferred, as shown in the bottom panel of Figure 14.6.

The results of the analysis are summarized in a clinical algorithm in Figure 14.7. The algorithm stratifies patients by pre-test probability as low (0.1–0.5), intermediate (0.51–0.76), and high (0.77–0.9), and shows the preferred sequence of tests and treatment. For example, for a patient with a low pre-test probability, a possibly malignant result on CT is followed by PET. If the PET is positive, surgery is the best option. If the PET is negative, needle biopsy is the best option to ensure the PET result is not a false negative. An algorithm is a good way to show the results of a complex analysis.

Recommended test sequence–possible malignant CT results																				
Next test after CT:	Biopsy		FDG-PET									Surgery						Surgery (no CT)		
Pretest Probability (%)	5	10	15	20	25	30	35	40	45	50	55	60	65	70	75	80	85	90	95	100
Post-test Probability (%)	10	20	28	35	42	48	54	59	64	69	73	76	80	84	87	90	93	95	98	100

Recommended test sequence–benign CT results																				
Next test after CT:	Watchful Waiting				Biopsy											FDG-PET		Surgery (no CT)		
Pretest Probability (%)	5	10	15	20	25	30	35	40	45	50	55	60	65	70	75	80	85	90	95	100
Post-test Probability (%)	<1	<1	1	2	2	3	3	4	5	6	7	8	10	13	16	20	26	36	54	100

Figure 14.6 Recommended test sequences and post-test probability after an initial CT scan for evaluation of a solitary pulmonary nodule. The **top panel** shows the preferred next test after a CT scan result that indicated a possibly malignant nodule. The pre-test probability (upper row of numbers) indicates the probability of cancer before the CT is performed. The post-test probability (lower row of numbers) indicates the probability of cancer after the CT result. For example, if the pre-test probability of cancer is 25%, the post-test probability after a positive CT is 42% and the preferred next action is PET scan. The **bottom panel** shows the preferred tests and post-test probability if the CT suggests the nodule is benign. As in the top panel, the pre-test probability (upper row of numbers) indicates the probability of cancer before the CT is performed. The post-test probability (lower row of numbers) indicates the probability of cancer after the CT result. CT = computed tomography; FDG-PET = 18-flourodeoxyglucose positron emission scanning. Adapted from Gould *et al.* (2003).

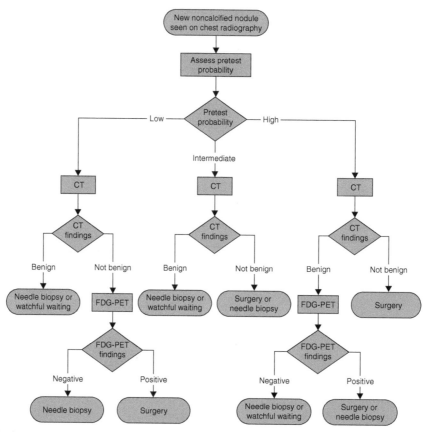

Figure 14.7 Algorithm for the evaluation of solitary pulmonary nodule, stratified by pre-test probability. The algorithm indicates the preferred strategy for the evaluation of a solitary pulmonary nodule for low, intermediate, and high pre-test probabilities of cancer. CT = computed tomography; FDG-PET = 18-flourodeoxyglucose positron emission scanning. Adapted from Gould *et al.* (2003).

14.3.8 Evaluate uncertainty

The sensitivity analyses showed that the pre-test probability of cancer, the sensitivity of CT, the diagnostic yield of biopsy, and the utility of watchful waiting could affect the preferred option at different stages of the management of the patient with a solitary pulmonary nodule.

Sensitivity analysis on one or two variables can provide key insights into the effects of uncertainty on decision making. However, for most analyses, the true value of many model parameters is uncertain. To address this problem, the analyst can perform probabilistic sensitivity analysis. **Probabilistic sensitivity analysis** evaluates the impact of uncertainty about many or all model parameters simultaneously. To do such an analysis, the analyst must estimate probability distributions for each important model parameter. In the probabilistic sensitivity analysis, the software randomly selects a value for each parameter from its distribution, and evaluates the model based on the chosen set of parameters to estimate costs, benefits, and cost-effectiveness. This process is then repeated 1000–10 000 times, each time with a new set of values for the model parameters, with each value chosen randomly from the probability distribution of the parameter. The result of the probabilistic sensitivity analysis is an estimate of costs, benefits, and cost-effectiveness (relative to the appropriate next-best strategy) for each decision option for each of 1000–10 000 runs of the model. With these results, the analyst can calculate the probability that the cost-effectiveness of a strategy is below a chosen threshold (say, $100 000 per QALY gained), accounting for the uncertainty in all model parameters chosen by the analyst. For example, if the cost-effectiveness of a decision option was less than $100 000 per QALY gained in 600 of 1000 model runs, then the probability of that strategy being cost-effective (for that threshold) would be 60%.

In our pulmonary nodule example, probabilistic sensitivity analysis indicated that for patients with low and high pre-test probabilities of cancer, strategies that included PET were cost-effective (at a threshold of $100 000 per QALY) in 77% and 99% of simulations, respectively.

14.3.9 Address ethical issues, discuss results

The important lesson from this example is that decision models can help us understand complex diagnostic and treatment problems. How to evaluate and treat a pulmonary nodule is complicated because the clinician can choose from several diagnostic tests, which can be done in different sequences, and from several treatment options. The analysis helped us choose the most effective and cost-effective strategies from among 40 clinically plausible options. The example also shows how the concepts of sensitivity, specificity, and pre-test and post-test probabilities are essential to understanding complicated real-world medical decision problems. The analysis did not raise specific ethical issues.

14.4 Calibration and validation of decision models

In the last two examples, we described how to construct and analyze complex models, first to analyze a public health problem (screening for HIV) and then for a complex diagnostic evaluation. An important question, which we did not address fully, is how we understand whether these models are predictive or valid. How do we assess whether they accurately reflect available empiric data? Over the last 15 years, substantial literature has developed on how to calibrate and validate decision models. The goals of calibration and validation are to ensure that models faithfully represent known empiric data, such as prevalence, incidence, the effectiveness of treatment, and the uncertainty in that data. Calibration and validation help the analyst and user see that the outcomes predicted by models align with available evidence applicable to the populations of interest, and to delineate the conditions under which the model is trustworthy for drawing conclusions. For published analyses intended to guide decision making, calibration and validation are essential parts of the analysis. Calibration of a complex model may require many months of work and computation. We provide here a brief, high-level overview.

The terms calibration and validation are not used consistently in the literature, and although sometimes used interchangeably, they are not synonymous. For our purposes, we consider **calibration** to be a set of techniques and methods to ensure that the model and its inputs incorporate and are consistent with available evidence and the accompanying uncertainty. A typical use of calibration would be the determination of the values of unobservable or unknown model parameters (for example, the speed of growth of undetected cancer) by matching the model output to closely replicate empiric data (for example, the incidence of cancer) (Goldhaber-Fiebert *et al.*, 2007, 2010; Vanni *et al.*, 2011). To do this usually involves using computational methods to assess many values of the unobserved (or unknown) parameters (the speed of growth of a cancer) to find sets of values for the parameters that result in the best match of the model outcomes to the outcomes observed in empiric data. For example, in a model to assess cancer screening, the model should accurately predict the cancer incidence observed in the population without screening. The calibration process would find values of model parameters such that the model accurately reproduces the observed incidence. The empiric data used to calibrate the model, such as incidence, prevalence, and mortality, are called calibration targets (Vanni *et al.*, 2011). In complex models, many parameters may require calibration and there may be more than 100 calibration targets. See for example, the study by Goldhaber-Fiebert *et al.* (2007) that reports the calibration of a cervical cancer model by using 1 000 000 simulations to choose 200 good-fitting parameter sets for 84 epidemiologic calibration targets.

Assessing the validity of a model is also important. There are several types of validity, including **face validity** (for example, do the structure and outcomes of the model make sense to experts), verification or **internal validity** (does the model work as intended), **cross-validity** (do the model results match the results from other models of the same problem), **external validity** (does the model match available evidence, such as a clinical trial that was not used in developing the model), and **predictive validity** (does the model predict the outcomes of future prospectively conducted experiments, such as clinical trials) (Eddy *et al.*, 2012). We note that validation of a model is done with respect to a specific set of research questions. A model may be valid to answer one question, or set of questions, but not others. For example, a model validated for addressing cervical cancer screening might not be valid to address questions about vaccination to prevent cervical cancer.

The purpose of calibration and validation is to provide additional confidence to both the analysts and the users that the model appropriately reflects relevant empiric data and is applicable for making decisions for the population of interest. Many analysts prefer Bayesian approaches to calibration (Menzies *et al.*, 2017, Jackson *et al.*, 2015). With this method, the analysts specify a joint prior probability density function for the parameters undergoing calibration. The calibration to empiric data produces an updated (or posterior) joint probability density function for the calibrated parameters. The analyst then uses these distributions to conduct analyses, including probabilistic sensitivity analyses.

To illustrate calibration and validation, we will use a cost-effectiveness analysis that evaluated the use of a drug to prevent the progression of chronic kidney disease (CKD) (Tisdale *et al.*, 2022). CKD is the ninth leading cause of death in the United States (Tisdale *et al.*, 2022). CKD usually progresses over many years and may lead to the need for kidney replacement therapy, such as dialysis. A large, double-blind, placebo-controlled randomized clinical trial showed that dapagliflozin, a sodium-glucose co-transporter-2 inhibitor, reduced progression of CKD, and reduced all-cause mortality (Heerspink *et al.*, 2020). The analysis we will discuss assessed the cost-effectiveness of the use of dapagliflozin to prevent the progression of CKD.

To assess the cost-effectiveness of the use of dapagliflozin required using data from many sources, including observational data about the progression of kidney disease and the results of the randomized trial that evaluated dapagliflozin for renal disease, called the dapagliflozin and prevention of adverse outcomes in chronic kidney disease (DAPA-CKD) trial (Heerspink *et al.*, 2020). The analysis assessed the use of dapagliflozin over the lifetime of a patient with CKD, which required developing and calibrating a model of the natural history of CKD to available evidence. Because the DAPA-CKD trial only followed patients for a few years, it was not suitable for developing a lifetime progression model. Kidney function is measured by the estimated glomerular filtration rate (eGFR), with an eGFR greater than $90\,ml/min/1.73\,m^2$ being normal, and stages of kidney disease defined by progressive reductions in the eGFR. For example, kidney failure requiring kidney replacement therapy is often defined as an $eGFR < 12\,ml/min/1.73\,m^2$.

The model included three unknown parameters that determined the long-term progression (natural history) of CKD: the annual rate of eGFR decline, the standard deviation of the eGFR decline, and the frequency with which individuals moved from one stage of kidney disease to another. To calibrate these parameters, we used calibration targets from three US longitudinal studies on nondiabetic mild-to-moderate CKD with long-term follow-up data on all-cause mortality and the incidence of key CKD outcomes. Calibration requires a criterion for the goodness-of-fit of model outcomes to empiric data, which can be a likelihood function in the case of Bayesian calibration, or other criterion with other approaches to calibration. We used a goodness-of-fit criterion based on the likelihood of the values of the three parameters given the empiric data of the calibration targets. Based on this calibration, our natural history model estimated a mean annual rate of decline of eGFR of $1.53\,ml/min/1.73\,m^2$. This rate of decline indicates that without treatment, we expect eGFR to decline by about $15\,ml/min/1.73\,m^2$ over a decade, which provides the basis for comparing the rate of decline when using dapagliflozin to the natural history of CKD.

We used several approaches to validate our model. We assessed face validity by extensive discussion with one of our collaborators who is a national expert in kidney disease, and a co-author of the DAPA-CKD trial. We conducted extensive sensitivity analyses and exploratory analyses under many different sets of assumptions to assess internal validity. For example, we explored both higher and lower effectiveness of dapagliflozin. Our analysis was the first cost-effectiveness analysis of the use of dapagliflozin for CKD. So, we had no other model-based analyses for comparison.

To assess external validity, we compared the modeled progression of the renal disease without dapagliflozin to available natural history data on long-term outcomes. To assess the external validity of the modeled treatment effect, we used the model to predict long-term outcomes incorporating the observed effectiveness from the DAPA-CKD trial and validated the results against the available evidence. To do this, we analyzed our model with a cohort of simulated patients that we designed to reflect the participants in the DAPA-CKD trial, including their age distribution, sex, and initial eGFR (Goldhaber-Fiebert *et al.*, 2010). We then compared the model output to the observed events in both the placebo and treatment arms of the DAPA-CKD trial. For each outcome, the model-based predictions matched well with the outcomes over the duration of the trial. We then compared longer-term outcomes from the model that incorporated data on response to dapagliflozin during the trial with expected outcomes based on available data. This validation exercise demonstrated that our model appropriately reflected the empiric data, which gave us confidence that it would be useful for assessing the cost-effectiveness of dapagliflozin over lifetimes with CKD.

In this section, we've discussed the evolving methods for calibrating and validating models. Calibration and validation are important components of good modeling practice. Moreover, the models may be used to formulate clinical and payment policies, so they must stand up to close scrutiny. We now turn to a different question: How can we use models for individual decision making?

14.5 Use of complex models for individual-patient decision making

Our example of the evaluation of a solitary pulmonary nodule illustrates the complexity of some medical decisions. The examples we have discussed show analyses that help inform clinical decisions, such as whether to screen for HIV or how to evaluate possible lung cancer. Although our lung cancer example showed the importance of the pre-test probability of cancer in choosing a management strategy, we did not discuss other characteristics of the patient that might be very important for individual patient decisions. For example, what if the patient had other illnesses that would increase the risk of surgery? And should older patients – who are at greater risk of death from other causes – be treated the same as younger patients? How should patients' utilities for the outcomes they may experience be incorporated into a decision? The sophisticated models we have discussed in this chapter each took more than a year and cost well over $100 000 to develop. Given the effort and expense, you might well ask how clinicians and patients could use these models for individual decisions. We now address this topic.

How to use decision models for patient-specific decision making is an active area of research. Computer-based programs that aim to help clinicians or patients make clinical decisions are called **decision support systems**. Among the many types of decision support systems, we will focus on a specific example: a prototype system that used the decision model we just discussed to help clinicians evaluate solitary pulmonary nodules. Systems like these seem promising, but whether they will prove useful in day-to-day clinical practice is a research question that requires further study.

14.5.1 The Alchemist decision support system

The Alchemist decision support system uses a modification of the model that we discussed in Section 14.3 to provide patient-specific decision support about the evaluation and management of pulmonary nodules. The decision support system, a prototype that is not in clinical use, was developed by Gillian Sanders, Michael Gould, and colleagues (see the paper by Sanders *et al.* (2000) for a description of a prototype for this system). The system had a Web-based interface that enables clinicians to enter information about a specific patient. This information is transmitted to a computer that runs the decision model using as model inputs the patient-specific information entered by the clinician.

The clinician first enters information that helps estimate the pre-test probability that the nodule is malignant, based on a clinical prediction model that uses the patient's age, size, location and appearance of the nodule, history of extrathoracic malignancy, and history of smoking. The clinician can also enter information about the patient that helps them assess the risks associated with diagnostic procedures. For example, an older patient, or a patient with breathing problems, might be at increased risk of complications of a needle biopsy.

The decision support system then runs the decision model using the inputs entered by the clinician. The output of the decision support system, transmitted back to the clinician via the Internet, is an analysis of the outcomes and costs associated with different management strategies, based on patient-specific information. The system generates a patient-specific algorithm, and tables that show health and economic outcomes, and cost-effectiveness, of different management strategies for the clinician's patient. Thus, Alchemist performs a real-time analysis adjusted for the clinical characteristics of the patient. The clinician could then use the model's results to help plan the next steps in the care of the patient.

Another important aspect of individual decision making is the incorporation of the patient's utilities for health outcomes into decisions. Although the Alchemist system, as designed, did not allow the user to input patient-specific utilities, the inclusion of utilities would be a straightforward extension. To incorporate patient-specific utilities, the clinician could assess a patient's utilities for the relevant outcomes using the techniques such as the standard gamble or the time tradeoff and enter them using the Web-based interface to the decision model.

14.5.2 Challenges for individual-patient decision making

A system such as Alchemist provides a mechanism for synthesizing the best available evidence and for incorporating patient-specific information in a formal decision-making framework. This approach has the potential to build on a comprehensive body of evidence and on the tools of decision making that you have studied in previous chapters.

However, developers and users face significant challenges in using models for individual decision support. The information available to tailor the probabilities of chance events, such as the mortality from surgery or a diagnostic procedure, may be limited. Fortunately, the analyst or clinician can use sensitivity analysis to decide which probabilities and utilities, if any, would change the expected utilities of the candidate management strategies and would therefore be important to obtain. For problems in which quality of life is an important determinant of the preferred treatment alternative, a patient-specific model would be improved by using the patient's utilities for the relevant health states. Models can alert clinicians to the importance of utilities for a specific problem and identify which outcomes are particularly important in terms of patients' utilities. In addition, a decision support system could provide instructions for assessing risk preferences if knowing them could make a difference in the ranking of alternative management strategies (as discussed in Chapter 7). Finally, for a decision support system that is used in practice, the developers would need a method for keeping the system current and for modifying both the structure and inputs to the model when new information or alternatives become available. Model maintenance would likely require ongoing funding, another potential challenge, especially if the decision support system is not proprietary.

The methodologic challenges are active areas of research. We note that even if we can meet these challenges, generally a model cannot capture all of the factors of a decision that are relevant for a specific patient. However, such systems are meant to be *aids* to judgment, not a substitute for it. Thus, the appropriate question is not whether a model can capture every relevant consideration, but whether the patient and clinician can make more informed decisions with the aid of a model-based analysis than without one. We believe that decision models have substantial potential to help make better-informed decisions.

Summary

In this chapter, we discussed how to choose among advanced modeling techniques, how to use a model to develop screening policy, how to analyze a complicated diagnostic problem, and how a model might be used as an aid for individualized decision making. The main goal of the chapter was to illustrate how analysts apply the concepts you learned in earlier chapters to real-world problems. Advanced decision models are now used in the development of clinical guidelines, to conduct cost-effectiveness analyses, and as the basis for analyses of complex screening, diagnostic, and therapeutic decisions.

Decision models are particularly useful for:

- Integrating evidence about alternatives, probabilities, and preferences.
- Illuminating tradeoffs between length of life, quality of life, risk, and costs.
- Describing the tradeoffs between harms and benefits in a formal framework that takes into account their probabilities and the patient's utilities for them.
- Identifying the key determinants of the effectiveness and cost-effectiveness of the strategies under consideration.

Although most clinicians will not be involved in the development of models like those in this chapter, they can apply the underlying concepts in daily clinical practice. These concepts can help clinicians understand when to order tests, how to interpret them, how to weigh harms and benefits, how to understand chance events and probability, and how to understand the role of patients' preferences (utilities) in decisions. As should be evident from the many examples in the book, good decisions do not always lead to good outcomes, and bad decisions do not always lead to bad outcomes. The play of chance is an inevitable part of medical decision making. But clinicians who understand the concepts covered in this book have a powerful framework for helping patients make decisions that increase the likelihood that they will have the outcomes that are most consistent with their preferences.

Bibliography

Barry, M.J., Wolff, T.A., Pbert, L. *et al.* (2023) Putting evidence into practice: an update on the U.S. Preventive Services Task Force methods for developing recommendations for preventive services. *Annals of Family Medicine*, 21(2), 165–171. doi: 10.1370/afm.2946.

This article provides an overview of how a national guideline development group makes recommendations, including the use of decision models.

Bendavid, E., Young, S.D., Bayoumi, A.M. *et al.* (2008) Cost effectiveness of HIV monitoring strategies in resource-limited settings – a Southern African analysis. *Archives of Internal Medicine*, **168**, 1910–18.

This study uses a microsimulation model to evaluate cost-effectiveness of management strategies for HIV.

Briggs, A., Weinstein, M., Fenwick, E. *et al.* (2012) Model parameter estimation and uncertainty analysis: a report of the ISPOR-SMDM modeling good research practices task force-6. *Medical Decision Making*, **32**(5), 722–32.

This paper provides best practices for parameter estimation and uncertainty analysis.

Caro, J., Briggs, A., Siebert, U., and Kuntz, K. (2012) Modeling good research practices – overview: a report of the ISPOR-SMDM modeling good research practices task force-1. *Medical Decision Making*, **32**(5), 667–77.

This paper provides an overview of a series of papers that describe best practices in modeling, developed by a joint task force of the International Society for Pharmacoeconomics and Outcomes Research (ISPOR) and the Society for Medical Decision Making (SMDM).

Eddy, D.M., Hollingworth, W., Caro, J.J. *et al.* (2012) Model transparency and validation: a report of the ISPOR-MDM Modeling research practices task force-7. *Value in Health*, **15**, 843–50.

This paper discusses approaches for model validation and transparency.

Felli, J.C. and Hazen, G.B. (1998) Sensitivity analysis and the expected value of perfect information. *Medical Decision Making*, **18**, 95–109.

This article introduces the concept of expected value of information, an important, advanced topic, not covered in the chapter.

Goldhaber-Fiebert, J.D., Stout, N.K., Ortendahl, J. *et al.* (2007) Modeling human papillomavirus and cervical cancer in the United States for analyses of screening and vaccination. *Population Health Metrics*, **5**(11) https://doi.org/10.1186/1478-7954-5-11.

This study reports calibration of a complex model of cervical cancer.

Goldhaber-Fiebert, J.D., Stout, N.K., and Goldie, S.J. (2010) Empirically evaluating decision-analytic models. *Value in Health*, **13**(5), 667–74.

This paper provides an overview of model calibration and validation.

Gould, M.K., Sanders, G.D., Barnett, P.G. *et al.* (2003) Cost effectiveness of alternative management strategies for patients with solitary pulmonary nodules. *Annals of Internal Medicine*, **138**, 724–35.

This study is the basis of the example in Section 14.3 of the chapter.

Heerspink, H.J.L., Stefánsson, B.V., Correa-Rotter, R. *et al.* (2020) Dapagliflozin in patients with chronic kidney disease. *New England Journal of Medicine*, **383**(15), 1436–46.

This randomized clinical trial provided the effectiveness evidence for the cost-effectiveness example in Section 14.4.

Jackson, C.H., Jit, M., Sharples, L.D., *et al.* 2015 Calibration of complex models through Bayesian evidence synthesis: a demonstration and tutorial. *Medical Decision Making*, **35**, 148–61.

This paper discusses a Bayesian approach to model calibration.

Joyce, V.R., Barnett, P.G., Bayoumi, A.M. *et al.* (2009) Health-related quality of life in a randomized trial of antiretroviral therapy for advanced HIV disease. *Journal of the Acquired Immunodeficiency Syndrome*, **50**, 27–36.

This study uses the time tradeoff, standard gamble, EQ-5D, and the health utilities index version 3 to assess the quality of life with HIV infection.

Karnon, J., Stahl, J., Alan, B. *et al.* (2012) Modeling using discrete event simulation: a report of the ISPOR-SMDM modeling good research practices task force-4. *Medical Decision Making*, **32**(5), 701–11.

This paper provides best practices for developing and analyzing discrete-event simulation models.

Knudsen, A.B., Rutter, C.M., Peterse, E.F.P. *et al.* (2021) Colorectal cancer screening: an updated modeling study for the U.S. Preventive Services Task Force. *Journal of the American Medical Association*, **325**(19), 1998–2011.

This article describes model-based analyses that informed the colorectal cancer screening guideline from the U.S. Preventive Services Task Force.

Long, E.F., Brandeau, M.L., and Owens, D.K. (2010) The cost effectiveness and population outcomes of expanded HIV screening and antiretroviral treatment in the United States. *Annals of Internal Medicine*, **153**, 778–89.

This study uses a dynamic compartmental model to assess population health and economic outcomes of expanded HIV screening and treatment.

Menzies, N.A., Soeteman, D.I., Pandya, A. *et al.* (2017) Bayesian methods for calibrating health policy models: a tutorial. *PharmacoEconomics*, **35**, 613–24.

This tutorial describes Bayesian methods for model calibration.

Owens, D.K. and Nease, R.F. (1997) A normative analytic framework for development of practice guidelines for specific clinical populations. *Medical Decision Making*, **17**,409–26.

This article demonstrates a method for tailoring guidelines to specific populations using expected value of information.

Owens, D.K., Whitlock, E.P., Henderson, J, *et al.* The U.S. Preventive Services Task Force (2016) Use of decision models in the development of evidence-based clinical preventive services recommendations: methods of the U.S. Preventive Services Task Force. *Annals of Internal Medicine*, **165**(7), 501–8.

This article describes how the U.S. Preventive Services Task Force uses decision models to aid in the development of practice guidelines.

Paltiel, A.D., Weinstein, M.C., Kimmel, A.D. *et al.* (2005) Expanded screening for HIV in the United States – an analysis of cost effectiveness. *New England Journal of Medicine*, **352**, 586–95.

This study evaluates HIV screening using a microsimulation model.

Petitti, D.B., Lin, J.S., Owens, D.K., *et al.* (2018) Collaborative modeling: experience of the United States Preventive Services Task Force. *American Journal of Preventive Medicine*, 54(1S1), S53–62.

This article describes the use of multiple independently developed models to aid in the development of practice guidelines.

Pitman, R., Fisman, D., Zaric, G.S. *et al.* (2012) Dynamic transmission modeling: a report of the ISPOR-SMDM modeling good research practices task force-5. *Medical Decision Making*, **32**(5), 712–21.

This paper provides best practices for developing and analyzing dynamic transmission models.

Roberts, M., Russell, L., Paltiel, A.D. *et al.* (2012) Conceptualizing a model: a report of the ISPOR-SMDM modeling good research practices task force working group-2. *Medical Decision Making*, **32**(5), 678–89.

This paper describes a conceptual framework for modeling and how to choose a modeling approach.

Sanders, G.D., Nease, R.F., and Owens, D.K. (2000) Design and pilot evaluation of a system to develop computer-based site-specific practice guidelines from decision models. *Medical Decision Making*, **20**, 145–59.

This paper describes an early version of the Alchemist decision support system.

Sanders, G.D., Bayoumi, A.M., Sundaram, V. *et al.* (2005) Cost effectiveness of screening for HIV in the era of highly active antiretroviral therapy. *New England Journal of Medicine*, **352**, 570–85.

This study is the basis of the example in Section 14.2 of the chapter.

Siebert, U., Alagoz, O., Bayoumi, A.M. *et al.* (2012) State-transition modeling: a report of the ISPOR-SMDM modeling good research practices task force-3. *Medical Decision Making*, **32**(5), 690–700.

This paper provides recommendations for the development, analysis, and reporting of state-transition models.

Tisdale, R.L., Cusick, M.M., Aluri, K.Z. *et al.* (2022) Cost-effectiveness of dapagliflozin for non-diabetic kidney disease. *Journal of General Internal Medicine*, https://doi.org/10.1007/s11606-021-07311-5.

This paper uses a model-based analysis to assess the cost effectiveness of a drug to prevent progression of chronic kidney disease. This study is the basis of the example in Section 14.4.

Vanni, T., Karnon, J., Madan, J. *et al.* (2011) Calibrating models in economic evaluation. A seven-step approach. *PharmacoEconomics*, **29**(1), 35–49.

This study provides on overview of methods for calibrating decision models.

Cost-effectiveness analysis

The purpose of this chapter is to help the reader understand how clinicians and policymakers can include the costs of medical care in decision making for patients and the populations they serve.

15.1   The clinician's conflicting roles: patient advocate, member of society, and entrepreneur

The clinician as an advocate for the patient. One of the clinician's roles in society is to be an advocate for the patient. Individual patients expect clinicians to do what is best for them, even when the needs of society conflict with the patient's needs. Thus, a woman with leukemia expects her clinician to write a letter protesting the refusal of the government health insurance program to pay the costs of an experimental treatment. At times, the needs of society conflict with the patient's needs. Thus, the government might reject the appeal saying that spending the money on programs to reduce premature birth is more important to the public than spending it on an unproven, costly treatment for the woman. Thus, both the patient and those who pay for health care have an interest in how a clinician practices medicine.

The problem is far more complex than an individual interaction between three parties: the clinician, the patient, and society. Society is an aggregation of individuals, and individuals' values may depend on whether they benefit from a patient care decision or whether it costs them money. The taxpayer who votes for a senator who promises to cut the cost of government health programs may one day become a beneficiary of those programs. The person who switches health insurance companies to save a few dollars in premium costs may eventually become ill and insist upon an expensive test that has little chance of altering the course of their care or their long-term outcomes.

So far, the focus of this book has been decision making for an individual patient. The reader has learned how to identify the decision alternative that maximizes the patient's expected utility, incorporating its effects on both length and quality of life. Some might view the clinician's role in society as making choices that maximize the patient's expected utility, even though doing so consumes resources that are no longer available for the care of others or may impose a significant financial burden on the patient. According to this view, it would be unethical to do slightly less than what would maximize your patient's utility in order to benefit someone else or to reduce the patient's financial burden of their care.

The experienced clinician will recognize that a rigid utility-maximizing perspective is unrealistic in practice. Imagine yourself in the following common situation:

The coronary care unit is full, and the head nurse has just called you about a patient in the emergency room with an acute myocardial infarction. They remind you that one of your patients has been in the coronary care unit for 2 days with a small myocardial infarction. The patient is doing well and has a much better outlook than the other patients in the coronary care unit. The head nurse says that the new patient in the emergency room will benefit much more from the coronary unit bed than your patient and asks you to move your patient to a vacant bed on a regular hospital floor.

Although unlikely, your patient might have a complication of myocardial infarction after transfer to a less intensively staffed part of the hospital, where a complication that might be handled successfully in the coronary care unit could prove fatal. If your sole motivation is to maximize your patient's expected utility, you would keep your patient in the coronary care unit for a few more days. However, recognizing that space in the coronary care unit is limited and that others have a right to access this resource, you agree to transfer your patient. This decision maximizes the expected utility of the population of acute myocardial infarction patients in the hospital – not just the patient under your direct care.

This example demonstrates that clinicians often make decisions that expose their patients to a slightly increased risk of harm in order to assure the best use of a shared resource. Physicians and their patients belong to a community of shared interest in good health.

The changing relationship between the payer, the clinician, and the patient. During the first half of the twentieth century, most patients bore the cost of illness from their savings. The clinician had to forgo expensive diagnostic tests or find alternatives to costly drugs depending on the patient's – or their family's – resources. In those days, physicians set their own fees and were free to charge what the patient could afford to pay, which could include accepting a nominal fee. The patient and the clinician were partners in trying to assure good care at a low cost because many patients had an urgent personal interest in minimizing the costs of their health care.

With the advent of access to health insurance for most people, health care costs became a shared concern because more costly care for some patients meant more costly insurance premiums for everyone. With health insurance, other people share in an individual patient's expenses. And so the costs of medical care have become a concern of groups of people rather than just the individual patient. In the relatively depersonalized environment created by health insurance, patients are less likely to ask the clinician about less expensive strategies that might involve greater uncertainty about the outcome.

The pendulum swings and the cost of health care is again a focus of attention for individual patients in the United States. To get insurance, the patient must usually agree to pay part of the cost of many services (co-payment) and often the patient pays all of the costs up to an amount (the deductible) above which the insurance pays most of the costs. Within a clinician's panel of patients, individual insurance plans and co-payments and deductibles may vary widely. Here, the clinician and the patient may work together to minimize costs to the patient – and the clinician must realize that a strategy to minimize out-of-pocket costs to one patient may not be the best strategy for the next patient, who has a different health insurance plan. Many clinical practices receive a lump sum to care for all the patient's health care needs, an arrangement that provides a strong incentive for clinicians to avoid unnecessary expenses. However, the clinician's role as patient advocate may conflict with the clinician's self-interest when the health plan pays a bonus to those who successfully control costs. In either situation, understanding the relationships between the costs of medical services and their benefits may help the clinician and the patient to make good decisions together, irrespective of the specifics of the insurance plan.

15.1.1 Principles of allocating scarce resources

There are several principles for allocating scarce health care resources:

- *Maximize health outcomes at any cost*: The clinician has a professional duty to maximize their patient's well-being. Expending additional resources may increase the chance of survival or improve the patient's quality of life, however slightly.
- *Minimize cost*: If taken to an extreme, this approach would often result in poor health outcomes and either reduced length and/or quality of life.
- *Maximize outcomes without exceeding the available resources*: Expend resources on health care if the additional cost for each additional unit of benefit is less than would be derived from using the money in another way.

The principal goal of this chapter is to describe a way to characterize decision alternatives that take both their costs and effectiveness into account. Such a cost-effectiveness analysis can help make decisions for allocating resources.

These resources may be owned jointly (by the clients of an insurance company) or individually (by a person who must make an out-of-pocket co-payment for a service covered partially by health insurance). Cost-effectiveness analysis can inform policymakers and individual patients.

15.2   Cost-effectiveness analysis: a method for comparing management strategies

Cost-effectiveness analysis is a method for comparing decision alternatives by their relative costs and effectiveness. It is an analytic tool for comparing the costs and effects of an intervention to at least one alternative. The results are expressed as a ratio of incremental cost to incremental effect, where "incremental" is the difference between the two interventions. In this chapter, health outcomes are the measure for comparing interventions, such as cases of a disease-prevented or quality-adjusted life years (QALYs) gained. *Cost-effectiveness analysis always compares strategies.* The incremental cost-effectiveness ratio (ICER) is calculated as the difference in costs between two compared alternatives (net costs), divided by the difference in their health outcomes (net effectiveness). The ICER estimates the additional cost of the intervention to buy one more unit of health.

When comparing two treatments, Treatment A and Treatment B, the incremental cost-effectiveness of Treatment A relative to Treatment B is:

$$\text{Incremental CE} = \frac{\text{Cost}(\text{Treatment A}) - \text{Cost}(\text{Treatment B})}{\text{Effectiveness}(\text{Treatment A}) - \text{Effectiveness}(\text{Treatment B})}$$

The incremental cost in the numerator represents the additional resources required from using Treatment A instead of Treatment B. The incremental effect in the denominator represents the additional health outcomes by using Treatment A rather than Treatment B.

Cost-effectiveness analysis comes into play when decision makers are trying to choose among several interventions, no intervention is both less expensive and more effective, and resources are limited. These choices should be based on a comparison of the health benefits, harms, and costs associated with the available alternatives. Cost-effectiveness analysis is designed to identify the way to spend on health that gives the most health for our health care dollars – as individuals or as a society.

15.2.1   Using cost-effectiveness analysis to set institutional policy: an extended example

Cost-effectiveness analysis may be used to set a policy that will affect the actions of others. Consider the problem of a prepaid group practice administrator who must decide between three strategies for managing the care of a patient with continuing pain from a kidney stone. A consultant has just presented the administrator with the following table:

Strategy	Cost	Life expectancy
A	$9400	19.60
B	$10 000	19.64
C	$10 000	19.28

The administrator notes right away that choosing between these strategies will require a compromise: Strategy A is the least expensive and Strategy B leads to the longest average survival. In deciding whether the additional effectiveness of Strategy B is worth its extra cost, the administrator calculates the incremental cost-effectiveness of Strategy B. Strategy B costs $600 more per patient than Strategy A and prolongs life 2 weeks (0.04 years) longer than Strategy A. The administrator is frustrated. The cost-effectiveness analysis clarified the problem, but it did not lead to an easy decision. To understand the administrator's dilemma, let us go back to the beginning and find out how the analysis was performed.

The administrator of a hospital-based group practice must decide whether to accede to the wishes of the chief of urology who has asked the hospital to purchase an instrument that dissolves kidney stones by ultrasonic waves. Kidney stones form in the kidney and eventually pass through the ureter to the urinary bladder, causing severe pain called renal colic. Occasionally, a stone does not pass into the bladder, and renal colic continues until the stone is removed surgically or dissolved. The urology chief proposes that all patients who do not pass their kidney stone within 48 hours should undergo treatment with high-energy ultrasonic waves to dissolve the stone. When this treatment is successful, fewer patients must undergo surgery to remove the kidney stone. Avoiding surgery will be especially important for patients whose risk of death from surgery is increased because of their poor medical condition.

The administrator asks the consultant to investigate this request. After investigation, the consultant comes up with the following facts:

- Fatality rate with surgery:
  - *Low-risk patients*: 2%
  - *High-risk patients*: 10%
- Success rate of treatment:
  - *Ultrasonic therapy*: 80% for all patients
  - *Surgery*: 100% for all patients who survive surgery
- *Prevalence of patients at high risk from surgery*: 20%
- Cost to the practice of treatments:
  - *Ultrasonic treatment*: $2000 (includes the purchase price of the ultrasound equipment amortized over its lifetime)
  - *Surgery*: $10 000

After hearing these facts, the administrator is convinced that the ultrasonic treatment may be beneficial to some patients but worries about the cost of purchasing the machine. Perhaps the surgeons could send patients who are too sick for surgery to a nearby hospital that has recently purchased an ultrasonic machine. Accordingly, the consultant investigates a resource-sharing arrangement whereby low-risk patients would have surgery locally and high-risk patients would be sent to the nearby hospital.

The administrator negotiates the following arrangement. The neighboring hospital will charge $4000 for an ultrasonic treatment. If the ultrasonic treatment fails, the patient will undergo surgery at the neighboring hospital, which will charge the practice $15 000 to perform the surgery.

The administrator asks the consultant to analyze the choice between:

- Surgery for all patients (the current mode of treatment);
- Ultrasonic treatment for all patients (with surgery if the ultrasonic treatment fails);
- Surgery for low-risk patients; ultrasonic treatments at the neighboring hospital for high surgical-risk patients and surgery if ultrasonic treatment fails.

The administrator asks the consultant to analyze the problem in terms of costs to the practice and length of life for the average kidney stone patient, who is 55 years old and has a 20-year life expectancy. The consultant uses the following sequence to perform the analysis.

I. **Define the problem to be solved and the objectives of the analysis**

The problem: In some patients with renal colic, a kidney stone does not pass spontaneously. Which of the three strategies for treating such patients should the administrator recommend for adoption by the practice?

The objectives: Predict the consequences of the three strategies by analyzing the expected costs and expected survival for 55-year-old patients. If possible, identify a dominant solution which will both maximize survival and minimize costs. If there is no dominant solution, use incremental cost-effectiveness analysis to characterize the decision alternatives.

II. **Define the consequences of each decision alternative**

The consultant represents the problem by a decision tree in which the probabilities and outcomes are those identified in the first phase of the investigation. The trees for each decision alternative are displayed separately (Figures 15.1, 15.2, and 15.3). The analyst chooses two outcomes: the patient's survival and the costs to the practice.

Treatment strategy 1: Surgery for all patients (the current mode of treatment)
Survival:
- *Immediate death due to surgery*: Life expectancy 0 years.
- *Survive surgery and live to one's normal life expectancy of 20 years.*

Treatment costs per patient:
- *Costs*: Surgery for all patients: $10 000.

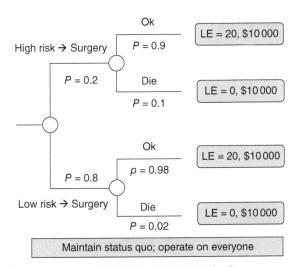

Figure 15.1 Outcomes of surgery within the practice for all patients with persistent renal colic.

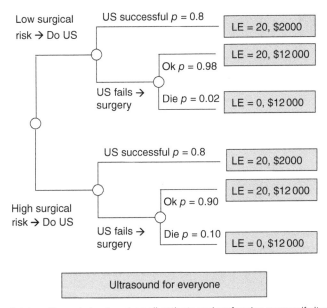

Figure 15.2 Outcomes of a strategy of doing ultrasonic treatment on all patients and performing surgery if ultrasonic treatment fails, both treatments done within the local practice.

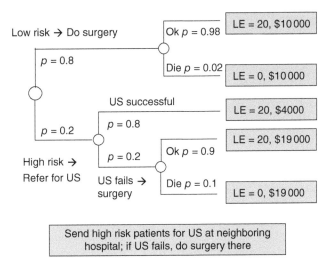

Figure 15.3 Outcome of doing surgery within the practice on low-risk patients with persistent renal colic and sending high-risk patients to a neighboring hospital for ultrasound treatment (and, if it fails, surgery at the neighboring hospital).

Treatment strategy 2: Purchase equipment for ultrasonic treatment. Perform ultrasonic treatment for all patients, with surgery if the treatment fails. All interventions to be performed within the practice;

Survival:
- *Immediate death due to surgery*: Life expectancy 0 years.
- *Survive surgery and live to one's normal life expectancy of 20 years.*
- *Successful ultrasound treatment*: Live to one's normal life expectancy of 20 years.

Treatment costs to the practice:
- *Outcome 1*: Ultrasound treatment successful: cost $2000.
- *Outcome 2*: Ultrasound fails. Total cost: cost of ultrasound $2000 + cost of surgery: $10000.

Treatment strategy 3: Surgery for all low-risk patients at local hospital; ultrasonic treatment at the neighboring hospital for patients with high surgical risk; surgery at the neighboring hospital if ultrasound fails.

Survival:
- *Immediate death due to surgery*: Life expectancy 0 years.
- *Survive surgery and live to one's normal life expectancy of 20 years.*
- *Successful ultrasound treatment at the neighboring hospital*: live to one's normal life expectancy of 20 years.

Treatment costs to the practice:
- *Outcome 1*: Surgery at a local hospital for low-risk patients: cost $10000.
- *Outcome 2*: Ultrasound at neighboring hospital; surgery at neighboring hospital if it fails. Total cost: cost of ultrasound $4000; cost of surgery: $15000.

III. Average out and fold back the decision tree

The results are shown in the following table:

Strategies	Expected cost	Life expectancy of patients
Strategy 1: surgery for everyone	$10000	19.28 years
Strategy 2: Buy ultrasound; use it for all patients	$4000	19.86 years
Strategy 3: Surgery for low-risk patients; Send high-risk patients to neighboring hospital for ultrasonic treatment	$9400	19.60 years

What does this analysis mean? To interpret it, examine each of the columns of the table in turn.

Expected cost: The expected cost of each of the three decision alternatives was obtained by averaging out and folding back, using cost as the measure of outcome.

	Operate on everyone	Buy ultrasound for your practice	Surgery for low-risk patients; high-risk patients to a nearby hospital for ultrasound
Expected cost	$10000	$4000	$9400

Interpretation: Purchasing the ultrasonic machine is the least costly alternative, presumably because most patients can be treated with ultrasound and do not require a $10000 surgical operation. Referral of all patients to the nearby hospital is expensive because of its high charges for ultrasound and surgery if needed.

Life expectancy: The life expectancy of the patients is obtained by averaging out and folding back the decision trees, using life expectancy as the measure of outcome.

	Operate on everyone	Buy ultrasound for your practice	High-risk patients are sent to a nearby hospital
Life expectancy	19.28 years	19.86 years	19.60 years

Interpretation: Purchasing the ultrasound machine leads to the longest expected length of life, presumably because fewer than 10% of the patients are subjected to the risk of death from surgery. In contrast, many more patients would undergo surgery with the other two decision alternatives.

Purchasing the ultrasonic machine for the practice leads to the lowest costs for the practice and the longest life expectancy for the patient. Since purchasing the ultrasound machine has the lowest cost and the best survival, it *dominates* the other choices. The hospital administrator is relieved to learn that they do not need to analyze the tradeoff between cost and survival.

As the administrator is about to place the order for the equipment for performing ultrasonic dissolution of kidney stones, they learn about a worldwide shortage of materials for a crucial part of the new version of the ultrasound machine. The company has shut down its production line and has no idea when this model will become available again. The alternative is to buy an older, more expensive model, which is less effective at dissolving kidney stones. The probability of successful treatment is only 0.50 with the older machine. The cost to the practice of each procedure will be $5000 using the older machine, rather than $2000. However, the neighboring hospital, which has the new ultrasound machine, can still offer the procedure for $4000. The consultant repeats the analysis after substituting the higher cost and reduced effectiveness of an ultrasound treatment using the older machine and presents the following table:

Strategies	Expected cost	Life expectancy of patients
Strategy 1: Surgery for everyone	$10 000	19.28 years
Strategy 2: Buy older model ultrasound; use it for all patients	$10 000	19.64 years
Strategy 3: Surgery for low-risk patients; send high-risk patients to the nearby hospital for ultrasound	$9400	19.60 years

The situation is now quite different. The least expensive alternative is different from the alternative that produces the longest life expectancy for patients. No strategy dominates. The administrator could choose based on either cost or survival but decides to use the ICER, which estimates the additional cost of an intervention to achieve one more unit of clinical outcome. The administrator must first choose which two alternatives to compare.

Strategy 1 is as costly as Strategy 2 and more costly than Strategy 3. Strategy 1 also leads to a shorter life expectancy than either Strategy 2 or 3. So, it is inferior to both. Therefore, the choice is between Strategy 2 and Strategy 3. Strategy 2 is more costly than Strategy 3 but more effective. So, choosing between them is difficult.

The administrator notes that patients' life expectancy will be slightly better if the practice buys its own ultrasound machine (Strategy 2). What will it cost the practice to choose Strategy 2 which will avoid the loss of life with Strategy 3, which involves doing surgery on all low-risk patients and the high-risk patients who fail ultrasonic treatments at the neighboring hospital? Would purchasing the ultrasonic machine be an extravagant departure from the hospital's usual management practices? How will the cost per year of life gained compare to other decisions that the practice has made recently? The average cost per procedure of buying the ultrasound machine is only $600 more than if high-risk patients are sent to the other hospital. The incremental cost-effectiveness of Strategy 2 (buying the ultrasonic machine) vs. Strategy 3 (surgery for low-risk patients; send high-risk patients to nearby hospital for ultrasound) is calculated as follows:

$$\text{Incremental CE} = \frac{\text{Cost}\left(\text{Strategy 2}\right) - \text{Cost}\left(\text{Strategy 3}\right)}{\text{LE}\left(\text{strategy 2}\right) - \text{LE}\left(\text{Strategy 3}\right)}$$

$$\text{Incremental CE} = \frac{\$10\,000 - \$9400}{19.64 \text{ years} - 19.60 \text{ years}} = \$15\,000 \text{ per year of life saved}$$

The improvement in life expectancy that can be obtained by buying the ultrasound machine will cost an additional $15 000 per additional year of life gained, which is consistent with past investments by the hospital. In fact, $15 000 per year of life saved compares very favorably to the cost-effectiveness of services that everyone seems to agree are an efficient use of resources. Clearly, this expenditure would be defensible in a presentation to the hospital board of trustees.

Cost-effectiveness analyses often express the gain to the patient as QALYs gained rather than life years saved. QALYs are life years in a health state multiplied by a measure such as the patient's utility for the quality of life in the health state. The topic of QALYs is explored further in Section 15.7

15.2.2 Flat-of-the-curve medicine

Often, one must choose from among several ways to use a service. For example, in screening for cancer of the cervix, one can obtain cervical cytology at any frequency. In practice, the typical frequency ranges from annual testing to testing every 3 years. To help analyze this problem, some investigators plot the cost of adopting each policy against its benefit (Figure 15.4). This analysis shows the small increment in effectiveness relative to the cost of more intensive

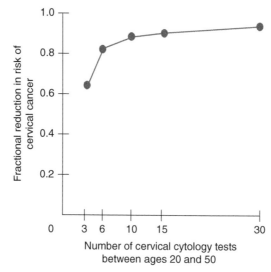

Figure 15.4 Incremental costs and incremental effectiveness of several methods for screening for hypothetical cancer.

screening for this hypothetical cancer. Practicing medicine with policies that provide a relatively small incremental benefit for the added cost is sometimes called "flat-of-the-curve medicine." How should one use the information in Figure 15.4 to choose a policy for cancer screening?

In principle, one should adopt the most intensive screening program that has a higher incremental cost-effectiveness than alternative uses for the resources. Cost-effectiveness analysis is a method for comparing decision alternatives, but to decide whether any alternative is cost-effective, a decision maker must have a criterion for cost-effectiveness. As noted in the preceding section, $50 000–$150 000 per QALY is often used. This, or any, threshold for calling a practice cost-effective has neither a theoretical basis nor a valid empirical rationale. The Second Panel on Cost-Effectiveness recommends against adopting one specific threshold for declaring a practice to be cost-effective. Instead, researchers should highlight how clinical or policy recommendations might change across a range of thresholds, which an organization could use to inform its resource allocation decision making (Neumann *et al.*, 2016). Cost–benefit analysis, our next subject, provides a direct approach for deciding if a program is worth undertaking.

15.3   Cost–benefit analysis: a method for measuring the net benefit of medical services

Definition of cost–benefit analysis: A comparison in which the costs and benefits of a service or services are both expressed in the same units.

To use cost–benefit analysis to compare different programs or policies, the analyst calculates net benefits by subtracting costs from benefits ($B–C$). Analysts also use the ratio of benefits to costs to compare policies, although net benefit provides a more easily explained meaning of the comparison: the gain or loss from an action, measured in units whose meaning is tangible.

15.3.1   The distinction between cost–benefit analysis and cost-effectiveness analysis

Many people have difficulty distinguishing between cost–benefit analysis and cost-effectiveness analysis. The distinction is quite subtle but important.

Cost-effectiveness analysis is helpful for comparing alternatives but is otherwise a limited measure for decision making. It can guide the choice between alternatives (pick the one with the most favorable incremental cost per QALY gained). However, to decide if either alternative is worth doing, one must choose an arbitrary threshold of cost-effectiveness. For example, you should have no difficulty choosing between a service whose cost per QALY gained is $1 000 000 and one whose cost per QALY gained is $100 000. To decide whether either of the services is worth its cost, you must first establish a definition of a service that is worth its cost (e.g., $50 000 per life year gained). A cost-effectiveness threshold is arbitrary because the unit of measure of costs (currency) is different than the unit for measuring effectiveness. Therefore, the units of cost-effectiveness do not have a natural, common-sense meaning that can serve as a framework for setting a threshold and convincing others that it is a reasonable basis for policy making.

This limitation becomes clearer when we contrast cost-effectiveness analysis with **cost–benefit analysis**, in which the measure of benefit and cost is monetary. Because the two measures have the same units (currency), the difference between them has the common-sense, real-world meaning of profit or loss, which is a natural criterion for deciding if a service is worth doing. Cost–benefit analysis has an important role to play when the benefits of a policy can be expressed in units of currency, and there are many valid applications in the policy field.

To summarize, cost–benefit analysis is one of several methods for deciding between alternatives, but its unique role is as a method for deciding whether a service is worth doing. Another advantage: choosing between policies with different outcomes is possible if the outcomes can be transformed into the same monetary measure, such as dollars.

15.3.2 Placing a monetary value on human life

Although cost–benefit analysis is potentially very powerful, it has one major drawback when applied to decisions that affect human health. Cost is usually expressed in units of currency (dollars, pounds, euro, or yen). Since the outputs of a service must also be in units of currency, the analyst faces a very difficult problem: how does one place a monetary value on health outcomes? The measure of the output of many medical policies is additional years of healthy life. Therefore, to apply cost–benefit analysis to medical problems, one must ask, "How does one place a monetary value on an additional year of life?" The methods for expressing the value of years of life in monetary terms are far from satisfactory. Here, we list several approaches.

How were past decisions valued? The size of an investment by society in a program designed to save lives and the number of lives actually saved is one measure of the value that society places on a life. However, these societal investments occur in a context that is unique to each occurrence. Generalizing from one such situation to another is risky.

The human capital method: This approach values a policy by its effect on the patient's lifetime earnings. A life saved at age 55 years means at least 10 more years of gainful employment. The monetary value of that period in the workforce can be calculated.

The human capital approach is widely used, although it has several deficiencies. By valuing everything by anticipated income, the human capital approach implies that the life of a person with a lifetime income of $100 000 is worth twice as much as a person with a lifetime income of $50 000. This notion may have validity in economic terms, but counter-examples are easy to imagine. The human capital approach also assumes that people are unwilling to pay more than their remaining lifetime earnings to postpone death. In fact, people with savings or a home might be willing to spend heavily from these reserves to postpone death. The next measure of the value of life is the amount that people are willing to pay to postpone death or avoid disability.

Willingness to pay: The willingness-to-pay method helps people express a value for life by saying how much they would be willing to pay for a program that would decrease the probability of a bad outcome by a stated amount.

- The subject might be told:
  - Suppose that the probability that you will die from a stroke is 0.01 during your remaining lifetime of 20 years. What is the most that you would be willing to pay over your lifetime for a program that would reduce this risk by 50%?
- *The subject might reply*: "$2000."

Interpretation: A lifetime probability of 0.01 is equivalent to a risk of 10 stroke deaths per 1000 individuals over 20 years. A reduction by 50% would eliminate 5 deaths per 1000 individuals over 20 years. Since 5 stroke deaths were avoided by 1000 people each paying $2000 (total $2 000 000) did not occur during those 20 years, 100 life-years would be gained, or $20 000 per life-year saved.

By asking such questions of a community sample, one can calculate the value that the populace places on saving a life. However, what one is willing to pay is likely to depend on the exact circumstances. The premise of the willingness-to-pay approach is that a person who is willing to pay $2000 to reduce the probability of death from a stroke by 5 strokes per 1000 individuals over 20 years would be willing to pay $400 000 ($2000 divided by 0.005) to avoid certain death from a stroke. Many would question that premise: reducing the probability of an outcome is not the same cognitively as completely avoiding a certain outcome.

Obtaining a consistent value for human life with the willingness-to-pay approach is difficult for other reasons. People's willingness to pay increases with the risk of death. Does this mean that the value that is placed on life depends on the risk of losing it? Wealthy people are generally willing to pay more for a program to reduce the risk of death than poor people. People are more willing to pay when they personally benefit from a program than when they are asked to pay for a program that will benefit others.

Clinicians may not accept the results of cost–benefit analysis because it is so difficult to develop a consensus opinion on the monetary value of a year of human life. Most clinicians who are interested in analyzing tradeoffs between clinical strategies use cost-effectiveness analysis. Perhaps policymakers should be paying more attention to the principal advantage of cost–benefit analysis: because the costs and benefits of a program are both measured in units of currency, they can express the tradeoff between them with a tangible measure that the public can understand (profit or loss, in units of currency).

15.3.3 Should clinicians take an interest in cost–benefit analysis?

The problems with applying cost–benefit analysis seem remote from daily practice. The individual clinician is not concerned with allocating effort between programs to improve the health of the community. The clinician's primary responsibility is to look after the interests of the patient. However, the choices open to the clinician may be affected by resource allocation decisions that are based on cost–benefit analysis. Policymakers must deal with such methods when they try to decide whether to allocate scarce government resources to screening programs to detect disease in young people or programs to treat chronic disease in old people. If clinicians want policymakers to listen to them, they should understand the methods that policymakers depend on and help them to apply these methods to the world of medical practice. That said, the foundations of cost–benefit analyses in health do not inspire confidence.

15.4 Methodological best practices for cost-effectiveness analysis

As described earlier, cost-effectiveness analysis provides a framework for considering the costs, benefits, and harms of available alternatives. Benefits can impact both mortality, and morbidity and can accrue differently to different sectors of society (i.e., to individual patients, caregivers, health systems, or populations). The time during which the harms, benefits, and costs may accrue can also vary. These complexities challenge both the analyst and the consumer of cost-effectiveness analyses. Because of its potential effects on public policy, maintaining public trust in cost-effectiveness analyses is important. A list of methodological best practices is an important part of the foundation of a scientific discipline. In 1993, the US Public Health Service convened a Panel of 13 nongovernment scientists and scholars with expertise in economics, clinical medicine, ethics, and statistics. Their charge was to review the state of cost-effectiveness analysis and to develop recommendations for the conduct and use of cost-effectiveness analysis in health and medicine. The resulting Gold Book (Gold 1996) published in 1996 by the original Panel on Cost-Effectiveness in Health and Medicine became the point of reference for doing cost-effectiveness analysis. Its recommendations guided the application of cost-effectiveness analysis for a generation of decision analysts, economists, and policymakers. Since 1996, the field of cost-effectiveness analysis and our learnings from the application of its methods have advanced significantly. The original Panel's efforts needed updating, and in 2016, the Second Panel on Cost-Effectiveness in Health and Medicine published their expanded recommendations (Neumann *et al.*, 2016).

The Second Panel on Cost-Effectiveness in Health and Medicine includes recommendations for the conduct, methods, and reporting of cost-effectiveness analyses. These recommendations seek to ensure the transparency of cost-effectiveness analyses so that decision makers can understand the tradeoffs of costs, harms, and benefits between strategies. Key recommendations for cost-effectiveness analysis include:

- All cost-effectiveness studies report a Reference Case analysis based on a health care sector perspective and another Reference Case analysis based on a societal perspective. The Reference Cases are defined by recommendations for components to consider for evaluation, methods to use, and elements for reporting. The Second Panel recommends that Reference Case analyses measure health effects in terms of QALYs. The purpose of standardizing methods and the various types of costs and benefits that are included in the Reference Case analyses is to enhance consistency across analyses performed by different decision analysts and thereby to help policymakers compare findings across studies.

- The results of the health care sector Reference Case analysis should be expressed as an ICER. The health care sector perspective should include health care sector (medical) costs reimbursed by third-party payers or paid for out-of-pocket by patients. Both types of medical costs include current and future costs, related and unrelated to the condition under consideration. So, for example, an analysis of treatments to prevent heart attacks would include the costs associated with the treatment itself and the downstream costs associated with heart disease but also the costs associated with other health conditions (e.g., cancer) that may occur only because the patient lives longer.

- The analysis should include an Impact Inventory Table that lists the health and nonhealth impacts of interventions included in the analysis. The main purpose of the Impact Inventory is to ensure systematic attention to all consequences, including those outside of the formal health care sector.
- Analysts should try to identify, quantify, and value nonhealth consequences that may affect the result of the analysis. For example, a treatment for children with autism would not only include clinical costs and benefits associated with the child's autism but also the impact of this treatment on the child's educational and employment trajectory.
- Analysts should clearly state the perspective of every analysis reported: the health care sector perspective, the societal perspective, or an additional perspective that the analyst considers to be important to the decisional context. Analysts should identify the primary decision maker(s) whose deliberations are the target of the analysis.
- Analysts should describe in clear and understandable language their conduct of the analyses. This directive applies especially to the assumptions of the model, and how the results change with alternative assumptions. Sensitivity analysis should describe the impact of the modeling assumptions that most strongly influence the results for different perspectives.

15.5   Reference case for cost-effectiveness analysis

As described above, the Second Panel on Cost-Effectiveness in Health and Medicine recommends that a cost-effectiveness analysis should be performed from the perspective of two Reference Cases. Each Reference Case follows the same set of standard methodological practices recommended by the Second Panel. One analysis takes a *health care sector perspective. The other takes* a *societal perspective.* From the health care sector perspective, we should include costs paid by third-party payers and out-of-pocket costs paid by patients (Table 15.1). The societal perspective incorporates all costs and all health effects regardless of who incurs the costs and who experiences the health effects. These should include informal health sector costs which are outside of the structured health care system but which may still add significant financial burden to patients and their families. Examples of such informal health sector costs include patient time costs (i.e., costs associated with patient time spent traveling to and from care, waiting for, and receiving care), unpaid caregiver costs, and transportation costs, as well as nonhealth care sector costs such as impacts on productivity, consumption, and those costs borne by social services, legal, education, housing, or the environment sectors. Health effects in both Reference Cases should be measured in QALYs.

Table 15.1 Cost components included in two reference case perspectives.

Reference case perspective	
Health care	*Societal*
Formal health care sector:* • Paid for by third-party payers • Paid for by patients out-of-pocket	Formal health care sector:* • Paid for by third-party payers • Paid for by patients out-of-pocket Informal health care sector: • Patient time • Unpaid caregiver time • Transportation costs Nonhealth care sectors: • Productivity • Consumption • Social services • Legal or criminal justice • Education • Housing • Environment • Other (e.g., friction costs)

* Includes current and future costs, related and unrelated to the condition under consideration.

Table 15.2 Impact inventory template.

Sector	Type of impact (List category within each sector with a unit of measure if relevant)*	Included in this reference case analysis from . . . perspective?		Notes on sources of evidence
		Health care Sector	Societal	
FORMAL HEALTH CARE SECTOR				
Health	*Health Outcomes (Effects)*			
	Longevity effects	☐	☐	
	Health-related quality-of-life effects	☐	☐	
	Other health effects (e.g., adverse events and secondary transmissions of infections)	☐	☐	
	Medical Costs			
	Paid for by third-party payers	☐	☐	
	Paid for by patients out-of-pocket	☐	☐	
	Future related medical costs (payers and patients)	☐	☐	
	Future unrelated medical costs (payers and patients)	☐	☐	
INFORMAL HEALTH CARE SECTOR				
Health	Patient time costs	NA	☐	
	Unpaid caregiver time costs	NA	☐	
	Transportation costs	NA	☐	
NONHEALTH CARE SECTORS (with examples of possible items)				
Productivity	Labor market earnings lost	NA	☐	
	Cost of unpaid lost productivity due to illness	NA	☐	
	Cost of uncompensated household production**	NA	☐	
Consumption	Future consumption unrelated to health	NA	☐	
Social services	Cost of social services as part of intervention	NA	☐	
Legal or criminal justice	Number of crimes related to intervention	NA	☐	
	Cost of crimes related to intervention	NA	☐	
Education	Impact of intervention on Educational achievement of population	NA	☐	
Housing	Cost of intervention on home improvements (e.g., removing lead paint)	NA	☐	
Environment	Production of toxic waste or pollution by intervention	NA	☐	
Other (specify)	Other impacts	NA	☐	

*Categories listed are intended as examples for analysts.
**Examples include activities such as housework; food preparation, cooking, and clean-up; household management; shopping; obtaining services; and travel related to household activity.
NA = not applicable
Published previously in Sanders et al. (2016).

15.6 Impact inventory for cataloguing consequences

The Second Panel on Cost-Effectiveness in Health and Medicine recommends the inclusion of an Impact Inventory Table in all cost-effectiveness analyses (Table 15.2). This Impact Inventory Table lists the health and nonhealth effects of a health care intervention to ensure that all consequences are considered, including those to patients, caregivers, social services, and others outside the health care sector. The Impact Inventory provides a framework for the analyst to organize the types of consequences to be considered in an analysis and to better ensure that all consequences, including the outcomes of the formal health care sector, are appropriately considered. An end user of the cost-effectiveness analysis can then use the information in the impact inventory table to better understand the applicability of the findings to their relevant population and any limitations of the simplifying assumptions on the true potential impact.

15.7 Measuring the health effects of medical care

To determine the cost-effectiveness of comparison strategies, we must quantify the impact of the available strategies on health outcomes. The Second Panel recommends that the Reference Case cost-effectiveness analyses should measure these health effects in terms of QALYs. QALYs allow an analyst to adjust the estimated life years for the various strategies by the health-related quality of life provided by those strategies. The Second Panel further recommends that we should incorporate QALYs that accrue both to the patient but then also to any additional people who are affected by the strategy such as informal caregivers. For determining the quality weights, these measures should be preference based such as the EQ-5D or the Health Utilities Index (HUI). These measures assume that a health state of "dead" has a score of 0.0 and a health state of "perfect health" has a score of 1.0. Health states which are less than perfect health will count as less than one full QALY.

EuroQol 5D (EQ-5D) is a validated preference-based system for measuring health status. The basis of EQ-5D is a person's responses to a questionnaire designed to elicit their status for each of the five dimensions of health (mobility, self-care, usual activities, pain and discomfort, and anxiety and depression) (EuroQol, 1990). The person chooses a response (no problem, moderate problem, and severe problem) for each dimension. The sum of the person's scores across the five dimensions is their EQ-5D health status score. The EQ-5D is available in many languages and the EQ-5D value sets have been constructed for various geographic locations. Similarly, the **HUI** is a validated preference-based system for measuring health status which is widely used to measure outcomes in QALYs (Furlong *et al.*, 2001). The HUI allows the user to quantify the health-related quality of life for several health states and thereby estimate health status scores. The current HUI3 includes eight attributes (vision, hearing, speech, ambulation, dexterity, emotion, cognition, and pain) and defines 972 000 unique health states. The HUI has been used in clinical and general populations, is available in many languages, and has been used throughout the world. There exist many population surveys using the HUI system, which provide reference data for interpreting HUI findings from clinical studies. Both the EQ-5D and HUI are widely used in cost-effectiveness analyses and allow the measurement of health effects for a population using QALYs. These measures of health status are not utilities as defined in Chapter 8.

For the Reference Case, the Panel recommends obtaining preferences from the community to foster comparability across studies. Although these community-based and generic measures should be used for the Reference Case, analysts may want to explore the impact of using estimates based on the patient or population with the target condition to aid in their decision making.

15.8 Measuring the costs of medical care

Cost-effectiveness analysis depends on accurate inputs. The most important concept is that the cost of an intervention should include both the costs of the intervention itself but then also the downstream costs (or savings) that occur because of the intervention. Such downstream costs may also include costs other than those incurred by the patient, including costs incurred outside of the health care sector. For example, a cost-effectiveness analysis of the use of an implantable cardioverter defibrillator includes not only the cost of the defibrillator itself but also the costs of all the care that occurs because the defibrillator was implanted, including follow-up visits and treatment of complications. It also includes costs incurred because the patient misses work for the implantation of the device, and for follow-up visits. It includes additional costs because the patient with the device lives longer and may therefore experience other health outcomes not associated with their risk of heart disease.

Specifically, the costs to incorporate into a cost-effectiveness analysis of an intervention include:
- Formal health care resources (including costs paid for by third-party payers and by patients out-of-pocket). These costs are the costs of the intervention itself and then the clinical costs that arise because of the intervention.
- Informal health care sector resources (including patient time spent traveling to and from care, waiting for, and receiving care, unpaid caregiver time, and transportation costs)
- Nonhealth care sector resources (including productivity, consumption, and costs borne by other sectors of the economy)

Of these costs, the health care resources are typically the best-defined component. However, for some interventions, other categories of costs may also be important. The Second Panel recommends including in the Reference Case for cost-effectiveness analyses some components (e.g., current and future medical costs and patients' out-of-pocket costs) in both the health care sector analysis and the societal perspective analysis. Other costs (e.g., time costs for patients and caregivers, transportation costs, productivity benefits, consumption costs, and other sector costs) should be included only in the societal Reference Case perspective (Table 15.1). This societal perspective therefore incorporates all costs and all health effects regardless of who incurs the costs and who experiences the effects. Given that medical care takes such a large share of many country's national incomes, it is important to evaluate a decision not only by how it affects health (through the health care sector perspective) but also by its effects beyond the health care sector (through the societal perspective).

Costs within the formal health care sector. The direct costs of care include the value of the resources used to provide an intervention. The analyst should define resources broadly and include current and future medical costs and patient's out-of-pocket costs. The direct costs include the cost of the intervention and the cost of its effects downstream (either good or bad). The analysis should account for all costs within the formal health care sector over the projected lifetime of the patient under each of the compared strategies.

Costs in the informal health care sector. The most obvious cost of an intervention is the cost of the intervention itself and the downstream costs associated with the patient's clinical visits or care. However, several additional "informal" costs within the health care sector may be substantial and should be considered. For example, informal costs are defined to include the cost of the patient's time for receiving treatment (e.g., taking unpaid leave from work), an informal (unpaid) caregiver's assistance to assist the patient during treatment or their future care trajectory, and transportation costs associated with getting treatment. Cost-effectiveness analyses performed from the health care system perspective do not include the costs incurred by the patient or caregiver. Therefore, they may have an inherent bias against interventions that rely on time inputs that are purchased and paid for by the health care sector and in favor of those that rely mostly on unpaid patient time or informal support (Neumann *et al.*, 2016; Russell, 2009). For example, consider two Treatments A and B which are equally effective. Next assume that Treatment A costs $10 000 and allows the patient to return to work the next day, while Treatment B costs $2000, but the patient must miss 4 weeks of work and requires caregiving from a family member during that time. From the health sector perspective, Treatment B would dominate Treatment A since it achieves the same effectiveness at a lower cost. From a societal perspective, however, the costs of missed time from work for the patient and their family member would be included and more accurately estimate the societal impact of the treatment decision. A societal perspective in a cost-effectiveness analysis is important, especially when informal costs are significant.

Costs outside of the health care sector

Productivity costs. Productivity costs include the costs from lost work due to illness or death. These costs to productivity occur when patients are not paid when they are receiving medical services and include wages that patients would have received but did not because illness prevented them from working. The Second Panel noted that effects on productivity are not measured by most preference-based measures (such as the EQ-5D or the HUI) or in the utility scores or quality-of-life weights (Neumann *et al.*, 2016). It, therefore, recommends that the productivity consequences of changes in health status be reflected in the numerator of cost-effectiveness ratios for Reference Case analyses conducted under the societal perspective while recognizing the possibility that this practice could lead to double counting if, in fact, the effects of illness on the patient's productivity reduce the patient's quality of life.

The calculation of productivity costs usually assumes that the patient is an average wage earner. Thus, analysts use average age- and gender-specific values for wages. While this approach facilitates doing a cost-effectiveness analysis, it may lead to systematic bias because wages – but not necessarily the value of time – vary by age and gender, which leads to undervaluing the time of the young, the elderly, and women. Therefore, the Second Panel recommends that the priority given to stratifying wage rates by age, sex, and/or disease conditions should depend on the needs of the decision makers who will use the analysis. The Panel recommends that if wages are stratified, the interpretation of the cost-effectiveness findings should include a discussion of the potential for systematic bias.

Other sector costs. The impact of health care interventions on resource use in sectors outside of health care should be estimated and incorporated into cost-effectiveness analyses to represent the societal perspective. For example, an intervention within a pediatric clinic which targets screening patients for food insecurity and providing resources to those in need will not only incur costs within the health care system but will also impact costs within the housing sector, the educational sector, and potentially the judicial sector. The valuation of the use of resources in these other sectors may be more difficult than in the health care sector, but they should be included explicitly in the Impact Inventory table for cost-effectiveness analysis. Cost-effectiveness analyses should include sensitivity analyses that present ICERs with and without these societal benefits.

Other cost categories. In addition to the health care sector costs and costs in other sectors, additional costs to be considered may include: future non-health care costs (costs incurred during added years of life due to an intervention or policy), friction costs (transaction costs associated with the replacement of a worker because of the impact of the illness and the intervention), transfer costs (costs which represent lost or improved access to resources due to an intervention), and fixed costs (costs which do not change despite increasing the number of intervention units served). When these other costs are substantial, they should be explicitly documented and included in the analysis that includes the societal perspective.

Discounting future costs. Some of the costs of an intervention may occur in the future. Most of us would rather pay $100 in 10 years' time rather than pay it today. If the interest rate on investments exceeds the rate of inflation, we should invest the $100 and earn interest for 10 years rather than paying the $100 today. Thus, the value or future cost depends on when it is incurred. The best way to avoid confusion is to estimate all future costs as if they had been incurred in the present. *Discounting* is the process of calculating the present value of money that will be spent in the future. The discount rate is the annual rate at which money is discounted. Following the recommendations of the Second Panel, in cost-effectiveness analyses from both the societal and the health care sector perspectives, the costs and health effects of all interventions should be discounted at the same rate of 3% but sensitivity analyses should be performed over a range of discount rates. The 3% discount rate may need revision over time as economic conditions change.

The present value of future expenses is given by the formula:

$$\text{Present Value} = \frac{\text{Future Value of Expense}}{\left(1 + \text{discount rate}\right)^t}$$

where t is the time when the future expenditure takes place.

Assuming a discount rate of 3%, the present value of a $1000 cost that is incurred 10 years from now is:

$$\text{Present Value} = \frac{\left(1000\right)}{\left(1 + 0.03\right)^{10}} = \$744$$

15.9   Interpretation of cost-effectiveness analysis and use in decision making

Although a cost-effectiveness analysis is a powerful method of evaluating the costs, benefits, and harms of available alternatives, it does not make the decision for patients, clinicians, health care systems, or policymakers. Rather a cost-effectiveness analysis provides information that these decision makers can use to inform their decision making by exploring the effects of the underlying uncertainties. Cost-effectiveness analyses are not a method of cost containment – they do not set the level of resources to be spent – but they can provide information that decision-makers can use to ensure that available resources are used as effectively as possible to improve health and provide value.

What is considered cost-effective depends on comparing the incremental cost-effectiveness threshold (or ICER) to some threshold value (e.g. $50 000/QALY or $100 000/QALY). The threshold depends on the decision maker, their available resources, and represents their willingness to pay for a unit of increased effectiveness (such as one QALY). There is no fixed threshold for defining cost-effectiveness and the decision-makers should consider a range of possible thresholds. How clinical or policy implications change with consideration of alternative thresholds is an important context for decision makers. The goals of cost-effectiveness analysis are (1) to aid decision makers in their efforts to enable people obtain the most health given available resources, and (2) to avoid wasting resources on interventions that provide little or no benefit, or actually do harm, while more beneficial interventions go underused. Cost-effectiveness analysis is not intended to deprive people or care, but rather to be transparent about the factors that influence the value of an intervention, so that decision makers are clear about the tradeoffs or costs, harms, and benefits of strategies. In a policy framework, it simply works to inform decisions by policymakers (insurance company medical directors, practice guideline panels, and large health systems) to ensure that available resources are used as effectively as possible to improve health.

15.10   Limitations of cost-effectiveness analyses

Like all models, cost-effectiveness analyses can play a useful role in decision making, but models are a simplification of reality and not complete decision making tools. Cost-effectiveness analyses are only as good as the underlying evidence that supports the analysis and the appropriateness of the underlying simplifying assumptions. But, acknowledging those limitations, they can be informative and powerful resources for decision makers. When performing cost-effectiveness analysis, analysts should provide a discussion of the limitations of the analysis and guide its users in interpreting and generalizing the results. Such limitations may include the relevance of the source populations for the data used in the analysis, assumptions that are based on expert opinion or lower-quality studies, failure to consider all plausible strategies or comparators, and simplifying assumptions about included costs and benefits. A cost-effectiveness analysis should discuss the potential effect of the limitations on the results. Sensitivity analyses are a powerful tool for explicitly assessing the impact of uncertainty about model parameters and simplifying assumptions in the decision models (see Chapter 7).

Summary

1. The clinician has an ethical obligation to be the patient's advocate. However, when resources are limited, the clinician will often have to take into account the needs of other patients or society as a whole when considering which strategies to implement for an individual patient.
2. Cost-effectiveness analysis is a method for comparing clinical strategies. The basis for comparison is the relationship between the costs of the available strategies and their clinical effectiveness.
3. Cost-effectiveness analysis is useful when a decision maker is trying to choose among several new or existing interventions, and resources are limited. Cost-effectiveness analysis is designed to identify the ways of spending on health care that provide the most health from our health care dollars.
4. Although cost-effectiveness analysis does not tell decision makers what option to choose, it provides them with a powerful framework for considering the various costs, benefits, and harms.
5. Reference cases for cost-effectiveness analyses should be performed both from a health sector perspective and from a societal perspective. For the latter, it is important to include all consequences of the strategies being considered, including those outside of the formal health care sector. Reference cases from these two perspectives with similar methodology for which costs and benefits to include, help with comparability of findings across studies.
6. Cost–benefit analysis measures the net benefits and costs in the same units (usually currency) and can therefore be used to decide if a strategy will be of net benefit to society.

Bibliography

Detsky, A.S. and Naglie, I.G. (1990) A clinician's guide to cost-effectiveness analysis. *Annals of Internal Medicine*, **113**(2), 147–54. https://doi.org/10.7326/0003-4819-113-2-147.

> Clinicians need to participate in policy making and dealing with scarce resources while advocating for their individual patient's needs and perspective. This article helps guide for understanding cost-effectiveness in setting funding priorities.

Drummond, M.F., Sculpher, M.J., Torrance, G.W. *et al.* (2005) *Methods for the Economic Evaluation of Health care programmes*. 3rd ed., Oxford University Press, Oxford.

> This is an excellent comprehensive textbook that covers a broad range of economic evaluations.

Eddy, D.M. (1980) *Screening for Cancer: Theory, Analysis, and Design*, Prentice-Hall, Inc., New Jersey.

> This book describes an influential mathematical model of cancer screening. The author's rigorous mathematical approach will be difficult for most readers, but the book is strongly recommended for the adventurous reader.

EuroQol, Group (1990) EuroQol – a new facility for the measurement of health-related quality of life. *Health Policy*, **16**(3), 199–208.

> Overview of the EuroQOL measurement instrument's development and guidance regarding implementation.

Furlong, W.J., Feeny, D.H., Torrance, G.W. and Barr, R.D. (2001) The health utilities index (HUI®) system for assessing health-related quality of life in clinical studies. *Annals of Medicine*, **33**, 375–84.

> Overview of the Health Utilities Index (HUI) system as a method to describe health status and obtain utility scores reflecting health-related quality of life.

Garber, A.M. and Phelps, C.E. (1997) Economic foundations of cost-effectiveness analysis. *Journal of Health Economics*, **16**(1), 1–31.

> The theoretical foundation, including ideas about choosing a cost-effectiveness threshold.

Gold, M., Siegel, J.E., Russell, L.B., and Weinstein, M.C. (1996) *Cost-Effectiveness in Health and Medicine*, Oxford University Press, New York.

Original bible for cost-effectiveness analysis in the U.S. Subsequently updated by the Second Panel work by Neumann and colleagues.

Neumann, P.J., Sanders, G.D., Russell, L.B. *et al.* (2016) *Cost-Effectiveness in Health and Medicine*, 2nd ed., Oxford University Press, New York, NY.

Revised edition of the Gold book. This book is written by the Second Panel on Cost Effectiveness in Health and Medicine which is a diverse panel of leaders in the field. Provides recommendations for conducting cost-effectiveness analyses and is considered the standard for performing such analyses.

Neumann, P.J., Kim, D.D., Trikalinos, T.A. *et al.* (2018) Future directions for cost-effectiveness analyses in health and medicine. *Medical Decision Making*, **38**(7), 767–77.

Overview of key topics for future research and policy as it relates to cost-effectiveness.

Owens, D.K., Qaseem, A., Chou, R., and Shekelle, P., for The Clinical Guidelines Committee of the American College of Clinicians (2011) High-value, cost-conscious health care: concepts for clinicians to evaluate benefits, harms, and costs of medical interventions. *Annals of Internal Medicine*, **154**, 174–80.

A tutorial that covers the concepts of cost-effectiveness analysis for clinicians.

Russell, L.B. (2009) Completing costs: patients' time. *Medical Care*, 47(7 Suppl 1), S89–93.

Paper which discusses the importance of patients' time as a cost of health and medical care and explains how to include it in costing studies.

Sanders, G.D., Neumann, P.J., Basu, A. *et al.* (2016) Recommendations for conduct, methodological practices, and reporting of cost-effectiveness analyses: second panel on cost-effectiveness in health and medicine. *JAMA*, **316**(10), 1093–103.

This article summarizes the recommendations of the Second Panel on Cost Effectiveness in Health and Medicine.

Sanders, G.D., Maciejewski, M.L., and Basu, A. (2019) Overview of cost-effectiveness analysis. *JAMA*, **321**, 1400–1.

Manuscript which provides an accessible overview for clinicians of cost-effectiveness analyses and the Second Panel's key recommendations.

Weinstein, M.C. and Stason, W.B. (1977) Foundations of cost-effectiveness analysis for health and medical practices. *The New England Journal of Medicine*, **296**, 716–21.

An excellent introduction to cost-effectiveness and cost-benefit analysis. The reference list contains many classic articles on measuring the monetary value of a human life.

Weinstein, M.C., Fineberg, H.V., and colleagues (1980) *Clinical Decision Analysis*, W. B. Saunders, Inc., Philadelphia, 228–65.

This book chapter explains how to measure the different types of health care costs.

Index

*Note: Page numbers in italics refer to Figures; those in **bold** to Tables.*

Medical Decision Making, Third Edition. Harold C. Sox, Michael C. Higgins, Douglas K. Owens, and Gillian Sanders Schmidler.
© 2024 John Wiley & Sons Ltd. Published 2024 by John Wiley & Sons Ltd.